Psychiatry Test Preparation and Review Manual

Commissioning Editor:
Susan Pioli

Project Development Manager:
Laura Anello

Project Manager:
Cheryl Brant

Design:
Stewart Larking

Marketing Manager:
Matt Latuchie

PSYCHIATRY TEST PREPARATION AND REVIEW MANUAL

J Clive Spiegel, MD

Clinical Assistant Professor
Department of Psychiatry and Behavioral Sciences
Montefiore Medical Center
Albert Einstein College of Medicine
Bronx, NY
USA

John M Kenny, MD

Clinical Instructor
Department of Psychiatry and Behavioral Sciences
Albert Einstein College of Medicine
Bronx Psychiatric Center
Bronx, NY

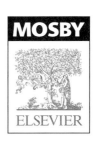

MOSBY
ELSEVIER

An affiliate of Elsevier Inc

First published 2007

ISBN-13: 978-0-323-04422-6
ISBN-10: 0-323-04422-0

British Library Cataloguing in Publication Data

A catalogue record for this book is available from the British Library

Library of Congress Cataloging in Publication Data.

A catalog record for this book is available from the Library of Congress

Notice

Medical knowledge is constantly changing. Standard safety precautions must be followed, but as new research and clinical experience broaden our knowledge, changes in treatment and drug therapy may become necessary or appropriate. Readers are advised to check the most current product information provided by the manufacturer of each drug to be administered to verify the recommended dose, the method and duration of administration, and contraindications. It is the responsibility of the practitioner, relying on experience and knowledge of the patient, to determine dosages and the best treatment for each individual patient. Neither the Publisher nor the author assume any liability for any injury and/or damage to persons or property arising from this publication.

The Publisher

ELSEVIER your source for books, journals and multimedia in the health sciences

www.elsevierhealth.com

Working together to grow libraries in developing countries

www.elsevier.com | www.bookaid.org | www.sabre.org

ELSEVIER | BOOK AID International | Sabre Foundation

The Publisher's policy is to use **paper manufactured from sustainable forests**

Printed in North America
Last digit is the print number: 9 8 7 6 5 4

Contents

Preface

Candidates facing their ABPN Part One Psychiatry examination or their Psychiatry Resident In-Training Examination (PRITE) have approached us many times asking if we can recommend good material or books with practice questions and comprehensive answer explanations. This recommendation has been a challenge because the question books available today have many deficiencies, the most notable of which is a lack of answer explanations that are thorough and helpful. Other volumes do not organize the practice questions into sample tests as we have chosen to do and this is where candidates will find this book really helpful, particularly in practicing test-taking technique and timing.

This volume serves as both test preparation and subject review not only for the ABPN Part One Psychiatry examination, but also for the PRITE exam, shelf exams in Psychiatry or Neurology, all three steps of the USMLE, and even the ABPN Psychiatry Recertification Examination. Candidates for any of these standardized tests will find this book extremely useful in helping prepare for their exam in Behavioral Medicine, Neurology, or both. We have a few simple suggestions to the candidate on how to maximize the benefit from this book. This book contains four practice tests, each with 150 multiple choice questions. Each test stands alone and mimics the actual ABPN Psychiatry Exam as far as the balance of subject matter is concerned. The multiple choice questions each have five answer choices with only one right answer. This is the only style of question currently used by the ABPN.

The actual ABPN Psychiatry exam is composed of two tests of about 210 questions each. The ABPN divides the material into approximately 65% Psychiatry and 35% Neurology. We have done the same in each of our four tests. Each individual test has about 95 Psychiatry questions and 55 Neurology questions. The questions cover a broad spectrum of material in both disciplines and approximate the composition of the actual ABPN exam. Candidates should give themselves one minute per question (two and a half hours to complete a 150-question test) and sit down undisturbed to do each test individually under test-taking conditions. Answers can then be checked with the answer key that follows each test. Studying can then be focused using the answer explanations that follow.

We have tried as much as possible to use each question as an opportunity to explain the right answer as well as the four wrong answers, which in most cases are equally important because wrong answers can also form the basis of their own question on an exam. To facilitate the candidate's studying, we have supplied a chapter reference at the end of each answer explanation. This will enable a candidate to go over the answer explanation and then easily go to a definitive and authoritative reference to learn more about the subject matter contained in the question. Most candidates will find that this volume is quite complete in and of itself and that further detailed review of many subjects will not prove necessary. We have used two authoritative references that we feel are the gold standard for the ABPN exam: *Kaplan and Sadock's Synopsis of Psychiatry: Behavioral Sciences/ Clinical Psychiatry*, ninth edition by Benjamin J. Sadock and Virginia A. Sadock, and *Neurology In Clinical Practice*, fourth edition by Bradley, Daroff, Fenichel and Jankovic. Each answer explanation in this volume has either a "K&S' reference (Kaplan and Sadock) or a "B&D' reference (Bradley, Daroff, et al.) following it. Candidates need only consult the appropriate chapter(s) in either volume to widen their knowledge base on any particular subject. Some candidates may find the latter text book to be unwieldy due to its two-volume size and that a more concise reference in Neurology may be better when studying to facilitate the ease and speed of looking up needed information. We can also recommend *Textbook of Clinical Neurology*, second edition by Christopher G. Goetz, which is considerably less detailed and less complete than *Neurology In Clinical Practice*, but may be simpler to consult while studying.

The candidate may find other references useful and we can certainly recommend *Neurology Secrets*, fourth edition, by Loren A. Rolak and *Psychiatry Secrets*, second edition, by James L. Jacobson and Alan M. Jacobson. These two volumes, which are high-yield guides that use a unique question and answer format, are very useful to help focus studying for standardized examinations in Psychiatry and Neurology. We hope that this volume serves as both practice material and study material for the candidate.

We would like to thank Susan Pioli and all those in the Psychiatry publishing division at Elsevier who gave us help and encouragement throughout the development of this book and without whose help this book would never have been possible.

J Clive Spiegel, MD
Manhasset, New York

John M Kenny, MD
Locust Valley, New York

Dedication

We would like to dedicate this book to our wives,
Jacqueline Hattem-Spiegel
And
Jennifer Halstead-Kenny
Without whose love, support, and understanding
This book would never have seen the light of day

Test Number ONE

1. A 16 year-old male suffers from irritable mood, increased energy, decreased need for sleep, and pressured speech. He was recently started on medication by his psychiatrist to control these symptoms. He comes into your office complaining of a significant worsening of his acne since starting this new medication. What drug was he started on?

    A. Oxcarbazepine
    B. Lorazepam
    C. Risperidone
    D. Lithium
    E. Lamotrigine

2. Which of the following is NOT true regarding bonding and attachment?

    A. Attachment lasts for life
    B. Attachment is the emotional dependence of an infant on his mother
    C. Bonding is the emotional attachment of a mother to her child
    D. Bonding is anchored by resources and security
    E. Poor attachments may lead to personality disorders

3. What is the best test for diagnosing Huntington's disease?

    A. Karyotype of chromosomes
    B. Serum ceruloplasmin
    C. Urine porphobilinogens
    D. Serum polymerase chain reaction (PCR)
    E. Cerebrospinal fluid (CSF) assay for 14-3-3 proteinase inhibitor protein

4. Lesions in the orbitofrontal region of the brain will present as a patient who is:
   A. Profane, irritable, and irresponsible
   B. Manic
   C. Depressed
   D. Apathetic
   E. Psychotic

5. A 65 year-old woman with schizophrenia believes that she is pregnant with God's child. She has been convinced of this for the past five years. When you confront her on this she tells you that she is certain that she is pregnant and that God is the father. She will not agree that this is not true. Her thinking is an example of which one of the following?
   A. Egomania
   B. Coprolalia
   C. Delusion
   D. Ailurophobia
   E. Obsession

6. A group of patients are looked at with regard to a risk factor for heart disease. They are divided into those who have the risk factor and those who do not. These groups are then followed for a number of years to see who does and who does not develop heart disease. This is an example of a:
   A. Cohort study
   B. Case-control study
   C. Clinical trial
   D. Cross-sectional survey
   E. Crossover study

7. Who developed the theory of "good enough mothering"?
   A. Piaget
   B. Freud
   C. Mahler
   D. Winnicott
   E. Erikson

8. A 47 year-old man presents to the emergency room in an acute state of disorientation, with tachycardia, ophthalmoparesis, diaphoresis, and ataxia. He dies in the hospital 48 hours later. Brain autopsy of this patient would reveal:
   A. Frontal and temporal lobe atrophy
   B. Substantia nigra depigmentation
   C. Hemorrhages in the ependyma of the third ventricle and superior vermis
   D. Diffuse Lewy bodies in cortex
   E. Subcortical white matter lesions perpendicular to the ventricles

9. Which of the following statements are TRUE concerning monoamine oxidase inhibitors (MAOIs)?
   A. MAOIs are not likely to cause orthostatic hypotension
   B. To switch between an MAOI and a SSRI you need a 3-day washout period
   C. Giving meperidine with an MAOI is contraindicated
   D. Lithium is contraindicated with MAOIs
   E. All MAOIs require adherence to a tyramine free diet

10. You are called to consult on an agitated patient on the medical unit. The patient is elderly, confused and pulling out her lines. You decide that she must be tranquilized for her own safety. Which one of the following drugs would be the best choice?
    A. Lorazepam
    B. Lithium
    C. Diazepam
    D. Aripiprazole
    E. Haloperidol

11. You are talking to one of your colleagues from surgery. He tells you about a post-operative patient that he is covering who keeps complaining of pain. He tells you that the patient was originally on intramuscular meperidine and was switched to the same dose of oral meperidine just yesterday. The patient has been complaining constantly and is getting the nursing staff upset. What do you think is responsible for this situation?
    A. The patient has low pain tolerance
    B. The patient has borderline personality disorder and is splitting the staff
    C. The patient has an intractable pain disorder
    D. The analgesic potency of oral meperidine is less than intramuscular meperidine
    E. The patient has a conversion disorder

12. A therapist gets assigned a new patient in his clinic. While looking at the materials the patient filled out in the waiting area he finds out that the patient has a substance abuse history. He immediately says "Stupid drug addicts, they're so annoying. They're such a waste of time. They never want to get better." This is an example of:
    A. Projection
    B. Transference
    C. Countertransference
    D. Resistance
    E. Confrontation

13. What is the likelihood of a patient acquiring Huntington's disease if his father is a carrier and has the illness?
    A. 25%
    B. 50%
    C. 75%
    D. 90%
    E. 100%

14. The following are all developmental tasks of middle adulthood, EXCEPT:
    A. Taking stock of accomplishments
    B. Reassessing commitments to family, work and marriage
    C. Using accumulated power ethically
    D. Engaging in risk-taking behavior
    E. Dealing with parental illness and death

15. A chronic schizophrenic has been taking medication for twenty years. Every morning he goes to his pill bottle and takes the pills his doctor prescribes. This is an example of:
    A. Primary prevention
    B. Secondary prevention
    C. Tertiary prevention
    D. Malingering
    E. Noncompliance

16. A patient with metastatic carcinoma of the lung presents with generalized muscle weakness and is found to have improved muscle strength with minimal exercise. The most likely diagnosis is:
    A. Myasthenia gravis
    B. Multiple sclerosis
    C. Guillain-Barré syndrome
    D. Polymyositis
    E. Lambert-Eaton myasthenic syndrome

17. Which one of the following tests does NOT detect psychotic thought processes?
    A. Draw a person test
    B. Minnesota multiphasic personality inventory (MMPI)
    C. Sentence completion test
    D. Thematic apperception test (TAT)
    E. Rorschach test

18. A patient presents with slowly progressive muscle weakness, fasciculations of arm muscles and tongue, difficulty swallowing and becomes wheelchair-bound. The diagnosis is amyotrophic lateral sclerosis. Postmortem studies of this patient's central nervous system would reveal:

    A. Nigrostriatal depigmentation and atrophy
    B. Frontal and temporal lobe atrophy
    C. Anterior horn cell degeneration
    D. Corpus callosum thinning and atrophy
    E. Dorsal column volume loss

19. All of the following are part of the ethical code of the American Psychiatric Association, EXCEPT:

    A. It is unethical to accept a commission for patient referrals
    B. It is unethical to have sexual relations with patients
    C. It is a psychiatrist's obligation to report other psychiatrist's unethical behavior
    D. Retiring psychiatrists must provide patients with sufficient notice of their retirement and make every reasonable effort to find follow up care for their patients
    E. Psychiatrists have an obligation to participate in executions

20. You are called by the medicine team to do a psychiatric consultation on a 90 year-old female with sepsis who is agitated, confused, disoriented and pulling out her lines. The medical team tells you that her mentation has been waxing and waning throughout the day. Your first consideration in approaching the case is:

    A. Determining capacity to refuse treatment
    B. Speaking to the patient's family
    C. Examining the patient's medication regimen
    D. Developing a therapeutic relationship with the patient
    E. Protecting the patient from unintended harm

21. Positive reinforcement, negative reinforcement, the operant, and the reinforcing stimulus are integral parts of what theory?

    A. Operant conditioning developed by Skinner
    B. Operant conditioning developed by Bandura
    C. Attribution theory developed by Hull
    D. Learned helplessness developed by Kandel
    E. Habituation theory developed by Pavlov

22. A seven year-old girl with staring spells and 3-per-second spike and wave activity on electroencephalogram (EEG) fails therapy with ethosuximide and has breakthrough spells. The next best medication of choice to treat this patient is:
    A. Phenytoin
    B. Divalproex sodium
    C. Phenobarbital
    D. Diazepam
    E. Carbamazepine

23. Episodes of sudden sleep onset, with sudden loss of muscle tone, followed by quick entry into rapid eye movement (REM) sleep are characteristic of which one of the following?
    A. Sleep changes associated with depression
    B. Sleep apnea
    C. Primary insomnia
    D. Narcolepsy
    E. Shift-work sleep disorder

24. All of the following neurotransmitters are associated with the inhibition of aggressive behavior, EXCEPT:
    A. Dopamine
    B. Norepinephrine
    C. Serotonin
    D. GABA
    E. Glycine

25. Which one of the following anticonvulsant agents needs rapid dosage increases early in therapy due to autoinduction of its own metabolism?
    A. Carbamazepine
    B. Divalproex sodium
    C. Phenytoin
    D. Phenobarbital
    E. Diazepam

26. Giving positive reinforcement intermittently at a variable schedule is the best way to prevent:
    A. Discrimination
    B. Generalization
    C. Extinction
    D. Respondent conditioning
    E. Transference

✓ 27. A young woman presents to the emergency room with a history of intractable seizures and mental retardation. You discover she has severe acne, skin depigmentation on her back and blotchy patches on her retinal surface on fundoscopic examination. The most likely diagnosis is:

A. Down's syndrome

B. Rett's disorder

C. Neurofibromatosus

D. Tuberous sclerosis

E. Williams' syndrome

28. Which one of the following drugs does NOT work by blocking the catabolism of acetylcholine?

A. Donepezil

B. Memantine

C. Tacrine

D. Rivastigmine

E. Galantamine

29. Which one of the following tests would be best used for testing executive function?

A. Thematic apperception test

B. Halstead-Reitan neuropsychological battery

C. Minnesota multiphasic personality inventory (MMPI)

D. Brief psychiatric rating scale (BPRS)

E. Trail making tests

30. You are asked as a psychiatrist to determine if a patient has the capacity to make a will. In order to make the will the patient must prove all of the following to you, EXCEPT:

A. He knows that he is making a will

B. He knows how the will distributes his property

C. He knows the nature of the property to be distributed

D. He knows who will inherit the property

E. He understands court procedure

31. All of the following are correct regarding the onset of puberty, EXCEPT:

A. Onset of puberty is triggered by the maturation of the hypothalamic-pituitary-adrenal-gonadal axis

B. Primary sex characteristics are those directly involved in coitus and reproduction

C. The average age of onset of puberty is 11 years of age for boys and 13 years of age for girls

D. Increases in height and weight occur earlier in girls than in boys

E. In adolescent boys testosterone levels correlate with libido

32. Sumatriptan (Imitrex) is contraindicated in patients with:
    A. Ischemic heart disease
    B. Kidney disease
    C. Obstructive pulmonary disease
    D. Inflammatory bowel disease
    E. Carcinoma

33. All of the following increase tricyclic antidepressant concentrations, EXCEPT:
    A. Clozapine
    B. Haloperidol
    C. Risperidone
    D. Cigarette smoking
    E. Methylphenidate

34. Which one of the following is TRUE regarding suicide?
    A. Completed suicide is most frequently related to bipolar disorder
    B. Adolescents most frequently succeed in committing suicide by hanging
    C. In recent years the suicide rate has increased dramatically among middle-aged adults
    D. Previous suicidal behavior is the best predictor of risk for future suicide
    E. Women successfully commit suicide more often than men

35. The classic stroke condition known as Gerstmann's syndrome can comprise all of the following symptoms, EXCEPT:
    A. Acalculia
    B. Right and left confusion
    C. Finger agnosia
    D. Alexia without agraphia
    E. Pure agraphia

36. Which one of the following is most appropriate for treatment with dialectical behavioral therapy?
    A. Histrionic personality disorder
    B. Borderline personality disorder
    C. Dependant personality disorder
    D. Schizoid personality disorder
    E. Obsessive-compulsive personality disorder

37. A 45 year-old woman with bipolar disorder complains of amenorrhea, galactorrhea, decreased libido and anorgasmia. She presents to the emergency room with an elevated serum prolactin level and is on risperidone 4 mg daily for bipolar disorder. On neurologic examination you discover decreased vision in both lateral visual fields. The most likely diagnosis is:

    A. Acute right parietal stroke
    B. Thalamic hemorrhage
    C. Pituitary macroadenoma
    D. Acute left parietal stroke
    E. Midbrain infarct

38. All of the following are true regarding the mental status examination, EXCEPT:

    A. Racing thoughts are considered part of thought process
    B. Blunted is a term used to describe affect
    C. Hallucinations are part of thought content
    D. Delusions are part of thought content
    E. Circumstantiality is part of thought form

39. A Malaysian man was brought into the emergency room after trying to commit suicide. The family describes an unusual course of events preceding the suicide attempt. The patient was depressed, preoccupied and brooding. He suddenly had an unprovoked outburst of rage in which he went around the neighborhood and indiscriminately maimed two people and three dogs. Two of the dogs died. Afterwards he had no memory of the episode and was exhausted. He then went into the kitchen of his home, picked up a knife and slit his wrists. The most appropriate diagnosis is:

    A. Koro
    B. Amok
    C. Piblokto
    D. Wihtigo
    E. Mal de ojo

40. An 80 year-old man with known vascular dementia presents to your emergency room with care givers complaining of new onset right hemiparesis and mutism. All of the following signs are compatible with this clinical presentation, EXCEPT:

    A. Meyerson's sign
    B. Right-sided Hoffman's sign
    C. Right-sided Babinski sign
    D. A positive palmomental reflex
    E. Complete loss of the gag reflex

41. Glutamate is all of the following, EXCEPT:
    A. One of the two major amino acid neurotransmitters
    B. An inhibitory neurotransmitter
    C. Involved in learning and memory
    D. The primary neurotransmitter in cerebellar granule cells
    E. A precursor of gamma aminobutyric acid (GABA)

42. Down's syndrome is associated with defects in chromosome 21. This is a feature also shared by:
    A. Turner's syndrome
    B. Klinefelter's syndrome
    C. Huntington's disease
    D. Alzheimer's disease
    E. Parkinson's disease

43. The diagnosis of brain death is compatible with all of the following, EXCEPT:
    A. Eyes fully open
    B. Absence of corneal reflexes
    C. Presence of oculovestibular reflexes
    D. Spontaneous activity seen on EEG
    E. Large, fixed pupils

44. Patients with compromised liver function should NOT use which one of the following drugs?
    A. Temazepam
    B. Diazepam
    C. Oxazepam
    D. Lorazepam
    E. Chlorazepate

45. Which one of the following is NOT an appropriate part of family therapy?
    A. Exploring family members' beliefs about the meanings of their behaviors
    B. Reframing problematic behaviors positively
    C. Focusing most of the session on the most dysfunctional member of the family
    D. Encouraging family members to interact differently and observe the effects
    E. Giving the family members things to think about and work on outside of sessions

46. Which one of the following statements is TRUE regarding neurotransmitters and anxiety?
    A. GABA has nothing to do with anxiety
    B. GABA, norepinephrine, and serotonin are associated with anxiety in some way
    C. Dopamine, glutamate, and histamine are associated with anxiety in some way
    D. Only acetylcholine is associated with anxiety
    E. Anxiety can be treated with injection of epinephrine

47. All of the following are used in treating myasthenia gravis, EXCEPT:
    A. Pyridostigmine
    B. Edrophonium chloride
    C. Plasmapheresis
    D. Intravenous immunoglobulin administration
    E. Thymectomy

48. You are called to evaluate a potentially delirious patient on a medical unit. As part of your workup you order an EEG. What do you expect to find on EEG if this is truly a delirium?
    A. 3-per-second spike and wave pattern
    B. Frontocentral beta activity
    C. Posterior alpha rhythm
    D. Generalized slow-wave activity consisting of theta and delta waves, with some focal areas of hyperactivity
    E. Right temporal spikes

49. Gower's maneuver or sign is typically seen in which one of the following neurologic conditions?
    A. Myasthenia gravis
    B. Multiple sclerosis
    C. Huntington's disease
    D. Duchenne's muscular dystrophy
    E. Myotonic dystrophy

50. All of the following antidepressants have strong sedative effects, EXCEPT:
    A. Trazodone
    B. Paroxetine
    C. Doxepin
    D. Clomipramine
    E. Mirtazapine

51. One of your patients of the opposite sex begins to act seductively and proceeds to ask you out for dinner. Which one of the following would be an appropriate response?

    A. Ignore the patient's advances
    B. Compliment the patient on the way she is dressed
    C. Tell the patient that you are seeing someone and therefore can't accept the offer
    D. Examine your own countertransference and explore the meaning of the patient's behavior
    E. Have sex with the patient and then make the patient find a new doctor

52. While on call one night in the emergency room, you are asked to evaluate a distraught couple that has been brought in by the police following a fight that started after the wife found out that her husband was wearing her panties to work. It turns out that he has been wearing women's undergarments for over a year because he finds this very sexually arousing. He has developed several fantasies imagining himself in women's undergarments. The most appropriate diagnosis for the husband is:

    A. Exhibitionism
    B. Fetishism
    C. Frotteurism
    D. Voyeurism
    E. Transvestic fetishism

53. A 48 year-old woman presents to your office with complaints of lancinating, brief, sharp pain to the left side of her face. The pain is short-lived and recurrent. It is triggered frequently by cold air touching her face. The pharmacologic treatment of choice for this condition would be:

    A. Divalproex sodium
    B. Clonazepam
    C. Carbamazepine
    D. Tiagabine
    E. Risperidone

54. A 75 year-old man presents to the emergency room with new onset headache, fever, vague joint pains and complaints of recent diminished vision. The first test of choice in this case is:

    A. Head CT scan
    B. MRI brain with diffusion-weighted imaging
    C. Lumbar puncture looking for CSF xanthochromia
    D. Serum sedimentation rate
    E. Carotid ultrasound looking for dissection

55. The concept that different mental disorders have different outcomes was pioneered by:
    A. Freud
    B. Bleuler
    C. Winnicott
    D. Kraepelin
    E. Kohut

56. A patient comes into your practice after referral from his primary care physician. He is convinced that he has cancer. He thinks that it hasn't been found yet, but is convinced that it is there. He remains convinced despite a full workup with negative results. Despite further reassurance by his doctors, he remains convinced that he has cancer. Which is the most appropriate diagnosis?
    A. Conversion disorder
    B. Hypochondriasis
    C. Body dysmorphic disorder
    D. Somatization disorder
    E. Briquet's syndrome

57. All of the following are characteristics of cluster headaches, EXCEPT:
    A. Attacks of short duration of 3 hours or less.
    B. Daytime attacks
    C. Male predominance
    D. Sharp, severe, retro-orbital pain
    E. Cyclical pattern of occurrence mainly in spring and fall seasons

58. All of the following are contraindications to bupropion, EXCEPT:
    A. Seizure
    B. Anorexia
    C. Use of a monoamine oxidase inhibitor (MAOI) in the past 14 days
    D. Head trauma
    E. Hypertension

59. All of the following should NOT be combined with monoamine oxidase inhibitors, EXCEPT:
    A. Meperidine
    B. Lithium
    C. Levodopa
    D. Selective serotonin reuptake inhibitors
    E. Spinal anesthetic containing epinephrine

60. All of the following can result in an acquired peripheral neuropathy, EXCEPT:
    A. Systemic lupus erythematosus (SLE)
    B. Toluene intoxication
    C. Acetaminophen overdose
    D. Vincristine therapy
    E. Epstein-Barr virus infection

61. All of the following are true regarding tricyclic antidepressants (TCAs), EXCEPT:
    A. Cigarette smoking decreases TCA levels
    B. Clozapine will increase TCA levels
    C. Methylphenidate will decrease TCA levels
    D. TCAs can have adverse cardiac effects
    E. TCAs have strong anticholinergic effects

62. Which one of the following antidepressants has the longest half-life?
    A. Fluvoxamine
    B. Paroxetine
    C. Citalopram
    D. Fluoxetine
    E. Sertraline

63. Self-mutilation is most common in which one of the following personality disorders?
    A. Borderline
    B. Narcissistic
    C. Histrionic
    D. Dependent
    E. Schizoid

64. A young man is admitted to the hospital with progressive proximal muscle weakness, generalized fatigue and a red nonpruritic rash to the face and body, especially around the knees and elbows. His workup should include screening for:
    A. Carcinoma
    B. Heart disease
    C. Intestinal bleeding
    D. Fibrotic lung disease
    E. Stroke

65. You are on call and get paged to go see a schizophrenic patient on the inpatient unit. The patient has a tremor, is ataxic and is restless. During the interview the patient vomits. The nurse tells you he has been having diarrhea and has been urinating very frequently. What question would be most useful to ask the patient?
    A. Can you count from 100 backwards by sevens?
    B. Where are you right now?
    C. Who is the current president?
    D. How much water have you been drinking recently?
    E. Are you HIV positive?

66. In what kind of schizophrenia is the onset late, the thought process more linear, and the outcome usually better?
    A. Paranoid
    B. Disorganized
    C. Catatonic
    D. Residual
    E. Undifferentiated

67. Which one of the following is NOT associated with good outcomes in schizophrenia?
    A. High premorbid functioning
    B. Little prodrome
    C. Early age at onset
    D. Acute onset
    E. Absence of family history of schizophrenia

68. During a workup you send a patient for an EEG. The results reveal shortened latency of rapid eye movement (REM) sleep, decreased stage IV sleep and increased REM density. These findings are most consistent with:
    A. Tumor
    B. Petit mal epilepsy
    C. Hepatic encephalopathy
    D. Delirium
    E. Depression

69. Homozygosity for which one of the following is believed to predispose patients to Alzheimer-type dementia?
    A. Tau
    B. Apolipoprotein E4
    C. Amyloid precursor protein
    D. Trisomy 21
    E. Presenelin

70. The following are all characteristics of narcissistic personality disorder, EXCEPT:
    A. Grandiosity
    B. Need for admiration
    C. Showing self-dramatization, theatricality, and exaggerated expression of emotion
    D. Preoccupation with fantasies of unlimited success, power and brilliance
    E. Interpersonally exploitative

71. The following are all criteria of post-traumatic stress disorder, EXCEPT:
    A. Re-experiencing the event
    B. Increased arousal
    C. Avoidance of stimuli associated with the trauma
    D. The duration of the disturbance is more than two months
    E. The person's response to the trauma involved intense fear or horror

72. After her mother died, Sarah felt extreme sadness, cried, blamed God, felt guilty, and became convinced that she was worthless and eventually tried to hang herself. Her diagnosis is:
    A. Normal bereavement
    B. Bipolar disorder
    C. Delusional disorder
    D. Anticipatory grief
    E. Pathological grief

73. The brains of patients with schizophrenia often reveal enlargement of the:
    A. Hippocampus
    B. Caudate
    C. Ventricles
    D. Corpus callosum
    E. Cerebellum

74. A 20 year-old patient comes into the emergency room while you are on call. She is 5 feet tall and has difficulty maintaining her body weight above 67 pounds. She has lost weight in the past by dieting and was encouraged by her progress. She continued to decrease food intake and increase exercising until her weight dropped below 63 pounds. At this time she is no longer having her menstrual periods. She comes to the emergency room with symptoms of peptic ulcer disease. Which one of the following would be considered the most important and urgent part of her initial medical workup?
    A. Bone scan
    B. Head CT scan
    C. Gastric emptying study
    D. Cholesterol level
    E. Serum potassium level

75. All of the following are true of delusional disorder, EXCEPT:

   A. It involves nonbizarre delusions that could happen in real life
   B. It may involve tactile hallucinations
   C. The erotomanic type involves another person of higher social standing being in love with the patient
   D. Daily functioning is markedly impaired
   E. The person's behavior is not markedly odd or bizarre

76. All of the following are true regarding female orgasmic disorder, EXCEPT:

   A. Female orgasmic disorder is the persistent absence of orgasm following a normal sexual excitement phase
   B. The incidence of orgasm in women increases with age
   C. Fears of impregnation or damage to the vagina as well as guilt are psychological factors involved in this disorder
   D. Female orgasmic disorder can be either life long or acquired
   E. Criteria include involuntary spasm of the vaginal musculature that interferes with intercourse

77. A patient presents to your office with a complaint of intense fear of going to social functions at her child's school. On further examination you note that she has fears that she will act in a way that will be humiliating or embarrassing. She is also made anxious by having to meet new people that she does not know. Your differential diagnosis of this patient should include which one of the following Axis II disorders?

   A. Borderline personality disorder
   B. Obsessive-compulsive personality disorder
   C. Narcissistic personality disorder
   D. Avoidant personality disorder
   E. Dependent personality disorder

78. Which one of the following anticonvulsant agents is known to cause hirsutism, facial changes and hypertrophy of the gingiva?

   A. Carbamazepine
   B. Valproate
   C. Phenobarbital
   D. Levetiracetam
   E. Phenytoin

79. A 52 year-old man is brought to the emergency room after being found by police prone on the edge of the sidewalk outside. He is moderately intoxicated with alcohol and unable to give an adequate history. Upon neurologic examination you discover that his right wrist and fingers are limp and he cannot lift them. He is also weak when he tries to extend his arm from a bent to straight position. He also has trouble turning his forearm over when it is placed palm down on a flat surface. The lesion in question here is most likely a(n):

   A. Radial nerve entrapment
   B. Ulnar nerve entrapment
   C. Median nerve entrapment
   D. Musculocutaneous nerve entrapment
   E. Suprascapular nerve entrapment

80. A patient comes into the emergency room complaining that twice during the past week he experienced a sudden loss of muscle tone. The first time occurred when he was told that his mother was diagnosed with cancer. The second came during a track meet while he was warming up before his turn to run. These episodes are most likely to be associated with which one of the following diagnoses:

   A. Sleep apnea
   B. Primary insomnia
   C. Primary hypersomnia
   D. Narcolepsy
   E. Circadian rhythm sleep disorder

81. Which one of the following is true regarding conversion disorder?

   A. It is intentionally produced
   B. It consists of complaints in multiple organ systems
   C. It involves neurologic symptoms
   D. It can be limited to pain
   E. It can be limited to sexual dysfunction

82. Which one of the following drugs is contraindicated in conjunction with therapy with levodopa/carbidopa in Parkinson's disease patients?

   A. Amitryptyline
   B. Fluoxetine
   C. Gabapentin
   D. Tranylcypromine
   E. Sertraline

83. Piaget's stage of concrete operations includes which one of the following?

   A. Identity versus role confusion
   B. Good enough mothering
   C. Conservation
   D. Inductive reasoning
   E. Object permanence

84. A 10 year-old child engages in sex play. This should be viewed as:
    A. A sign of homosexuality
    B. A sign of hormonal imbalance
    C. The result of excessive television viewing
    D. Normal development
    E. Premature development

85. You see a child in the clinic who has fragile X syndrome. You would expect him to have all of the following, EXCEPT:
    A. Mental retardation
    B. Long ears
    C. Narrow face
    D. Arched palate
    E. Short palpebral fissures

86. What would you expect from 18 month-old children with secure attachments after their parents leave them alone with you in a room?
    A. They would try to bring the parents back into the room
    B. They would immediately run to you and sit on your lap
    C. They would become more inquisitive
    D. They would not notice the parents' absence
    E. They would become aggressive and violent

87. Which one of the following agents is a potent cytochrome P-450 inhibitor and can dangerously increase levels of lamotrigine in patients?
    A. Phenytoin
    B. Diazepam
    C. Valproate
    D. Phenobarbital
    E. Gabapentin

88. You are introduced to a child with a physical deformity. When would you predict that the deformity would have the greatest psychological impact on the child?
    A. Infancy
    B. Preschool
    C. Elementary school age
    D. Early adolescence
    E. Adulthood

89. Which one of the following is a specific inhibitor of monoamine oxidase type B (MAOI-B)?
    A. Moclobemide
    B. Phenelzine
    C. Tranylcypromine
    D. Selegiline
    E. Befloxatone

90. Which one of the following will produce a hypodopaminergic state when used chronically?
    A. Heroin
    B. PCP
    C. Alcohol
    D. Amphetamines
    E. Cocaine

91. The anticonvulsant agent valproic acid can cause which one of the following problems in the fetus of pregnant patients?
    A. Spina bifida
    B. Macrocephaly
    C. Hypertelorism
    D. Oligohydramnios
    E. Intrauterine growth retardation

92. Which one of the following agents is a dopamine agonist?
    A. Haloperidol
    B. Pergolide
    C. Quetiapine
    D. Buspirone
    E. Fluphenazine

93. A 25 year-old man is brought to see you because of change in personality following a boating accident. He fell off of his boat and landed head first on the dock. He was previously friendly, happy, and high functioning. Now his speech is pressured and his mood is labile. He has been irresponsible at work and has been fired from his job. His memory is intact. Which one of the following brain areas did he damage?
    A. Temporal lobe
    B. Occipital lobe
    C. Basal ganglia
    D. Substantia nigra
    E. Frontal lobe

94. Which one of the following inhibits norepinephrine reuptake?
    A. Haloperidol
    B. Ziprasidone
    C. Chlorpromazine
    D. Olanzapine
    E. Aripiprazole

95. Which one of the following has mixed dopamine agonist-antagonist properties?
    A. Haloperidol
    B. Ziprasidone
    C. Chlorpromazine
    D. Olanzapine
    E. Aripiprazole

96. Damage to which one of the following brain areas is most likely to present with depression?
    A. Occipital lobe
    B. Right prefrontal cortex
    C. Left prefrontal cortex
    D. Right parietal lobe
    E. Left parietal lobe

97. Which one of the following brain areas is characteristically serotonergic?
    A. Ventral tegmental area
    B. Substantia nigra
    C. Nucleus accumbens
    D. Cerebellum
    E. Raphe nuclei

98. A patient presents to your office with a history of wing-flapping coarse tremor of the upper extremities, ataxia and a rapidly progressive confusional state developing over several months. The test of choice to diagnose this patient is:
    A. Serum ACE level
    B. Chromosomal analysis for CAG triplet repeats
    C. Serum ceruloplasmin level
    D. Lumbar puncture and CSF titer for oligoclonal bands and myelin basic protein
    E. Edrophonium hydrochloride testing (Tensilon test)

99. A patient comes into the emergency room high on cocaine. Which one of the following brain regions would you expect to be most active in terms of the reward he is experiencing from the drug?

   A. Neocortex
   B. Substantia nigra
   C. Nucleus accumbens
   D. Locus ceruleus
   E. Raphe nuclei

100. What is the therapeutic focus of motivational enhancement therapy?

   A. Anger
   B. Depression
   C. Medical comorbidity
   D. Ambivalence
   E. Environment

101. You are teaching a class to a group of first year psychiatric residents. You review some of the psychological tests with them and describe their use. One of the anal-retentive types in the front row asks which of the tests has the highest reliability. Your answer is?

   A. Wechsler adult intelligence scale
   B. Thematic apperception test
   C. Draw a person test
   D. Minnesota multiphasic personality inventory
   E. Projective personality assessment

102. Freud is best associated with which one of the following?

   A. Learning theory
   B. Mesolimbic dopamine theory of positive psychotic symptoms
   C. Conflict theory
   D. Self psychology
   E. Drive theory

103. The most common cause of intracerebral hemorrhage is:

   A. Hypertension
   B. Intracranial tumors or metastases
   C. Disorders of coagulation (coagulopathies)
   D. Vascular malformations
   E. Trauma

104. How would Beck describe the problem found in depression?
    A. Learned helplessness
    B. Not good enough mothering
    C. Neurochemical imbalance
    D. Cognitive distortion
    E. Lack of social skills

105. A Type I error occurs when:
    A. The null hypothesis is rejected when it should have been retained
    B. The null hypothesis is retained when it should have been rejected
    C. There is false rejection of a difference that was truly significant
    D. The probability of an event occurring is 0
    E. The probability of an event occurring is 1

106. The process by which a patient in a clinical trial has an equal likelihood of being in a control group versus an experimental group is:
    A. Probability
    B. Risk
    C. Percentile rank
    D. Power
    E. Randomization

107. A 32 year-old man who is HIV positive presents to the emergency room with mild fever to 101°F, headache, stiff neck, photophobia and lethargy. His CD4 count is zero and he has a highly elevated viral load. The most useful immediate diagnostic test for his current condition would be:
    A. Head CT scan with contrast
    B. MRI of the brain with and without gadolinium
    C. Lumbar puncture for CSF analysis and India ink staining
    D. Chest radiography and blood cultures
    E. Serum cold agglutinin assay

23

108. The probability of finding a true difference between two samples is:
    A. Probability
    B. Risk
    C. Percentile rank
    D. Power
    E. Randomization

109. The number of people who have a disorder at a specified point in time is:
    A. Probability
    B. Risk
    C. Point prevalence
    D. Power
    E. Randomization

110. To diagnose anorexia nervosa, the patient must be below what percentage of normal body weight?
    A. 85%
    B. 65%
    C. 93%
    D. 50%
    E. 75%

111. How long after taking PCP can it still be found in the urine?
    A. 1 day
    B. 2 days
    C. 5 days
    D. 8 days
    E. 10 days

112. Which one of the following is associated with the amyloid precursor protein?
    A. Wilson's disease
    B. Schizophrenia
    C. Alzheimer's disease
    D. Bipolar disorder
    E. Huntington's disease

113. A patient you put on carbamazepine has weakness and a rash. Which lab test would you order first?
    A. Liver profile
    B. Electrolytes, BUN, creatinine, glucose (Chem-7)
    C. Complete blood count
    D. Thyroid function tests
    E. VDRL

114. An initial workup of a patient with anorexia nervosa should include all of the following diagnostic tests, EXCEPT:
    A. Complete blood count
    B. Chem-7
    C. Thyroid function tests
    D. Electrocardiogram
    E. Head CT scan

115. The test of choice to diagnose human central nervous system prion disease is:
    A. Serum assay for 14-3-3 proteins
    B. CSF assay for 14-3-3 and tau proteins
    C. EEG
    D. MRI of the brain with and without gadolinium
    E. Head CT scan with contrast

116. Which eye findings are common in schizophrenia?
    A. Failure of adduction
    B. Failure of accommodation
    C. Pupillary dilatation
    D. Abnormal smooth pursuit saccades
    E. Weakness of the third cranial nerve

117. A patient on risperidone comes into your office and reports that she intends on going to her gynecologist because she hasn't been having her menstrual periods. She has taken a pregnancy test and it was negative. Which lab test would you order?
    A. Lumbar puncture
    B. Risperidone level
    C. Complete blood count
    D. Liver profile
    E. Prolactin level

118. A 20 year-old man comes into the emergency room. He has superficial cuts on his arms, legs and abdomen. He reports being very depressed and feels that his neighbors are out to harm him. His most likely diagnosis is:
    A. Dysthymic disorder
    B. Schizoaffective disorder
    C. Borderline personality disorder
    D. Bipolar disorder
    E. Adjustment disorder with mixed anxiety and depressed mood

119. Which one of the following conditions has the highest prevalence?
    A. Depressive disorders
    B. Anxiety disorders
    C. Schizophrenia
    D. Dementia
    E. Substance abuse

120. Which one of the following has the greatest co-morbidity with pathological gambling?
    A. Schizophrenia
    B. Posttraumatic stress disorder
    C. Agoraphobia
    D. Major depressive disorder
    E. Intermittent explosive disorder

121. A couple comes into the emergency room. The wife says that her husband has become convinced that she is cheating on him, and that it is not true. He has been following her, smelling her clothing, going through her purse, and making regular accusations. He does not meet criteria for a mood disorder. He denies other psychotic symptoms. Medical and substance abuse history are negative. What is his diagnosis?

    A. Schizophrenia
    B. Major depressive disorder with psychotic features
    C. Delusional disorder
    D. Delirium
    E. Shared psychotic disorder

122. Which one of the following disorders presents with the patient being preoccupied with having a given illness based on misinterpretation of bodily sensations?

    A. Somatoform disorder
    B. Factitious disorder
    C. Conversion disorder
    D. Pain disorder
    E. Hypochondriasis

123. A patient asks you about the data proving that alcoholism is hereditary. During your discussion, the patient asks you the following question: "The study of which group most strongly supports the heredity of alcoholism?" Your answer is:

    A. Siblings
    B. Cousins
    C. Parents
    D. Mothers-daughters
    E. Adopted siblings

124. A patient falls down on the floor of your office. He states that he has a terrible headache. He begins to hyperventilate. He has asynchronous tonic-clonic movements on both sides of his body. He is not incontinent, and is not injured. He is conscious the whole time. What is the most likely explanation for this presentation?

    A. Complex seizure
    B. Simple seizure
    C. Psychogenic seizure
    D. Myoclonus
    E. Carpal tunnel syndrome

125. The lesion that produces the classic signs of internuclear ophthalmoplegia in multiple sclerosis is most often found in the:
   A. Superior colliculus
   B. Medial longitudinal fasciculus
   C. Inferior colliculus
   D. Nucleus of the third nerve
   E. Nucleus of the sixth nerve

126. Which form of schizophrenia occurs later, and results in less decline in cognitive functioning as compared to the others?
   A. Disorganized
   B. Paranoid
   C. Catatonic
   D. Undifferentiated
   E. Residual

127. A middle-aged man comes to you with the complaint that he cannot stop gambling. He has wasted tens of thousands of dollars in casinos and his wife just left him. He has also been fired from his job because he misses so much work to gamble. Where would his diagnosis best fit in the following choices?
   A. Personality disorders
   B. Psychotic disorders
   C. Anxiety disorders
   D. Substance abuse disorders
   E. Impulse control disorders

128. An 8 year-old boy is getting beaten up at school because of his social interactions. He talks at the other children rather than to them. He is obsessed with cats. His cognitive and language development are appropriate. His diagnosis is:
   A. Conduct disorder
   B. Oppositional defiant disorder
   C. Attention deficit-hyperactivity disorder
   D. Autism
   E. Asperger's disorder

129. An 8 year-old boy is getting beaten up at school because of his lack of social interactions. He talks at the other children rather than to them. He is obsessed with cats. His cognitive and language development are significantly impaired. His diagnosis is:
   A. Conduct disorder
   B. Oppositional defiant disorder
   C. Attention deficit-hyperactivity disorder
   D. Autism
   E. Asperger's disorder

130. A subjective sense that the environment is changed or unreal is:
    A. Depersonalization
    B. Derealization
    C. Fugue
    D. Amnesia
    E. Anosognosia

131. A young patient presents to your office with dementia. He has been involved in heavy drug use. He has used heroin, PCP, LSD, amphetamines and inhalants. If you were to postulate which most likely caused his dementia, which one would you choose?
    A. Heroin
    B. LSD
    C. PCP
    D. Amphetamines
    E. Inhalents

132. Which is the best matched pair among the following?
    A. Family therapy—seclusion and restraint
    B. Vocational assessment—social skills training
    C. Assertive community treatment—psychoanalysis
    D. ADHD—ECT
    E. Psychiatric rehabilitation—social skills training

133. All of the following are clinical features highly suggestive of multiple sclerosis, EXCEPT:
    A. Optic neuritis
    B. Worsening with elevated body temperature
    C. Fatigue
    D. Steady progression from initial onset
    E. Lhermitte's sign

134. A 20 year-old woman comes to the emergency room with hypokalemic alkalosis, enlarged parotids, hypotension and Russell's sign. What diagnosis do you suspect?
    A. Psychosis
    B. Major depressive disorder
    C. Bulimia
    D. Inhalant induced euphoria
    E. HIV

135. While on call in the emergency room you receive a phone call from emergency medical services (EMS) to say that they are bringing in a patient who is highly intoxicated and behaviorally out of control. The patient's friend told EMS that he has been taking amphetamines. If this is true, what is the most prominent psychiatric symptom you would expect to see?
    A. Hallucinations
    B. Suicidal tendencies
    C. Disorganized speech
    D. Paranoia
    E. Anxiety

136. A 29 year-old woman has begun hearing voices since seeing her child hit by a car three weeks ago. She has become irritable, fearful, and is not sleeping well. The most likely diagnosis is:
    A. Schizophrenia
    B. Acute stress disorder
    C. Dysthymic disorder
    D. Bipolar II disorder
    E. Adjustment disorder with depressed mood

137. Children with depression often present with which one of the following?
    A. Urinary incontinence
    B. Violence
    C. Irritability
    D. Hallucinations
    E. Delusions

138. A patient comes into the clinic carrying a diagnosis of schizoid personality disorder. To confirm this diagnosis, you would look for which one of the following?
    A. Bright, revealing clothing
    B. Grandiosity
    C. Paranoia
    D. Lack of close relationships
    E. Magical thinking

139. If you apply your abilities solely for the patient's well being, and do no harm to the patient, you are said to have:
    A. Beneficence
    B. Malignancy
    C. Justice
    D. Validity
    E. Autonomy

140. All of the following are true of Tourette's syndrome, EXCEPT:
    A. The course is usually not progressive
    B. Symptoms increase in times of stress
    C. Initial symptoms may decrease, increase, or persist
    D. Vocal tics are done to intentionally provoke others
    E. Medication can be helpful

141. On your drive in to work you wonder if you will encounter any violent patients during your day. If you encounter the following types of patients today, which group of patients is the most likely to attack you?
    A. Bipolar patients
    B. Schizophrenic patients
    C. Borderline patients
    D. Substance abusers
    E. Major depressive disorder patients

142. What is the best indicator that a patient has the ego strength for psycho-dynamic psychotherapy?
    A. Diagnosis
    B. Age
    C. Quality of relationships
    D. Gender
    E. Mental status examination

143. T2-weighted MRI brain imaging of a patient reveals the scan pictured below. The patient is a 36 year-old woman who presented to the emergency room with recurrent episodes of unilateral arm and leg weakness and numbness with gait instability. The treatment of first choice in this case would be:
    A. Intravenous ceftriaxone administration
    B. Intravenous immunoglobin therapy
    C. Plasmapheresis
    D. Sublingual aspirin and intravenous heparin therapy
    E. Intravenous corticosteroid therapy

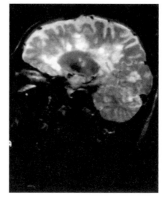

144. A patient with borderline personality disorder and past suicide attempts calls you after a fight with her boyfriend. She has been cutting herself since the fight and is hearing voices. What is the best level of care for this patient at this time?

A. Inpatient hospitalization
B. Outpatient therapy
C. Speak to her again in 5 days
D. Extended inpatient stay (1+ months)
E. Group therapy session

145. A 75 year-old woman is referred to your practice by an internist for depression. On initial examination you discover that the patient has recently just recovered from a heart attack. Which one of the following medications would be the best choice for this patient?

A. Amitryptiline
B. Doxepin
C. Buproprion
D. Methylphenidate
E. Citalopram

146. All of the following are classic characteristics of neurofibromatosus type 1 (von Recklinghausen's disease), EXCEPT:

A. Café au lait spots and cutaneous neurofibromas
B. Bilateral acoustic schwannomas
C. Optic gliomas
D. Lisch nodules
E. Axillary or inguinal freckling

147. The sign that best differentiates between delirium and dementia is:

A. Sleep disturbance
B. Hallucinations
C. Disorientation to place
D. Violent behavior
E. Alteration of consciousness

148. What is the first step towards treating a 23 year-old medical student who comes to your office with a complaint of insomnia?

A. Prescribe zolpidem
B. Prescribe benzodiazepines
C. Prescribe diphenhydramine
D. Restrict the use of the bed to sleep and intimacy only
E. Obtain a sleep study

149. What is the American Psychiatric Association's position on therapy to change the sexual orientation of homosexuals?
     A. This type of therapy should be encouraged
     B. Homosexuality is a medical disorder
     C. Only teens should be treated, before they become sexually active
     D. There is little data showing negative outcomes of such therapy
     E. No existing data supports doing this therapy

150. A 20 year-old college student is brought into the emergency room after a party. He has tenting of the skin on the backs of his hands, is nauseated and vomits, acts seductively towards the nursing staff, and thinks the security guards are out to kill him. He tells you: "The one with the red hair is out to slay me." The emergency medical technician tells you the patient apparently collapsed while dancing at a "rave". What substance has he most likely taken?
     A. Cannabis
     B. Ketamine
     C. Diacetylmorphine
     D. Methylenedioxyamphetamine
     E. Some form of volatile inhalant

Answers

Test Number **ONE**
ANSWER KEY

1	D	51	D	101	A
2	D	52	B	102	E
3	D	53	C	103	A
4	A	54	D	104	D
5	C	55	D	105	A
6	A	56	B	106	E
7	D	57	B	107	C
8	C	58	E	108	D
9	C	59	B	109	C
10	E	60	C	110	A
11	D	61	C	111	D
12	C	62	D	112	C
13	B	63	A	113	C
14	D	64	A	114	E
15	C	65	D	115	B
16	E	66	A	116	D
17	B	67	C	117	E
18	C	68	E	118	C
19	E	69	B	119	B
20	E	70	C	120	D
21	A	71	D	121	C
22	B	72	E	122	E
23	D	73	C	123	E
24	A	74	E	124	C
25	A	75	D	125	B
26	C	76	E	126	B
27	D	77	D	127	E
28	B	78	E	128	E
29	E	79	A	129	D
30	E	80	D	130	B
31	C	81	C	131	E
32	A	82	D	132	E
33	D	83	C	133	D
34	D	84	D	134	C
35	D	85	E	135	D
36	B	86	A	136	B
37	C	87	C	137	C
38	C	88	D	138	D
39	B	89	D	139	A
40	E	90	E	140	D
41	B	91	A	141	D
42	D	92	B	142	C
43	C	93	E	143	E
44	B	94	B	144	A
45	C	95	E	145	E
46	B	96	C	146	B
47	B	97	E	147	E
48	D	98	C	148	D
49	D	99	C	149	E
50	B	100	D	150	D

44

ANSWER EXPLANATIONS

Question 1. D. Several cutaneous side effects are possible with lithium including acne, follicular and maculopapular eruptions. Alopecia has also been reported. Major side effects of lithium include gastrointestinal complaints, tremor, diabetes insipidus, hypothyroidism, weight gain, cardiac arrhythmia and edema. Lamotrigine is an anticonvulsant that is also used for mood stabilization. Side effects can include Stevens-Johnson syndrome, anemia, thrombocytopenia, liver failure, and pancreatitis. Lorazepam is a benzodiazepine, which causes sedation, respiratory suppression, and has a high addictive potential. Risperidone is an antipsychotic that can cause extrapyramidal side effects, neuroleptic malignant syndrome, metabolic syndrome, gastrointestinal upset, increased salivation and lactation, among others. Oxcarbazepine is an anticonvulsant that may cause leukopenia, thrombocytopenia, Stevens-Johnson syndrome, and several other side effects. With the exception of lithium, the other choices do not worsen acne.
K&S Ch. 3

Question 2. D. Attachment, which is the emotional dependence of the infant on his mother, involves resources and security, because the infant depends on the mother for these things. Attachment theory was developed by John Bowlby, and says that a secure attachment between mother and child affects the child's ability to form healthy relationships later in life. Attachment occurs when there is a warm intimate and continuous relationship between child and mother. The attachment gives the infant a feeling of security. Bonding is the mother's feelings for her infant. In bonding, the mother does not rely on her baby for food and protection. Therefore bonding does not involve resources and security. It is thought that bonding occurs with skin to skin contact between infant and mother. All other choices given are true regarding attachment theory.
K&S Ch. 4

Question 3. D. Serum polymerase chain reaction (PCR) is the test of choice to examine the number of trinucleotide repeats (>35 in adults and >50 in children) in order to diagnose Huntington's disease (HD). The HD gene resides on the short arm of chromosome 4 at 4p16.3. A chromosomal karyotype can reveal only macroscopic defects in chromosomes such as deletions, translocations, or trisomies. Serum ceruloplasmin, when low, is diagnostic of Wilson's disease. Urine porphobilinogens and aminolevulinic acid, when detected in urine in excessive amounts, are diagnostic of acute intermittent porphyria. Creutzfeld-Jakob disease is diagnosed by cerebrospinal fluid assay for 14-3-3 proteinase inhibitor proteins.
B&D Ch. 77

Question 4. A. Orbitofrontal lobe lesions cause patients to appear profane, irritable, and irresponsible. When presented with cases that involve personality changes, one should suspect pathology in the frontal lobes. Also, deficits in executive functioning usually involve the frontal lobes. Medial frontal lesions cause apathy, characterized by limited spontaneous movement, gesture, and speech. Left frontal lesions can cause depression. Right frontal lobe lesions can cause mania.
K&S Ch. 3

Question 5. C. This is an example of a delusion, which is a fixed false belief that is not accepted by members of the same cultural background. Delusions may be mood congruent or mood incongruent. They may have themes that are bizarre, persecutory, paranoid, grandiose, jealous, somatic, guilty or erotic. Coprolalia is the compulsive utterance of obscene words, as seen in Tourette's disorder. Egomania is a pathological self preoccupation. Ailurophobia is a dread of cats. An obsession is the pathological persistence of an irresistible thought or feeling that can not be eliminated from consciousness and is associated with anxiety.
K&S Ch. 8

Question 6. A. This is a description of a cohort study, in which a well-defined population is followed over a period of time. Cohort studies are also known as longitudinal studies. Cohort studies provide direct estimates of risk associated with a suspected causative factor. A case-control study is a retrospective study that examines persons without a particular disease. In a clinical trial, specially selected patients receive a course of treatment, and another group does not. Patients are assigned to either group on a random basis. The goal is to determine the effectiveness of the treatment. Cross-sectional surveys describe the prevalence of a disease in a population at a particular point in time. Crossover studies are a variation of the double-blind study in which the placebo and treatment groups switch at some point in the study.
K&S Ch. 4

Question 7. D. Although all of the choices contributed to our understanding of child development, it is Winnicott who developed the concept of good enough mothering. This concept is based on the understanding that the mother plays a vital role in bringing the world to the infant and offering empathic anticipation of the infant's needs. If she does these things well enough the baby will move towards the development of a healthy sense of self. Piaget described stages of cognitive development consisting of sensorimotor, preoperational thought, concrete operations, and formal operations. Freud was the founder of psychoanalysis, giving us the oral, anal, phallic and latency stages of development. Mahler developed stages of separation-individuation to describe how children develop identity that is separate from their mothers. Her stages were normal autism, symbiosis, differentiation, practicing, rapprochement and object constancy. Erikson developed an 8-stage life cycle. The stages are trust vs mistrust, autonomy vs shame and doubt, initiative vs guilt, industry vs inferiority, identity vs role diffusion, intimacy vs self absorption, generativity vs stagnation, and integrity vs despair and isolation.
K&S Ch. 2&6

Question 8. C. The clinical picture presented is that of Wernicke's encephalopathy. Classically seen in alcoholics, the clinical triad is that of mental confusion, ophthalmoplegia and gait ataxia. The usual brain autopsy finding is that of microhemorrhages in the periventricular gray matter, particularly around the aqueduct and third and fourth ventricles. Frontal and temporal lobe atrophy is consistent with Pick's dementia. Parkinson's disease would result in depigmentation of the pars compacta of the substantia nigra in

the midbrain. Diffuse Lewy bodies can be seen in both Parkinson's disease and Alzheimer's disease. Subcortical white matter lesions perpendicular to the ventricles (also called Dawson's fingers) are consistent with a demyelinating disease such as multiple sclerosis.
B&D Ch. 63

Question 9. C. Monoamine oxidase inhibitors (MAOIs) increase levels of biogenic amine neurotransmitters (serotonin, norepinephrine, and dopamine) by preventing their degradation. There are two types of MAO enzyme, MAO-A which breaks down serotonin, norepinephrine, and dopamine, and MAO-B which breaks down dopamine. It is contraindicated to give meperidine with an MAOI. Because these drugs increase intra-synaptic levels of biogenic amine neurotransmitters they should not be given with other drugs that do the same. There have been reports of death in patients given MAOIs and meperidine simultaneously. Patients should inform each of the doctors that they are seeing that they are taking an MAOI. Lithium can be given with MAOIs. When switching a patient from a selective serotonin reuptake inhibitor to an MAOI you need to allow a 14-day washout (28 days for fluoxetine). This is because the combination of these drugs in the system at the same time can potentiate a serotonin syndrome. Orthostatic hypotension is a major side effect of the MAOIs. Other side effects include weight gain, edema, sexual dysfunction, and insomnia. Moclobemide and selegiline are reversible MAO-A inhibitors and because they only weakly potentiate the pressor effects of tyramine they do not require a tyramine free diet at low doses.
K&S Ch. 36

Question 10. E. The best choice for tranquilizing agitated patients is haloperidol. Given that the patient in question is elderly, starting with a small dose of haloperidol would be appropriate. Benzodiazepines should be avoided in cases of suspected delirium, which based on the question stem is a concern for this patient. Hence answer choices A and C are out. A benzodiazepine given to a delirious patient can worsen the delirium and further disinhibit the patient making them more agitated. In general one should use great caution in giving benzodiazepines to the elderly, and when used, they should be given in small doses. Aripiprazole, an atypical antipsychotic, only comes in oral form which would likely be unfeasible in an acutely agitated patient. Other atypical antipsychotic drugs that come in intramuscular injectable form such as olanzapine or ziprasidone would be appropriate choices. Lithium is not standardly used to tranquilize patients. It is a mood stabilizer used in the treatment of bipolar disorder and can only be administered orally.
K&S Ch. 10

Question 11. D. Oral meperidine has lower analgesic potency than intramuscular meperidine; therefore the same dose of the oral agent will not cover pain as well as the same dose of the intramuscular agent. There is no reason to suspect that the patient has low pain tolerance or a pain disorder as she is only very recently post-operative and would be expected to be in pain. There is no evidence of a personality disorder given. Conversion disorder presents with neurological symptoms which are not solely limited to pain and as such this is not a conversion disorder.
K&S Ch. 12

Question 12. C. This is an example of countertransference, which refers to the conscious and unconscious feelings the therapist has towards the patient. Transference refers to the feelings the patient has towards the therapist. Resistance is when ideas that are unacceptable to the patient are prevented from reaching awareness. The term is usually used in reference to therapy where the patient withholds relevant information, remains silent, is late, or misses

appoinments. Confrontation is addressing an issue that the patient does not want to accept. Projection is reacting to unacceptable inner impulses as if they were outside the self. It may often take the form of perceiving one's own feelings in another and then acting on that perception.
K&S Ch. 6

Question 13. B. Huntington's disease is transmitted by an autosomal dominant inheritance pattern. If one parent is an affected carrier, the likelihood of transmission to any given child is 50%. The protein huntingtin is coded on the short arm of chromosome 4. The gene contains an expanded trinucleotide repeat sequence of CAG (normally less than 29 repeats occur).
B&D Ch. 77

Question 14. D. Middle adulthood spans the years between ages 40 and 65. At the end of early adulthood people review the past and decide what the future will hold for them. In their occupation they start to see differences between early aspirations and what they have actually achieved. In middle adulthood people take stock of accomplishment, reassess commitment to family, work, and marriage, use power ethically, and deal with the illness of their parents. Hence, all of the choices are life tasks faced in middle adulthood except risk-taking behavior. This takes place traditionally in adolescence. Adulthood typically begins with selecting a mate, deciding on an occupation, and achieving independence and self sufficiency.
K&S Ch. 2

Question 15. C. This is an example of tertiary prevention. Primary prevention is when a clinician does something to prevent the onset of a disease. This is done by reducing causative agents, reducing risk factors, increasing host resistance, or interfering with the transmission of a disease. Secondary prevention is when one identifies a disease in its early stages and seeks prompt treatment. Tertiary prevention involves reducing deficits caused by an illness in order to obtain the highest possible level of functioning. The other answer choices have nothing to do with prevention. Malingering is consciously faking illness for secondary gain. Noncompliance is a term that refers to not following a doctor's instructions.
K&S Ch. 4

Question 16. E. Lambert-Eaton myasthenic syndrome (LEMS) is a paraneoplastic abnormality of presynaptic acetylcholine release, often described in conjuction with small cell lung carcinoma. The likely mechanism is immune-mediated, directed against voltage-gated calcium channels. The clinical hallmark of the disorder is generalized weakness with initial improvement in strength after minimal exercise. The electromyogram (EMG) reveals a classic decrementing to 3 Hz stimulation in muscles of the hands or feet. Multiple sclerosis would be expected to cause numerous different deficits, motor, sensory, or both, that are diffuse in space and time. Guillain-Barré syndrome, also known as acute inflammatory demyelinating polyneuropathy (AIDP), is a rapidly occurring demyelinating disease that can present with ascending pain, paralysis, sensory loss, or any combination of these symptoms. The clinical hallmark of AIDP is a loss of deep tendon reflexes in the extremities. The test of choice is EMG and nerve conduction studies which usually reveal loss of H reflex and decreased nerve conduction velocities. Polymyositis is an inflammatory disease of the muscle.
B&D Ch. 84

Question 17. B. This question is really asking which of the choices is not a projective test, as one of the purposes of a projective test is to detect psychosis. The only choice that is not a projective test is the Minnesota multiphasic personality inventory (MMPI), which is a self-report inventory used to assess personality and areas of psychopathologic functioning. The draw

a person test consists of the patient being asked to draw a person. The level of detail is thought to correlate with intelligence and developmental level. Then the patient is asked to draw a person of the opposite sex. The patient is then questioned on what they drew. The assumption is that the drawing represents the expression of the self or the body in the environment. The sentence completion test consists of asking the patient to complete a series of incomplete sentences. The tester focuses attention on strong affect, repeated answers, humor, or unusual responses. The thematic apperception test is a series of pictures shown to a patient. The patient then generates a story to explain the pictures. The patient's most accepted and conscious traits and motives are attributed to the character closest to the patient in sex, age, and appearance. More unconscious or unacceptable traits are attributed to those characters most unlike the patient. The Rorschach test is a series of 10 inkblots that serve as inspiration for free association. The patient's responses to each card are recorded and closely interpreted.
K&S Ch. 5

Question 18. C. Amyotrophic lateral sclerosis (ALS) is a disorder of the upper and lower motor neurons. The spinal cord lower motor neurons are also known as the anterior horn cells. These classically degenerate in ALS and can be demonstrated on autopsy. Callosal thinning and atrophy are hallmarks of multiple sclerosis. Frontotemporal atrophy can be seen in Pick's dementia. Nigrostriatal depigmentation is a result of Parkinson's disease. Dorsal column pathology can be seen in vitamin B12 deficiency polyneuropathy with loss of vibration and joint position sensation.
B&D Ch. 80

Question 19. E. It is considered unethical for psychiatrists to participate in executions. According to the American Psychiatric Association, it is unethical to accept commission for patient referrals. It is unethical to have romantic or sexual relationships with patients. Psychiatrists are expected to report the unethical behavior of other psychiatrists. When retiring, the psychiatrist needs to give patients sufficient notice and make an effort to find them follow-up care. The above are ethical issues often questioned on standardized exams.
K&S Ch. 58

Question 20. E. This patient is clearly delirious based on the description. While all of the other choices are logical steps, the first and most important is protecting the patient from harm. In this case that would involve sedating the patient before she gets harmed as a result of her own agitation. This is a good rule to keep in mind whenever dealing with an agitated patient. The first responsibility is to keep both patient and staff from getting harmed.
K&S Ch. 10

Question 21. A. The use of positive and negative reinforcement is part of operant conditioning developed by Skinner. In operant conditioning the animal is active and behaves in a way that produces a reward. Learning occurs as a consequence of action. The desired behavior reaps a positive reward. An undesired behavior gets a negative reward. Bandura is a proponent of social learning theory, which says we learn through modeling others and through social interaction. Attribution theory says that people are likely to attribute their own behavior to situational causes, and the behavior of others to personality traits. This then affects their feelings and behavior. Hull did work in the neurophysiologic aspects of learning, developing a drive reduction theory of learning. Learned helplessness is a model for depression developed by Seligman, in which an organism learns that no behavioral change can influence the environment. The organism becomes depressed

and apathetic because no matter what it does its environmental circumstances never change. Kandel studied habituation and sensitization in snails. Habituation theory says that an animal can learn to stop responding to a repeated stimulus. Sensitization theory says that an organism can be taught to respond more easily to a stimulus, or be made more sensitive to that stimulus. Pavlov developed classical conditioning. In classical conditioning, a neutral stimulus is paired with one that evokes a response so that eventually the neutral stimulus comes to evoke the same response. He did the classic experiments with dogs salivating when hearing their master's footsteps.
K&S Ch. 4

Question 22. B. Ethosuximide is the treatment of choice for uncomplicated absence seizures, the clinical presentation depicted in this question. Failing ethosuximide, the next best choice would be valproic acid, which has efficacy in partial complex, primary generalized and absence seizure types. Carbamazepine would be a very poor choice to treat absence seizures, as it is ineffective in absence seizures and may even worsen the condition. Phenobarbital is not indicated for use in absence seizures. Diazepam is useful only for emergencies such as status epilepticus and usually in rectal, intramuscular, or intravenous forms. Phenytoin is indicated for partial and generalized tonic-clonic seizures; not for absence seizures.
B&D Ch. 73

Question 23. D. The description in this question is that of narcolepsy. Narcolepsy consists of irresistible attacks of refreshing daytime sleep that occur daily for three months or more. The sudden loss of muscle tone described is known as cataplexy. One also sees increased intrusion of rapid eye movement (REM) sleep into the transition between sleep and wakefulness causing hypnopompic (while awakening) and hypnagogic (while falling asleep) hallucinations, as well as sleep paralysis. This disorder can be dangerous as it can lead to automobile or industrial accidents. Treatments can involve stimulants such as amphetamines, methylphenidate (Ritalin), or modafinil (Provigil), as well as structured napping times during the day. Modafinil is a non-stimulant medication FDA-approved for narcolepsy. Its mechanism of action is on histamine neurons in the reticular activating system in the pons. Sleep changes associated with depression include early morning awakening and difficulty falling asleep. Sleep apnea presents with daytime irritability and drowsiness with prominent snoring at night. Primary insomnia is characterised by difficulty initiating or maintaining sleep, or nonrestorative sleep for at least one month. Shift-work sleep disorder is a type of circadian rhythm sleep disorder that occurs in those that repeatedly and rapidly change their work schedules. This can lead to somnolence, insomnia, as well as somatic problems such as an increased likelihood of peptic ulcer.
K&S Ch. 24

Question 24. A. Dopamine is associated with the induction of aggression. Serotonin is associated with decreased aggression. In particular, the cerebrospinal fluid levels of 5-HIAA, a major serotonin metabolite, have been shown to be inversely correlated with the frequency of aggression. GABA is the major inhibitory neurotransmitter of the brain and is associated with decreased aggression. Norepinephrine is associated with decreased aggression and its functions are thought to be connected to that of serotonin, particularly in mood disorders. Glycine is an inhibitory neurotransmitter, and as such is not associated with increased aggression. As a general rule, it is thought that cholinergic and catecholaminergic mechanisms seem to be involved in the induction of aggression, and serotonin and GABA seem to inhibit such behavior.
K&S Ch. 3&4

Question 25. A. Carbamazepine induces its own metabolism. This effect decreases its 24-hour half-life by at least 50% during the first three to four weeks of therapy. Increments in dosages after the first few weeks of therapy are often necessary to maintain therapeutic serum levels. None of the other mentioned anticonvulsants have this unique pharmacokinetic profile.
B&D Ch. 73

Question 26. C. This question reviews aspects of both operant and classical conditioning. In classical conditioning a neutral (or conditioned) stimulus is repeatedly paired with one that evokes a response (the unconditioned stimulus), such that the neutral stimulus comes to evoke the response. In operant (Skinnerian) conditioning, a random behavior is reinforced with reward. Initially, every desirable response is rewarded which enables the behavior to be learned. Giving positive reinforcement intermittently and variably is the best way to prevent a behavior from going extinct. Extinction occurs when the conditioned stimulus is constantly repeated without the unconditioned stimulus until the response evoked by the unconditioned stimulus eventually disappears. Generalization is the transfer of a conditioned response from one stimulus to another. For example, the dog that learned to salivate to a bell now salivates to the sound of a cabinet being opened. Discrimination is recognizing and responding to differences between similar stimuli. For example, a dog can be trained to respond differently to two similar bells. Transference that takes place during psychotherapy can be thought of as a form of stimulus generalization. Respondent conditioning is just another term for classical conditioning.
K&S Ch. 4

Question 27. D. Tuberous sclerosis is an autosomal dominant neurocutaneous disorder with a prevalence of about 1 in 6000–9000 individuals. The classic neurologic features of the disease are seizures, mental retardation and behavioral problems. Cutaneous lesions include the ash leaf spot (hypomelanotic macule), adenoma sebaceum (facial angiofibromas) and shagreen spots (irregularly shaped, often raised or textured skin lesion on the back or flank). Retinal hamartomas can be observed in many patients. Neuropathologic lesions include subependymal nodules and cortical hamartomas. Down's syndrome, or trisomy 21, frequently results in early onset Alzheimer's type changes in the brain including neurofibrillary tangles and cholinergic deficits. Rett's disorder, a pervasive developmental disorder seen only in girls, involves deceleration of head growth from ages 5 months to 4 years, loss of purposeful hand skills and development of stereotyped hand movements between ages 5 months and 2.5 years, loss of social engagement and acquired impairment in expressive and receptive language skills. Although seizures can be observed in up to 75% of Rett's patients, there are typically no skin lesions associated with the disorder. Neurofibromatosus has two types: NF1, classic von Recklinghausen's disease, with café au lait spots (6 or more to make the diagnosis), subcutaneous neurofibromas, axillary freckling, Lisch nodules (pigmented iris hamartomas), optic nerve glioma, neurofibromas and schwannomas. NF1 is caused by a mutation of the 60 exon NF1 gene on chromosome 17q. NF2 is caused by a mutation of the NF2 gene on chromosome 22. NF2 patients have few cutaneous lesions. The diagnostic hallmark of NF2 is bilateral vestibular (VIII nerve) schwannomas. Williams' syndrome is an autosomal dominant mental retardation syndrome that occurs by a hemizygous deletion including elastin locus chromosome 7q11-23. Patients with the disorder have short stature, unusual facial features that include depressed nasal bridge (an upturned nose), broad forehead, widely spaced teeth, elfin-like facies, as well as thyroid, renal and cardiovascular anomalies. Psychiatric symptoms include anxiety, hyperactivity, hypermusicality. Seizures and skin lesions are not observed in Williams' syndrome.
B&D Ch. 71

Question 28. B. The mechanism described is that of the cholinesterase inhibitors used in Alzheimer's disease. By potentiating cholinergic transmission, these drugs cause modest improvement in memory and goal-directed thought. These drugs include medications such as tacrine, donepezil, galantamine and rivastigmine. All of the answer choices in this question are cholinesterase inhibitors except for memantine. Memantine is also used for Alzheimer's dementia, but works by binding to N-methyl-D-aspartate (NMDA) receptors, acting as an antagonist and thereby slowing calcium influx into cells. The slowing of calcium influx halts cell destruction.
K&S Ch 36

Question 29. E. Of the tests listed, the only one that tests executive function is the trail making test. The trail making test involves connecting letters and numbers in order, alternating between letters and numbers (i.e., connect A-1-B-2-C-3 etc.) Another acceptable answer would be the Wisconsin card sorting test, but is not an answer choice. The Wisconsin card sorting test evaluates abstract reasoning and flexibility in problem solving. The thematic apperception test is used to test normal personality and involves showing pictures and having the patient come up with stories. The patient's most accepted and conscious traits and motives are attributed to the character closest to the patient in sex, age, and appearance. More unconscious or unacceptable traits are attributed to those characters most unlike the patient. The Halstead-Reitan battery helps find the location of brain lesions as well as differentiate between those who are brain damaged and those who are neurologically intact. It consists of a series of 10 tests. The Minnesota multiphasic personality inventory (MMPI) is a personality assessment used to find areas of psychopathologic functioning. It consists of more than 500 statements to which the patient must respond "true", "false" or "cannot say". The brief psychiatric rating scale (BPRS) is used to assess the severity of psychosis in schizophrenia.
K&S Ch. 5

Question 30. E. The first four choices are all very important pieces in determining whether a person can make a will, including whether or not the person knows he is making a will. In order to have the capacity to make a will, three things are needed. The first is the ability to understand the nature and extent of one's property. The second is that one must know that one is making a will. The third is that one must know to whom the property will be bequeathed. The last answer choice is part of the McGarry instrument which determines whether someone is competent to stand trial. It has nothing to do with making a will.
K&S Ch. 57

Question 31. C. The average age of onset of puberty is 11 years for girls and 13 years for boys. All other answer choices are true. The onset of puberty is triggered by maturation of the hypothalamic-pituitary-adrenal-gonadal axis. This leads to secondary sex characteristics such as enlarged breasts and hips in girls and facial hair and lowered voice in boys. Primary sex characteristics are those involved in coitus – the external genitals and reproductive organs. Increases in height and weight occur earlier in girls than in boys. Sex hormones increase slowly through adolescence and correlate with bodily changes. Follicle stimulating hormone (FSH) and leutinizing hormone (LH) increase through adolescence, being above normal adult values by age 17 or 18. Testosterone seems to increase around age 16 or 17 and then stabilize at adult levels in males.
K&S Ch. 2

Question 32. A. Sumatriptan (Imitrex) is an anti-migraine medication indicated for acute, abortive therapy of migraine headache. All drugs in the triptan class act as potent agonists at 5-HT 1B and 5-HT 1D receptors. Although these

receptors reside principally on intracranial blood vessels, they may have an effect on the coronary arteries as well and could theoretically cause vasoconstriction, vasospasm and acute myocardial infarction. Therefore, these agents are contraindicated in patients with coronary ischemic heart disease, as well as with uncontrolled hypertension.
B&D Ch. 75

Question 33. D. Antipsychotic drugs and methylphenidate increase tricyclic antidepressant (TCA) concentrations through their interaction with the cytochrome p450 system. Other drugs that increase TCA concentrations include acetazolamide, aspirin, cimetidine, thiazides, fluoxetine and sodium bicarbonate. Cigarette smoking decreases their concentration through its action on the 1A2 enzyme. Other drugs that decrease TCA concentrations include ascorbic acid, lithium, barbituates, and primidone.
K&S Ch. 36

Question 34. D. Completed suicide is most often associated with depression, not bipolar disorder. Adolescents most frequently commit suicide with guns, not by hanging. In recent years the suicide rate has gone up dramatically among adolescents, not among middle-aged adults. Previous suicide attempts are the best predictor of future risk of suicide. This is a very important factor which should be taken into account whenever taking a patient history. Men successfully commit suicide three times more often than women. Another factor contributing to completed suicides is age. For men, the highest risk period is after 45 years of age. For women, the highest risk period is after 55 years of age. Married people are less likely to commit suicide than single or widowed people. As far as religion is concerned, rates of suicide among Roman Catholics are less than those for Protestants or Jewish people. With race, whites are more likely to commit suicide than others, especially white males. Physical health may play a role. Thirty-two per cent of people who commit suicide have seen a doctor within the past six months. With regard to occupation, the higher a person's social status, the higher the rate of suicide. A fall in social status also increases the risk.
K&S Ch. 34

Question 35. D. Alexia without agraphia is seen with lesions involving the splenium of the corpus callosum. Gerstmann's syndrome usually involves left parietal lobe damage. The clinical picture is the classic tetrad of acalculia, agraphia (without alexia), right and left confusion and finger agnosia (the inability to name the thumb, index, middle, ring and pinky fingers when called upon to do so). The lesion in Gerstmann's syndrome localizes to the left angular gyrus.
B&D Ch. 57

Question 36. B. Dialectical behavioral therapy (DBT) is a form of therapy developed by Marsha Linehan for the treatment of borderline personality disorder. The therapist is supportive and directive. Specific exercises are performed to help solve problems and improve interpersonal skills. The focus of therapy is on reducing impulses to self-mutilate.
K&S Ch. 35

Question 37. C. The clinical picture portrayed in this question is that of hyperprolactinemia induced by dopamine blockade in the tuberoinfundibular system by a neuroleptic medication. Conventional neuroleptics and risperidone can increase the volume of pituitary microadenomas by blocking dopamine and increasing serum prolactin levels. When an adenoma grows beyond 1.5 cm in diameter it can encroach on the medial portion of both optic nerves outside of the sella turcica. This optic nerve involvement results in the classic clinical sign of bitemporal hemianopsia. Appro-

43

priate treatment would be the discontinuation of the offending drug and possibly administration of bromocriptine. Some adenomas require surgical intervention if they are unresponsive to medication therapy.
B&D Ch. 58

Question 38. C. The mental status examination is the description of the patient's appearance, speech, actions, and thoughts during the interview. All of the choices are correct with the exception of C. Content of thought includes such things as delusions, preoccupations, obsessions, compulsions, phobias, suicidality and homicidality. It is a common mistake to put hallucinations in the thought content section of the mental status exam. Hallucinations are false sensory perceptions and fall under the category of perception. The categories of the mental status examination are appearance, psychomotor activity, attitude, mood, affect, speech, perception, thought content and process, consciousness, orientation, memory, concentration, attention, reading and writing, visuospatial ability, abstract thought, information and intelligence, impulsivity, judgment and insight, and reliability.
K&S Ch. 7

Question 39. B. This is a clear description of the Malaysian cultural syndrome of Amok. It consists of a sudden rampage including homicide and/or suicide, which ends in exhaustion and amnesia. Koro is an Asian delusion that the penis will disappear into the abdomen and cause death. Piblokto occurs in female Eskimos of northern Greenland. It involves anxiety, depression, confusion, depersonalization, derealization, ending in stuporous sleep and amnesia. Wihtigo is a delusional fear displayed by Native American Indians of being turned into a cannibal through possession by a supernatural monster, the Wihtigo. Mal de ojo is a syndrome found in those of Mediterranean descent involving vomiting, fever, and restless sleep. It is thought to be caused by the evil eye.
K&S Ch. 14

Question 40. E. The patient has clearly suffered a left hemispheric stroke, possibly in the middle cerebral artery territory. Any hemispheric stroke that involves the corticospinal tract can result in an appearance of contralateral Babinski and Hoffman's signs. The Babinski sign is the upward motion of the big toe and fanning of the other toes when the plantar surface of the foot is stroked upwardly from bottom to top with a noxious stimulus or blunt instrument like the butt of a reflex hammer. The Hoffman's sign is positive when the adduction of the thumb is noted upon a fast downward flick being administered to the index or middle finger of the same hand. Hoffman's sign is equivalent to the Babinski sign except it is in the upper extremity. The palmomental reflex and Meyerson sign are two of the classic so-called frontal release signs. The palmomental reflex is positive when the chin muscle contracts as the thenar eminence of the palm contralateral to the brain lesion is stroked with a blunt instrument. Meyerson sign is the presence of a persistence of the glabellar reflex of blinking upon confrontation of the forehead by tapping with a finger. The blinking normally should extinguish after several taps of the forehead, but in the presence of frontal lobe damage, the response does not extinguish as rapidly. Complete loss of the gag reflex would be expected only in a devastating stroke involving the brain stem or complete brain death.
B&D Ch. 57

Question 41. B. Glutamate is the major excitatory neurotransmitter in the brain. Glutamate is the precursor to gamma aminobutyric acid (GABA). The major inhibitory neurotransmitters are GABA and glycine. Glutamate works on the N-methyl-D-aspartate (NMDA) receptor as well as four types of non-NMDA receptors. The NMDA receptor is bound by PCP. Glutamate is thought to be very important in learning and memory. Glutamate is also

important in the theory of excititoxicity, which postulates that excessive glutamate stimulation leads to excessive intracellular calcium and nitric oxide concentrations and cell death. Under stimulation of the NMDA receptor by glutamate has been found to cause psychosis, therefore glutamate is thought to play some role in schizophrenia, although the exact nature of that role is yet unclear. Locations for glutamate in the brain include cerebellar granule cells, striatum, hippocampus, pyramidal cells of the cortex, thalamocortical projections, and corticostriatal projections.
K&S Ch. 3

Question 42. D. Alzheimer's disease has been associated with defects in chromosome 21. The gene for amyloid precursor protein is found on the long arm of chromosome 21. This protein plays a significant role in the development of Alzheimer's disease. These defects have been shown to run in families. Some studies have shown as high as 40% of Alzheimer's patients have a positive family history for the disease. Turner's syndrome results from a missing sex chromosome -XO. The result is absent or minimal development of the gonads. No sex hormones are produced. Individuals with Turner's syndrome are female, but with no secondary sex characteristics and an absence or minimal development of the gonads. Klinefelter's syndrome is the presence of an extra chromosome, making the patient XXY. They have a male habitus because of the presence of the Y chromosome, but because of the extra X chromosome they do not develop strong male characteristics. They have small underdeveloped genitals. They are infertile, and can develop breast tissue during adolescence. Huntington's disease results from the expansion of trinucleotide repeat sequences at chromosome 4p16.3. The disease typically presents with dementia and chorea. Parkinson's disease results from the loss of dopaminergic neurons from the substantia nigra. It can present with dementia as well as a clear pattern of symptoms including shuffling gait, pill-rolling tremor, and masked facies. Other than Alzheimer's the other diseases listed have nothing to do with chromosome 21.
K&S Ch. 10

Question 43. C. The diagnosis of brain death can be made only in the complete absence of the brainstem reflexes (i.e., absent gag, fixed pupils, absent oculocephalic and oculovestibular reflexes, absent corneal reflexes). The eyes may either be open or closed in the presence of brain death. The EEG pattern need not be flat line to diagnose brain death. There have been known cases of preserved cortical function and hence positive activity on EEG despite a complete lack of brainstem functioning.
B&D Chs 5&61

45

Question 44. B. Of the drugs listed, diazepam is the one that needs oxidative metabolism by the liver. The other four are safe choices for patients with compromised liver function because they have no active metabolites or do not need oxidation by the liver. Patients with hepatic disease and elderly patients are at particular risk from adverse effects due to the benzodiazepines, especially if repeated high doses are given. Benzodiazepines should be used with caution in anyone with a history of substance abuse, cognitive disorders, renal disease, liver disease, central nervous system depression, or myasthenia gravis.
K&S Ch. 36

Question 45. C. All of the answer choices are reasonable things to do with a family in family therapy, except focusing most of the attention on the most dysfunctional member. The focus of the therapy should be on the whole family as a system, in which everyone plays a role. The problems that the family are having should not be treated as one person's fault.
K&S Ch. 35

Question 46. B. The neurotransmitters associated with anxiety are norepinephrine, serotonin, and gamma aminobutyric acid (GABA). Poor regulation of norepinephrine is thought to be involved in anxiety disorders. Noradrenergic neurons are found primarily in the locus ceruleus. Stimulation of the locus ceruleus increases anxiety, and ablation of the locus ceruleus blocks anxiety responses. Serotonin is also thought to be involved in anxiety, although its role is less clear. Serotonergic drugs have shown a clear propensity to decrease anxiety. Serotonergic neurons are located primarily in the raphe nuclei in the pons. The role of GABA in anxiety is clearly supported by the strong effect that benzodiazepines have on lessening anxiety. Benzodiazepines enhance the effect of GABA at the GABA receptor, thus decreasing anxiety. Those neurotransmitters not directly associated with anxiety include dopamine, glutamate, histamine, and acetylcholine. There is no evidence as yet that these neurotransmitters play a role in the pathophysiology of anxiety. Injection of epinephrine would worsen anxiety.
K&S Ch. 3

Question 47. B. Myasthenia gravis (MG) is an autoimmune neurologic disorder involving the production of autoantibodies against postsynaptic nicotinic acetylcholinergic receptor sites on muscle. There is passive transfer of the offending antibodies to the fetus across the placenta. The clinical picture is that of diplopia, dysarthria, dysphagia and other signs and symptoms of bulbar palsy, fatigue and muscle weakness. Mental status and cognition are usually intact. Deep tendon reflexes are generally preserved. There is a relationship between MG and thymoma. About 10% of patients with MG have thymoma. Edrophonium chloride (Tensilon), a short-acting cholinergic agent, is used to diagnose the disorder clinically and pyridostigmine (Mestinon) is used to treat the disorder on an ongoing basis. Other diagnostic tests include electromyography (EMG) and nerve conduction studies, which reveal a classic decrementing upon rapid repetitive muscle stimulation. Serum antibody levels can also be titered. Other therapeutic modalities include steroids, plasmapheresis, intravenous immunoglobulin (IVIG) administration, immunosuppressive agents, for example, azathioprine (Imuran).
B&D Ch. 84

Question 48. D. Generalized slow activity consisting of theta and delta waves with focal areas of hyperactivity is the EEG pattern of delirium. An important characteristic of this pattern is that the rhythm is slowed. Choice A is the pattern for absence seizures. This is a commonly asked pattern on exams. Choice B is normal adult drowsiness. Choice C is a normal pattern seen when the eyes are closed. Upon awakening, the posterior alpha rhythm is replaced by random activity. Right temporal spikes, choice E, are significant for a seizure focus. In addition to the above information, the appearance of delta waves is considered abnormal and should raise concern regarding a structural lesion, except if the patient is asleep.
K&S Chs 3&10

Question 49. D. Gower's maneuver or sign is a classic bedside indicator of muscular dystrophy or myopathy. Usually seen in children, the sign is present when a patient gets up from the floor or a chair by using the hands because of muscle weakness in the legs. Duchenne's is called a dystrophinopathy because it is an autosomal recessive hereditary disease of muscle due to a lack of dystrophin, a protein found in muscle membrane. Duchenne's is the most common of the childhood muscular dystrophies. Muscular weakness is usually greater proximally. Other features include diminished deep tendon reflexes (except the Achilles reflex), elevated CPK, mental retardation in about one third of cases and enlarged muscles, due to fat infiltration, particularly the calves.
B&D Ch. 85

Question 50. B. The tricyclic antidepressants (TCAs), trazodone, and mirtazapine are all sedating drugs. Sedation is a common effect of the TCAs and can be a welcome one if the patient isn't sleeping well. The most sedating of the TCAs are amytriptiline, trimipramine and doxepin. The least sedating are desipramine and protriptyline, with other TCAs falling between these two groups in the amount of sedation they cause. Trazodone is an antidepressant that can be extremely sedating. For this reason it is sometimes used independently for insomnia. Trazodone can also cause priapism, in which case the patient should be switched to another medication. The SSRIs and SNRIs in general are not very sedating.
K&S Ch. 36

Question 51. D. The appropriate response to this situation is to examine your own behavior and countertransference. You should then share your observations about the patient's behavior with the patient and examine the meaning of the patient's behavior. Answer choice A is a bad idea as ignoring the problem will not make it go away. Flirting with the patient is inappropriate and having sex with the patient is a violation of ethics which is strictly forbidden for psychiatrists. Revealing personal information is also not appropriate for the therapist to do and does not address the patient's underlying motivations.
K&S Chs 35&58

Question 52. B. This is an example of fetishism. In fetishism, a person, usually a male, obtains sexual arousal from an inanimate object such as women's undergarments, a glove, a shoe, etc. This needs to go on for at least six months to qualify for the diagnosis, and often involves sexual fantasies involving the object. Exhibitionism involves being sexually aroused by exposing one's genitals to a stranger. Frotteurism involves becoming sexually aroused by touching and rubbing against a nonconsenting person. Voyeurism is a pattern of obtaining sexual arousal from watching an unsuspecting person who is naked, disrobing, or engaged in sexual activity. Transvestic fetishism is a pattern of sexual arousal from cross-dressing, usually seen in a heterosexual male. The answer to this question is not transvestic fetishism because the patient was wearing women's undergarments only under his normal male work clothes. He was not going to work in a dress with makeup and high heel shoes. It is not dressing like a woman that arouses him, but a fantasy connected with an inanimate object, namely the panties.
K&S Ch. 21

47

Question 53. C. The case above describes trigeminal neuralgia (*tic douloureux*). It is usually unilateral in about 90% of cases. It usually affects the upper two branches of the fifth nerve (V2 and V3). Treatments of choice are carbamazepine (Tegretol) and oxcarbazapine (Trileptal), which modulate pain centrally and peripherally. About 75% of patients respond to carbamazepine therapy. Other treatments include gabapentin (Neurontin), tricyclic antidepressants, tiagabine (Gabitril), opioid analgesics, nonsteroidal anti-inflammatory agents, lidocaine patches and benzodiazepine sedatives. Some patients opt for an invasive intervention, radiation therapy in the form of stereotactic gamma-knife treatment to alleviate the pain.
B&D Ch. 75

Question 54. D. This is the classic clinical picture of temporal (also called giant-cell) arteritis, a systemic vasculitis of the medium-sized vessels. Women are affected more often than men (about 3:1). The disease occurs in the elderly, usually over 50 years of age. Clinically, the disease can present as new onset or change in headache with fever, fatigue, myalgia, night sweats, weight loss, and jaw claudication (tiredness upon chewing). About 25% of patients have polymyalgia rheumatica. The temporal artery can demonstrate tenderness to palpation with induration and diminished or absent pulse. The most feared complication is irreversible and sudden vision loss as a result of central retinal artery occlusion. The initial test of choice is the serum erythrocyte sedimentation rate (ESR), which is virtually always elevated. Temporal artery biopsy is the gold-standard diagnostic test of choice in the face of an elevated ESR. The treatment of choice is prednisone. Brain imaging would not reveal the abnormality. Lumbar puncture for cerebrospinal fluid xanthochromia is done to diagnose subarachnoid hemorrhage. Carotid dissection does not involve systemic constitutional symptoms, but usually presents with ipsilateral stroke-like deficits due to arterial embolization.

B&D Ch. 75

Question 55. D. The concept that mental disorders have different outcomes was pioneered by Emil Kraepelin. He was the first to differentiate between the course of chronic schizophrenia, and that of manic psychosis. He used the term *dementia praecox* borrowing it from the work of French psychiatrist Morel. Eugen Bleuler later renamed it as schizophrenia and stressed that it need not have a deteriorating course. Winnicott was one of the central figures in the school of object relations theory. He developed the concepts of the "good enough mother" and the "transitional object". Sigmund Freud is the founder of classic psychoanalysis. Heinz Kohut is best known for his writings of narcissism and self psychology.

K&S Ch. 13

Question 56. B. This is a clear case of hypochondriasis. The patient believes that he has a specific serious disease despite a negative workup and the reassurance of his doctors. Conversion disorder is when a patient has a neurologic symptom which is attributed to psychological conflict and cannot be explained medically. Body dysmorphic disorder is preoccupation with an imagined defect in appearance. Often slight physical imperfections cause markedly excessive concern. Somatization disorder (also known as Briquet's syndrome) is a condition where a patient has multiple physical complaints involving several organ symptoms. These symptoms can not be explained by a medical diagnosis. The symptoms are not intentionally produced. Symptoms can include pain, sexual symptoms, gastrointestinal symptoms, and pseudoneurological symptoms.

K&S Ch. 17

Question 57. B. Cluster headache is a rare type of headache occurring in ≤ 0.5% of the population. Sufferers are usually males in their twenties and thirties. Most sufferers experience episodic cycles of four to twelve weeks' duration that are predominant in the spring and fall seasons. Attack periods can be considered chronic, that is lasting one year or more without remission or with remission periods of less than two weeks' duration. Attacks can last anywhere from fifteen minutes to three hours in duration. They can occur as often as eight times a day, or as infrequently as once every other day. The attacks are generally nocturnal. Alcohol consumption is a common trigger. The attacks are excruciatingly painful and retro-orbital in location. Pain can radiate to the teeth, neck and temporal regions and can be accompanied by ipsilateral autonomic symptoms. Patients prefer moving their head or pacing rather than lying still. Abortive therapies include oxygen by nasal cannula at eight to ten liters per minute, sumatriptan subcutaneous injection and ergotamine. Prophylactic therapies include prednisone, verapamil, divalproex sodium, methysergide and lithium.

B&D Ch. 75

Question 58. E. Seizure, anorexia, head trauma, and use of a monoamine oxidase inhibitor (MAOI) in the past 14 days are all contraindications to using

bupropion, because of the propensity of bupropion to lower the seizure threshold. One does not want to use this medication in a situation where the seizure threshold may already be lowered, or a seizure focus is present. The medication can also cause weight loss, so use in those who are under-weight is not a good idea. It can also lead to increased rates of seizures in patients with eating disorders. Although it can increase blood pressure in some patients, it does not cause hypertensive crises and is not contraindicated in patients with high blood pressure. Hypertension is a strong concern when using venlafaxine because of its ability to potentiate hypertensive crisis. Bupropion is also used for smoking cessation. Waiting for 14 days when switching to or from an MAOI is a hard and fast rule to prevent drug–drug interactions which could lead to a serotonin syndrome. Bupropion is not associated with sexual side effects in the way that the selective serotonin reuptake inhibitors are.
K&S Ch. 36

Question 59. B. Lithium and phentolamine are not contraindicated with monoamine oxidase inhibitors (MAOIs). Meperidine and selective serotonin reuptake inhibitors (SSRIs) can not be given at the same time as MAOIs and this often comes up on standardized tests. There should be a 14-day washout period between giving an SSRI and an MAOI. Levodopa and spinal anesthetics containing epinephrine are also part of a long list of medications that should not be mixed with a MAOI.
K&S Ch. 36

Question 60. C. There are numerous causes of acquired peripheral neuropathy. The more notable causes include: vincristine and INH therapies, excess B6 therapy, inhalant abuse such as toluene or nitrous oxide, heavy metal poisoning, hydrocarbon exposure, B12 deficiency, niacin deficiency, and complications of mononucleosis (Epstein-Barr virus infection). Autoimmune diseases such as lupus can also cause peripheral neuropathy. Acetaminophen overdose dose not generally affect the peripheral nervous system.
B&D Ch. 82

Question 61. C. Of all of the answer choices, the only one that is not true is C. Methylphenidate will increase tricyclic antidepressant (TCA) levels, as will some antipsychotics. Smoking decreases TCA levels. Antipsychotics and methylphenidate increase TCA concentrations through their interaction with the cytochrome p450 system. Other drugs that increase TCA concentrations include acetazolamide, aspirin, cimetidine, thiazides, fluoxetine and sodium bicarbonate. Cigarette smoking decreases their concentration through induction of the 1A2 enzyme. Drugs that decrease TCA concentrations include ascorbic acid, lithium, barbituates, and primidone.
K&S Ch. 36

Question 62. D. Of the selective serotonin reuptake inhibitors, fluoxetine has the longest half life, lasting 1–2 weeks, fluvoxamine has the shortest, lasting about 15 hours. All others have half lives of about 1 day.
K&S Ch. 36

Question 63. A. Self-mutilation is most often associated with borderline personality disorder. Borderline patients often use this behavior to express anger, elicit help from others, or numb themselves to overwhelming affect. They have tumultuous interpersonal relationships and strong mood swings. They can have short lived psychotic episodes. Their behavior is often unpredictable. They can rarely tolerate being alone, and are known for splitting people into all good or all bad categories. They lack a consistent sense of identity.
K&S Ch. 7

Question 64. A. The clinical picture depicted in this question is that of dermatomyositis. Dermatomyositis is an autoimmune disease that affects skin and muscle. Skin rash appears generally with the onset of muscle weakness. The rash is classically purplish and is mainly seen on the face and eyelids. It can also appear on the neck, elbows and the knees which are often reddened and indurated. Serum CPK levels are often elevated. Needle electromyography (EMG) demonstrates myopathy and muscle irritability, with fibrillations, positive sharp waves and increased insertional activity. The hallmark finding on muscle biopsy is perifascicular atrophy and 'ghost' fibers. There is a strong relationship between dermatomyositis and occult neoplasm in up to 50% of patients with the disorder. The usual neoplasm is carcinoma and can be in the lung, breast, stomach or ovary most typically. A cancer workup is essential in patients found to have dermatomyositis, including chest radiography, rectal and vaginal exams, hematologic studies and testing for occult blood in stool.
B&D Ch. 85.

Question 65. D. The case presented in this question is a common description of water intoxication. Symptoms include tremor, ataxia, restlessness, diarrhea, vomiting, polyuria, and eventual stupor. This is a problem that can be found in up to 20% of patients with chronic schizophrenia. When found, these patients need close monitoring of their electrolytes, and in many cases must be water restricted with close monitoring of their intake and output. The electrolyte disturbances that result from drinking enormous quantities of water can become serious medical issues and in some cases prompt medical hospitalization. Although the other questions could be useful in doing a thorough evaluation, the patient's symptoms and psychiatric diagnosis should suggest water intoxication.
K&S Ch. 13

Question 66. A. This question stem describes paranoid schizophrenia. In paranoid schizophrenia, there are delusions and hallucinations most prominently, but specific behaviors suggestive of disorganized or catatonic schizophrenia are absent. The onset is usually later than other types of the disease, and they show less regression of their mental facilities and emotional responses. Disorganized schizophrenia has early onset and poor outcome. It is marked by a regression to primitive, disinhibited, and unorganized behavior and absence of catatonic symptoms. Patients display prominent thought disorder and their contact with reality is poor. Catatonic schizophrenia consists of negativism, rigidity, posturing, and alteration between stupor and excitement. Patients often exhibit stereotypies, mannerisms, and waxy flexibility. Residual schizophrenia presents with evidence of a schizophrenic disturbance with absence of a complete set of active symptoms and an absence of adequate symptoms to qualify as one of the other types of schizophrenia. It can consist of emotional blunting, social withdrawal, eccentric behavior, illogical thinking and mild loosening of associations.
K&S Ch. 13

Question 67. C. All of the answer choices are associated with good outcomes except early age of onset. The older the patient is at onset, the better the prognosis. Good prognostic indicators for schizophrenia include late onset, obvious precipitating factors, acute onset, good premorbid functioning, mood disorder symptoms, being married, family history of mood disorders, good support systems, and positive symptoms. Poor prognostic factors include young onset, no precipitating factors, insidious onset, poor premorbid functioning, withdrawn or autistic-like behavior, being single, divorced or widowed, family history of schizophrenia, poor support systems, negative symptoms, neurological symptoms, history of perinatal trauma, no remissions in early years, many relapses, and history of assaultiveness.
K&S Ch. 13

Question 68. E. The findings given in this question are descriptors of sleep patterns one would find in depression. One might also find increased awakening during the second half of the night and increased length of the first rapid eye movement (REM) sleep episode. Electroencephalography can be used to evaluate sleep, but in clinical psychiatry, it is most often used to separate temporal lobe seizures from pseudoseizures and to distinguish dementia from pseudodementia caused by depression. The other answer choices given are clear distractors. Tumor is unrelated to sleep changes and could potentially show up on an EEG as a seizure focus, but we have no history here of either seizures or seizure focus on EEG. Petit mal epilepsy has a classic 3-per-second spike and wave pattern, which is clearly not mentioned in the question. Hepatic encephalopathy would cause a delirium, making answer choices C and D very similar. EEG patterns in delirium would show generalized slow activity, i.e. theta and delta waves, with possible areas of hyperactivity. Hepatic encephalopathy often shows on EEG as bilaterally synchronous triphasic slow waves. None of that is mentioned in the question, as we are solely talking about sleep patterns. Therefore E is the only reasonable answer.
K&S Ch. 15

Question 69. B. The genetics of Alzheimer's dementia (AD) are the subject of ongoing research. A positive family history of the disorder is found in about one-quarter of cases. This type of Alzheimer's dementia is further classified as familial AD or FAD. The most significant genetic risk factor is believed to be homozygosity for the inheritance of the E4 allele of apolipoprotein E (apo E). Other less significant risks may be mutations in Presenelin 1 (on chromosome 14) and Presenelin 2 (on chromosome 1) proteins and amyloid precursor protein (APP). Apo E4 genotyping may be useful in patients with cognitive deficits as it points very strongly to the clinical diagnosis of AD. Neurofibrillary tangles are a neuropathologic hallmark of AD and a major component of these tangles is the microtubule-associated protein, tau. Abnormal hyperphosphorylation of tau results in the destruction of the neuronal cytoskeleton and the aggregation of tangles. Trisomy 21 (Down's syndrome) predisposes patients to early onset of Alzheimer's dementia in as many as 90% of cases. Neuropathologic findings in these cases are identical to those seen in elderly patients. The reason for the early onset of the condition in Down's patients is believed to be overexpression of the APP gene and thus increased β-amyloid deposition.
B&D Ch. 72

Question 70. C. The answer choices are all characteristics of narcissism, except C. Answer choice C describes characteristics of histrionic personality disorder. Histrionic personality disorder is marked by a pattern of excessive emotionality and attention seeking. Narcissism is marked by grandiosity, need for admiration, and lack of empathy.
K&S Ch. 27

Question 71. D. For posttraumatic stress disorder (PTSD) the duration of the disturbance must be at least one month. All other answer choices are correct. In PTSD the person was exposed to an event that involved either actual or threatened death or injury or a threat to their or others' physical integrity. Their response involves intense fear, helplessness, or horror. The event is re-experienced as flashbacks or recurring dreams. Patients may act or feel as if the event was recurring. If they perceive things that remind them of the event, they are caused intense psychological distress and show physiological reactivity. Patients with PTSD often spend great energy avoiding stimuli that remind them of the event. They can also demonstrate a numbing of general responsiveness as shown by inability

51

to remember certain aspects of the trauma, loss of interest in significant activities, feelings of detachment from others, restricted affect, and feelings of a foreshortened future. They also show signs of increased arousal such as problems with sleep, irritability and outbursts of anger, poor concentration, hypervigilance, and excited startle response.

K&S Ch. 16

Question 72. E. Uncomplicated grief is often manifested as a state of shock, numbness or bewilderment. It may be followed by sighing or crying. This may lead to weakness, decreased appetite, weight loss, problems concentrating, and sleep disturbances. This is all considered part of normal grief. Once a person begins to manifest worthlessness, suicidality, excessive guilt, hallucinations, or psychomotor retardation the grief is no longer normal. Pathological grief can take many forms ranging from absent or delayed grief, to excessively intense or prolonged grief, to psychosis and suicidality. Anticipatory grief is expressed in advance of a loss deemed to be inevitable. This grief ends at the time when the loss occurs, regardless of what happens after. The grief may intensify as time goes on and the person moves closer and closer to the loss, and turn to acute grief when the loss occurs. Delusional disorder and bipolar disorder are unrelated to the information in the question stem.

K&S Ch. 2

Question 73. C. Numerous neuropathologic abnormalities accompany schizophrenia on both a microscopic and macroscopic level. Hippocampal neurons can be atrophic. Lamina III neurons in the hippocampus can be disorganized and scattered. This is not solidly replicated in neuropathologic specimens. One of the most replicable findings is enlargement of the cerebral ventricular system, particularly the lateral ventricles. This finding has been extensively replicated over numerous neuropathologic specimens. Other affected areas include the thalamus and the dorsolateral prefrontal cortex.

K&S Ch.3

Question 74. E. The patient presented in this question is a clear case of anorexia nervosa. No single laboratory test can diagnose the disease, but a battery of tests is needed to properly evaluate the patient medically. Tests to order include serum electrolytes, renal function tests, thyroid function tests, glucose, amylase, complete blood count, electrocardiogram, cholesterol, dexamethasone suppression test, and carotene. Of these, one of the most important tests is the serum potassium level. Eating-disorder patients can commonly become hypokalemic, develop a hypokalemic hypochloremic alkalosis and have cardiac complications including arrhythmias and sudden death. Osteoporosis can be found in anorexic patients, but a bone scan is not a vital initial procedure. A head CT scan is not warranted. Delayed gastric emptying can occur with eating disorders, but a study to prove such is not urgent. Cholesterol is often increased in these patients, but again, not urgent.

K&S Ch. 23

Question 75. D. All of the answer choices regarding delusional disorder are true except D. You do not have to have impairment of daily functioning to qualify for delusional disorder. The most prominent feature of the disorder is delusions. These delusions can be paranoid, grandiose, erotic, jealous, somatic, or mixed. These patients lack significant mood symptoms and they lack the bizarre delusions found in schizophrenia. "I'm being followed by the police" is a nonbizarre delusion, because it is possible that it could be true. "I'm being tracked by aliens" is a bizarre delusion and is not possible. The primary medication treatment is with antipsychotics, in addition to individual therapy, and sometimes family therapy.

K&S Ch. 14

Question 76. E. Female orgasmic disorder is the persistent absence of orgasm in women following a normal excitement phase. It is based on the clinician's judgment that the women's orgasmic capacity is less than would be reasonable for her age, sexual experience, and adequacy of sexual stimulation she receives. The overall prevalence is thought to be somewhere around 30 percent. It is true that the incidence of orgasm increases with age, attributed to less psychological inhibition and more experience. Psychological factors, like those listed in answer choice D, may play a role. It can be either lifelong or acquired depending on whether the patient has ever had an orgasm at any point in life. Answer choice E refers to vaginismus, which is an involuntary contraction of the outer third of the vagina preventing intercourse. It can occur following rape, or in women with psychosexual conflicts.
K&S Ch. 21

Question 77. D. The case described in this question is consistent with social anxiety disorder (social phobia). It involves certain specific social situations which provoke intense anxiety because of fear of embarrassment or humiliation. An important differential to consider would be avoidant personality disorder. In this disorder there is a pervasive pattern of social inhibition, feelings of inadequacy, and hypersensitivity to negative evaluation. It leads to the avoidance of other people unless the sufferer is sure that he is going to be liked. Avoidant personality disorder leads to restraint of intimate relationships for fear of being shamed or ridiculed. These patients often view themselves as socially inept or personally unappealing. They avoid jobs with significant interpersonal contact. Very importantly, they desire the closeness and warmth of relationships but avoid them for fear of rejection. Borderline personality disorder is characterized by a pattern of instability of interpersonal relationships, self-image, and affect, as well as marked impulsivity. Obsessive-compulsive personality disorder is defined by a pervasive pattern of preoccupation with orderliness, perfectionism, and mental and interpersonal control, at the expense of flexibility, openness, and efficiency. Narcissistic personality disorder is defined by a pattern of grandiosity, need for admiration, and lack of empathy. Dependent personality disorder is defined by a pervasive need to be taken care of that leads to submissive and clinging behavior and fears of separation.
K&S Ch. 27

Question 78. E. Phenytoin (Dilantin sodium) is notorious for causing hirsutism in women, facial dysmorphism and gingival hypertrophy. The drug can also cause cerebellar atrophy when taken over a long period of time, resulting in cerebellar signs and symptoms, such as ataxic gait and dysmetria of the extremities. Carbamazepine has the distinction of inducing its own metabolism. It can also cause rash that can lead to Stevens-Johnson syndrome. Another side effect of carbamazepine includes hyponatremia by antidiuretic hormone-like effect. It can also cause leukopenia and toxic hepatitis. Valproate can cause leukopenia, liver failure, weight gain, hair loss, fetal neural tube defects such as spina bifida and polycystic ovary syndrome. Levetiracetam is an anticonvulsant with minimal side effects. One of the more worrisome, but infrequent side effects of levetiracetam is agitation or hyperactivity. Phenobarbital is a barbiturate anticonvulsant and shares the side effects of that class: central nervous system depression, sedation, respiratory compromise and depression. Phenobarbital can of course be deadly in overdose.
B&D Ch. 73

Question 79. A. The clinical picture depicted in this question is known as a "Saturday night palsy", which is synonymous for a radial nerve entrapment. Entrapment of the radial nerve at the axilla often results from prolonged armpit compression when the arm is draped over the edge of a chair or when a

patient is on crutches. A radial nerve palsy of this kind results in weakness of the extensor muscles of the wrist and fingers, triceps weakness and supinator weakness. Such compression injury usually resolves in one to two months. Ulnar nerve entrapment can occur either at the elbow or at the wrist. Elbow trauma may result in ulnar nerve entrapment in the cubital tunnel. Other causes include arm compression during surgery under general anesthesia. Ulnar nerve compression results in weakness of the flexor carpi ulnaris, intrinsic hand muscles and fourth and fifth finger deep flexor weakness. Median nerve entrapment at the wrist can result in a classic carpal tunnel syndrome. This is the most common of the entrapment neuropathies. Tenosynovitis of the transverse carpal ligament places pressure on the median nerve in the tunnel resulting in nocturnal hand paresthesias of the thumb, index and middle fingers. There may be sensory loss, thenar atrophy and a positive Tinel's sign, in about 60% of cases. Tinel's sign is positive when percussion of the nerve over the wrist results in paresthesias in the median nerve territory. Flexing the hand at the wrist for about one minute or more is called the Phalen's maneuver and can result in similar paresthesias. Injury to the median nerve is sustained with use of handheld vibrating tools and repetitive forceful use of the hands and wrists compromising the carpal tunnel. The diagnostic test of choice for carpal tunnel syndrome is needle electromyography (EMG) and nerve conduction studies which reveal delayed sensory latency across the wrist in 70–90% of cases. Musculocutaneous nerve injury can occur with brachial plexus injuries such as by shoulder dislocation, compression to the shoulder during surgical anesthesia or by repetitively carrying heavy objects over the shoulder (carpet carrier's palsy). Biceps and brachialis weakness is the hallmark of musculocutaneous nerve injury. The suprascapular nerve is a pure motor nerve of the brachial plexus. Entrapment injury can occur after repetitive forward traction at the shoulder. Diffuse aching pain in the posterior shoulder is a usual symptom. EMG demonstrates denervation of the infraspinatus and supraspinatus muscles.
B&D Ch. 82

Question 80. D. The case described shows loss of muscle tone in times of extreme emotion or physical exertion. This is found in association with narcolepsy. In narcolepsy, there are irresistible attacks of sleep that occur daily. They are characterized by either cataplexy, which is the loss of muscle tone described above, or the recurrent intrusions of rapid eye movement (REM) sleep into the transition between sleep and wakefulness, causing hypnopompic or hypnogogic hallucinations or sleep paralysis. Sleep apnea is a medical condition which can be either central or obstructive and leads to snoring, daytime drowsiness and irritability. It can have negative long term cardiac consequences as well. Primary insomnia is difficulty initiating or maintaining sleep, or nonrestorative sleep for at least one month. It is independent of any known physical or medical condition. It is often treated with benzodiazepines or zolpidem. Primary hypersomnia is excessive sleepiness for 1 month as demonstrated by prolonged sleep episodes at night or daily sleep episodes during the day. Treatment consists of stimulants such as amphetamines and the non-stimulant modafinil (Provigil). Sodium oxybate (Xyrem) is FDA-approved for cataplexy associated with narcolepsy. Xyrem is essentially a synthetic analog of gamma hydroxybutyrate (GHB) which is a drug of abuse notorious for being used as a date rape drug. Circadian rhythm sleep disorder is a persistent pattern of sleep disruption resulting from a mismatch between the sleep-wake cycle of the environment and the circadian sleep-wake pattern. It can be specified as delayed sleep phase type, jet lag type, or shift work type. Modafinil has a specific FDA indication in shift-work sleep disorder, as well as narcolepsy, obstructive sleep apnea and idiopathic hypersomnia.
K&S Ch. 24

Question 81. C. Conversion disorder usually involves neurologic symptoms. Multiple organ system complaints are found in somatization disorder. If symptoms are limited to pain, it is a pain disorder, not a conversion disorder. If symptoms are limited to sexual dysfunction, it is a sexual disorder, not conversion disorder. Conversion disorder symptoms are not intentionally produced.
K&S Ch. 17

Question 82. D. The monoamine oxidase (MAO) type A inhibitors are contraindicated with levodopa/carbidopa repletion therapy. Monamine oxidase inhibitors are postsynaptic enzymatic metabolizers of dopamine. Concomitant use of MAO-A type inhibitors and levodopa/carbidopa can result in poor response to the levodopa repletion therapy and worsening of parkinsonian symptoms. MAO inhibitors need to be discontinued two weeks prior to the initiation of levodopa repletion therapy to avoid a negative interaction. The antidepressants in the selective serotonin reuptake inhibitor class (fluoxetine and sertraline, among others) are not contraindicated with levodopa repletion therapy. Tricyclic antidepressants are also safe with levodopa repletion, as is gabapentin.
B&D Ch. 77

Question 83. C. Piaget proposed four stages of cognitive development. They were the sensorimotor stage, the stage of preoperational thought, the concrete operations stage, and the formal operations stage. During the concrete operations stage the child begins to deal with information outside of himself and to see things from other's perspectives. He also develops conservation, which is the idea that though objects may change, they can maintain characteristics that allow them to be recognized as the same (example: different leaves may be different shapes and colors but are all leaves). The concept of reversibility is also understood at this stage. It says that things can change form and shape and then go back again (example: ice to water to ice.)
K&S Ch. 4

Question 84. D. By two to three years of age, almost all children have a concept of being either male or female. Infants begin exploring their genitalia by fifteen months of age. Children also develop interest in other's genitals leading to exploration and exhibition. Sexual curiosity and sex play increase during puberty, but are normally present before puberty. They are not a sign of anything abnormal, nor is it a result of television, homosexuality, hormonal imbalance, or premature development.
K&S Ch. 21.

Question 85. E. Short palpebral fissures are found in children with fetal alcohol syndrome, not fragile X syndrome. Fragile X syndrome presents with mental retardation, long ears, narrow face, short stature, hyperextendable joints, arched palate, macro-orchidism, seizures and autistic features. There is a high rate of attention deficit-hyperactivity disorder, and learning disorders. It is the second most common cause of mental retardation. It results from a mutation of the X chromosome.
K&S Ch. 38

Question 86. A. In normal attachment, a child at 18 months of age would use a transitional object in the absence of the mother. There would be less anxiety at separation than in pervious stages, but it would not be completely gone. The child would try to master strange situations when the mother was nearby. There is object permanence. It is not until 25 months of age that the child would be expected to tolerate the mother's absence without distress. In the situations described in the other answer choices, the child would be scared, not violent. The child would not immediately run to you as he would have some stranger anxiety. He would not feel safe enough in the mother's absence to become more inquisitive. The child would definitely notice the mother's absence.

K&S Ch. 4

Question 87. C. Valproate is the classic inhibitor of cytochrome P-450 3A4 which causes inhibition of enzymatic clearance of lamotrigine. Doses of lamotrigine need to be lowered and generally started at lower doses when administered concomitantly with valproic acid, to avoid lamotrigine toxicity. The other agents noted in this question do not have cyp-450 3A4 inhibitory properties in this fashion.

K&S Ch. 36

Question 88. D. It is during adolescence that children move away from the family and the friend group provides the most important relationships. During this time, any deviation in appearance, dress, or behavior can lead to a decrease in self-esteem. For this reason the child would most likely suffer the most psychological impact from a deformity during adolescence.

K&S Ch. 2

Question 89. D. Whereas some monoamine oxidase inhibitors (MAOIs) work on both MAO-A, and MAO-B, selegeline works solely on MAO-B. MAO-A is involved in the metabolism of serotonin and norepinephrine. MAO-B is involved in the metabolism of phenylethylamine. Both are involved in the metabolism of dopamine. MAO-A in the gastrointestinal tract is involved in the metabolism of tyramine. If you block these enzymes, tyramine is not broken down and can lead to hypertensive crisis.

K&S Ch. 36

Question 90. E. Cocaine blocks dopamine reuptake from the synaptic cleft, leading to increased levels of dopamine. When chronically used, this disturbance of normal dopamine metabolism leads to depletion of dopamine. Cocaine has also been shown to be associated with decreased levels of cerebral blood flow. Patients recovering from cocaine addiction show a drop in neuronal activity and a decreased activity of dopamine which can persist for up to a year and a half after stopping the drug.

K&S Ch. 12

Question 91. A. Neural tube defects are the most worrisome fetotoxic side effects of valproic acid in the pregnant patient. The classic presentation is that of fetal spina bifida. With formation of the neural tube early in gestation, spina bifida can usually be detected by fetal ultrasound in the first trimester. The other noted problems are not attributable to side effects of valproic acid.

K&S Ch. 36

Question 92. B. Dopamine agonists are newer agents used to treat Parkinson's disease. The classic agents of this class available for use in the United States are pergolide, bromocriptine, pramipexole and ropinirole. Ropinirole is now also indicated in restless legs syndrome and is one of the treatments of choice for that disorder. Worrisome side effects of the dopamine agonists include hallucinations, sedation and orthostatic hypotension. There is a much lower incidence of dyskinesias with the dopamine agonists than with levodopa therapy. Haloperidol and fluphenazine are conventional antipsychotic agents and hence are dopamine antagonists. Quetiapine is a second-generation atypical antipsychotic that has dopamine antagonist properties as well. Buspirone is approved for generalized anxiety disorder and is a 5-HT 1A partial agonist.

B&D Ch. 77

Question 93. E. The frontal lobes are the seat of executive functioning. They also play a large role in the personality. Damage to the orbitofrontal region can cause disinhibition, irritability, mood lability, euphoria, lack of remorse, poor judgment, and distractability. Damage to the dorsolateral frontal regions leads to extensive executive functioning deficits. Damage to the medial frontal region leads to an apathy syndrome.
K&S Ch. 3

Question 94. B. Ziprasidone (Geodon) stands alone as the one atypical antipsychotic that inhibits serotonin and norepinephrine reuptake. All of the atypical antipsychotics block the serotonin 2A and dopamine D2 receptors. The reuptake inhibition seen with ziprasidone however, is unique, as is its blockade of the serotonin-1A receptor.
K&S Ch. 36

Question 95. E. Aripiprazole (Abilify) is the only antipsychotic that can work as both a partial dopamine agonist-antagonist. It is postulated to work on positive symptoms of schizophrenia by blocking dopamine, and negative symptoms of schizophrenia by being an agonist at dopamine receptors in the prefrontal cortex. All of the other antipsychotics available only block dopamine receptors. This blockade of dopamine receptors in the frontal cortex theoretically leads to a worsening of negative symptoms by the medication, particularly by the typical antipsychotics.
K&S Ch. 36

Question 96. C. The prefrontal cortices influence mood differently. If one activates the left prefrontal cortex mood is lifted. If the right prefrontal cortex is activated, mood is depressed. Therefore a lesion to the left prefrontal cortex would cause depression, and a lesion to the right prefrontal cortex would cause euphoria and laughter. The parietal and occipital lobes are not the predominant lobes involved in emotion.
K&S Ch. 3

Question 97. E. The raphe nuclei of the brainstem, predominantly in the pons, are the major sites of serotonergic cell bodies. The ventral tegmental area, substantia nigra, and nucleus accumbens are all dopaminergic areas and are parts of the major neuronal pathways involved in the pathophysiology of schizophrenia. The cerebellum is a distracter.
K&S Ch. 3

Question 98. C. The clinical picture depicted in this vignette is that of Wilson's disease. Wilson's disease is an autosomal recessive disorder of abnormal copper metabolism. It is linked to the q14-21 (ATP7B) region of chromosome 13. Prevalence is about 1 in 30 000. The disorder results in a problem with incorporation of copper into ceruloplasmin and with diminished biliary excretion of copper. This results in excessive deposition of copper in the brain, with a predilection for the basal ganglia. The most useful laboratory test is serum ceruloplasmin which is most often decreased to less than 20 mg/dL (normal range is 24–45 mg/dL). The most frequent neurologic manifestations are parkinsonism, flapping tremor, ataxia, dystonia and bulbar signs such as dysphagia and dysarthria. Signs of liver failure are usually present. The treatment of choice is penicillamine, a copper-chelating agent, which in many cases can reverse the deficits of the disease. Serum ACE level (angiotensin converting enzyme) would be a screening test for sarcoidosis. Chromosomal analysis for CAG triplet repeats by polymerase chain reaction (PCR) would be the test of choice for Huntington's disease. Lumbar puncture for cerebrospinal fluid oligoclonal bands and myelin basic protein would be a useful supportive test (in addition to brain and/or

spinal cord MRI) for multiple sclerosis. The Tensilon test is for the diagnosis of myasthenia gravis.
B&D Ch.77

Question 99. C. The mesolimbic pathway of dopaminergic neurons, starting at the ventral tegmental area and projecting to the nucleus accumbens is thought to be highly involved in the sense of reward one gets from cocaine use, and is a major mediator of cocaine's effects. It is very involved in amphetamine's effects as well. The locus ceruleus of the brainstem contains a high number of adrenergic neurons, and mediates the effects of opiates and opioids.
K&S Ch 12

Question 100. D. The therapeutic focus of motivational enhancement therapy is on the patient's ambivalence toward staying off of their drug of abuse. It is a type of therapy specifically used with patients addicted to drugs of abuse.
K&S Ch. 35

Question 101. A. Of the many psychological tests used today, the reliability of the Wechsler Adult Intelligence Scale (WAIS) is among the highest. Retesting of people, even at later ages, rarely reveals higher IQ scores. The scores are consistent and repeatable. As such it is the most reliable of the choices given. It also has a very high validity in identifying mental retardation and predicting future school performance. There is also a childhood version of the same test, the Wechsler Intelligence Scale for Children (WISC).
K&S Ch. 5

Question 102. E. Freud's drive theory focused on basic instincts or drives that motivated human behavior. These drives were libido and aggression. In Freud's model, a drive has four parts. The "source" is the part of the body from which the drive comes. The "impetus" is the amount of intensity of the drive. The "aim" is any action that discharges the tension. The "object" is the target of the action. The other theories listed have nothing to do with Freud. Self psychology is the theory of Kohut. Learning theory cannot be attributed to any one individual, but has many theories and contributors. Conflict theory is a distracter, as is the mesolimbic dopamine theory.
K&S Ch. 6

Question 103. A. Numerous studies have shown the principal cause of intracerebral hemorrhage (ICH) to be hypertension. Chronic hypertension likely causes lipohyalinosis of the small intraparenchymal arteries and microaneurysms of Charcot and Bouchard that rupture due to increased vascular pressure. ICH accounts for about 10% of all strokes. The most common area of predilection for ICH is the putamen in about one-third of cases, followed by the thalamus in about 10–15% of cases. The other choices listed in this question are all less-frequent causes of ICH.
B&D Ch. 57

Question 104. D. Aaron Beck is the originator of cognitive behavioral therapy (CBT). In this theory, patients' assumptions affect their cognitions, which in turn affect their mood. As such, it would be cognitive distortion that Beck would most likely find as the cause of depression. The other answer choices may be things to which other theorists attribute depression, or are totally unrelated answer choices included to distract.
K&S Ch. 35

Question 105. A. A type I error occurs when the null hypothesis is rejected when it should have been retained. It is the equivalent of saying that a true difference exists between two samples when the difference is due solely to chance.
K&S Ch. 4

Question 106. E. Randomization is the process by which each patient in a clinical trial has an equal chance to be assigned to a control group or an experimental group. This process protects against selection bias. Power is the probability of finding the difference between two samples. It is the probability of rejecting the null hypothesis when it should be rejected. Probability is the likelihood that an event will occur. A probability of 1 means it will occur, a probability of 0 means that it will not. Risk is a distracter.

K&S Ch. 4

Question 107. C. The clinical picture here is that of cryptococcal meningitis in an AIDS patient with severe immunocompromise. About 10% of AIDS patients develop this infection by the encapsulated yeast *Cryptococcus neoformans*. CD4 count is generally less than 200/μL. Although MRI of the brain is a good test, in this case the results would be nonspecific. The scan might demonstrate meningeal enhancement with gadolinium, suggesting a subacute or chronic meningitis. There may also be multiple small abscesses seen on scan due to fungal invasion of the Virchow-Robin spaces surrounding meningeal vessels. Hydrocephalus due to obstruction of cerebrospinal fluid (CSF) flow may also be seen. In rarer cases a mass lesion, or cryptococcoma, with surrounding edema can be seen, due to consolidation of the infection. The most important immediate test is the lumbar puncture. Opening pressure should be measured and is usually elevated. CSF is most often colorless and clear. CSF analysis can reveal a leucocytosis of 50–1000 cells/mm^3 with lymphocytic predominance. CSF protein is usually elevated from 50–1000 mg/dL. India ink staining of CSF viewed under the microscope will quickly reveal an identifiable capsule and budding yeasts and requires no special laboratory machinery or testing. CSF cryptococcal antigen assay is indeed more sensitive than India ink staining and should concomitantly be done, as it is now readily available in most centers. Chest radiography would only be helpful with a suspicion of lung involvement or pulmonary symptoms. Blood cultures are generally negative in fungal infection and should only be done if concomitant bacterial infection is suspected. Amphotericin B intravenous administration is the treatment of choice for central nervous system fungal infections. The problem with Amphotericin B is a high rate of up to 80% renal toxicity as a side effect.

B&D Ch. 59

Question 108. D. Power is the probability of finding the difference between two samples. It is the probability of rejecting the null hypothesis when it should be rejected. Randomization is the process by which each patient in a clinical trial has an equal chance to be assigned to a control group or an experimental group. This process protects against selection bias. Probability is the likelihood that an event will occur. A probability of 1 means it will occur, a probability of 0 means that it will not. Risk is a distracter.

K&S Ch. 4

Question 109. C. The number of people who have a disorder at a specific point in time is the point prevalence. It is calculated by dividing the number of people with the disorder at that time by the total population at that time. Randomization is the process by which each patient in a clinical trial has an equal chance to be assigned to a control group or an experimental group. This process protects against selection bias. Power is the probability of finding the difference between two samples. It is the probability of rejecting the null hypothesis when it should be rejected. Probability is the likelihood that an event will occur. A probability of 1 means it will occur, a probability of 0 means that it will not. Risk is a distracter.

K&S Ch. 4

Question 110. A.   One of the main criteria for anorexia is a failure to maintain body weight at or above 85% of what would be expected for the person's height and age. Other criteria include a fear of becoming fat, even though the person is underweight, problems in the way one's body is experienced, and undue influence of body weight on self-esteem. Anorexic patients also deny the seriousness of their being underweight, and often have amenorrhea. There are two types of anorexia, the restricting type, and the binge eating/purging type.
K&S Ch. 23

Question 111. D.   PCP can be found in the urine up to 8 days after use. Some other drugs of note include: cannabis – up to 4 weeks, cocaine – up to 8 hours, and heroin – up to 72 hours.
K&S Ch. 7

Question 112. C.   Amyloid precursor protein is the protein that makes up the amyloid plaques found in the brain in Alzheimer's disease. The protein is encoded by a gene found on chromosome 21. The amyloid deposits found in Alzheimer's disease are the hallmark of the disease's neuropathology. Wilson's disease is the result of abnormal copper metabolism, not amyloid. Schizophrenia, bipolar disorder, and Huntington's disease have nothing to do with amyloid.
K&S Ch. 10

Question 113. C.   A complete blood count (CBC) would be the first test to order because of the risk of significant side effects on the hematopoietic system. Carbamazepine can cause decreased white blood cell count, agranulocytosis, pancytopenia, and aplastic anemia. Carbamazepine also has a vasopressin-like effect and can cause water intoxication and hyponatremia. Carbamazepine interacts significantly with the cytochrome P-450 system and as such has many interactions with many drugs. Great care should be taken when prescribing carbamazepine with other medications.
K&S Ch. 36

Question 114. E.   Because the starvation associated with anorexia effects a multitude of organ systems, a battery of tests is warranted when working up the disease. These include electrolytes, renal function tests, thyroid tests, glucose, amylase, complete blood count, electrocardiogram, cholesterol, carotene level and a dexamethasone suppression test. There is not an indication for a head CT, as one would not find changes on the head CT of an anorexic patient that would differentiate it from a normal head CT.
K&S Ch. 23

Question 115. B.   Creutzfeldt-Jakob disease (CJD) is one of a number of human spongiform encephalopathies and is associated with prion infection. The worldwide incidence of CJD is about 0.5 to 1 in one million per year. A new variant was thought to have developed during the later nineties resulting from consumption of meat from cattle infected with bovine spongiform encephalopathy. The clinical picture is that of a prodromal period of vegetative symptoms such as asthenia and sleep and appetite disturbances. This is followed by the onset of a rapidly progressive dementia with deficits in memory, concentration, depression, self-neglect and personality changes. The condition progresses to global dementia over time and death typically occurs from two to seven months after onset of symptoms. The diagnostic test of choice today is lumbar puncture with cerebrospinal fluid assay of 14-3-3 and tau proteins, the specificity and sensitivity of which exceed 90%. CT scans of the brain are useless as they remain normal in a majority of cases. There may be atrophy seen on CT scan with ventricular enlargement, but this is nonspecific and diagnostically unhelpful. MRI of the brain may reveal atrophy with symmetrical

increased signal intensity in the basal ganglia, which is again not particularly helpful in diagnosing CJD. Electroencephalogram is more helpful and is expected to reveal a characteristic one to two cycle-per-second triphasic sharp wave pattern superimposed on a background of electrical depression. This pattern is seen in up to 80% of cases at some point during the course of the illness.
B&D Ch. 59

Question 116. D. Disorders of smooth visual pursuit and disinhibition of saccadic eye movements are commonly found in patients with schizophrenia. This has been proposed by some as a trait marker for schizophrenia, because it is found regardless of medication use and is also present in first degree relatives. It is thought that the eye movement disorders are the function of pathology in the frontal lobes.
K&S Ch. 13

Question 117. E. Many of the antipsychotic medications block dopamine in the tubero-infundibular tract. Because of this dopamine blockade, the patient develops an elevated prolactin level. That elevated prolactin level leads to galactorrhea and amenorrhea. In the case given, the risperidone is the most likely cause of the patient's symptoms. You would want to check the serum prolactin level and adjust the risperidone dose, or consider switching the patient to another medication.
K&S Ch. 7

Question 118. C. Patients with borderline personality disorder have frequent mood swings. They can develop short-lived psychotic episodes. They often cut or mutilate themselves to elicit help from others, to express anger, or to numb themselves to strong affect. Both men and women can have borderline personality disorder, though it is more common in women. The other answer choices do not fit the case as well as borderline personality disorder. Schizoaffective disorder patients do not usually self-mutilate. Dysthymic disorder is not consistent with psychotic symptoms. There is no description of mania, so bipolar disorder is unlikely. There is no acute stressor so adjustment disorder doesn't fit well. Whenever a question involves cutting or self-mutilation, strongly consider borderline personality disorder.
K&S Ch. 27

Question 119. B. Of the choices given, the highest prevalence is for anxiety disorders. Over 30 million people in the United States have an anxiety disorder. About 17.5 million have depression. About 2 million have schizophrenia. About 5 million have dementia. About 12.8 million use illicit drugs.
K&S Ch. 4

Question 120. D. There is an association between pathological gambling and mood disorders, particularly major depressive disorder (MDD). There is also an association with panic, obsessive-compulsive disorder and agoraphobia, but the association with MDD is greater. Criteria for pathological gambling include preoccupation with gambling, gambling increased sums of money to obtain excitement, being unsuccessful at stopping or cutting back, gambling to escape dysphoric mood, lying to significant others about gambling, loss of important relationships over gambling, committing illegal acts in order to gamble, relying on others to pay the bills because of money lost gambling, and a desire to keep going back to break even.
K&S Ch. 25

Question 121. C. This is a case of delusional disorder. In delusional disorder the patient has nonbizarre delusions (i.e., they could be true, but are not). They do not meet criteria for schizophrenia. Their functioning in day to day life is relatively preserved. It may take various forms, such as erotomanic type, grandiose type, jealous type, persecutory type, somatic type, or mixed type. This patient does not meet criteria for schizophrenia. There are no mood symptoms, so this rules out depression. He is not confused, disoriented, and waxing and waning in consciousness, so this rules out a delirium. The wife is not a partner in the delusions, she thinks there is something wrong with him, so this rules out a shared psychotic disorder. Given all of this, the correct answer is delusional disorder.

K&S Ch. 14

Question 122. E. Hypochondriasis involves being convinced that one has a serious disease based on misinterpretation of bodily sensations. The preoccupation with having the illness persists despite reassurance by doctors. It causes clinically significant impairment in functioning. Somatoform disorders is a general category that includes somatization disorder, conversion disorder, hypochondriasis, body dysmorphic disorder, and pain disorder. Facticious disorder is when a patient feigns illness for primary gain (i.e., benefits of the sick role). Conversion disorder is the development of a neurological deficit as a result of psychological conflict. Pain disorder is the presence of pain as the predominant clinical focus, where the pain is thought to be substantially mediated by psychological factors.

K&S Ch. 17

Question 123. E. There are multiple studies that all point to a genetic predisposition for alcoholism. The studies that separate environmental from genetic factors are some of the most convincing. Studies of adoptees clearly demonstrate that children whose biological parents were alcoholics are at increased risk for alcoholism, even when brought up by adopted families where neither parent has an alcohol problem. In addition, children whose biological parents do not have an alcohol problem are not more likely to become alcoholic if raised in a home with parents who have alcohol problems.

K&S Ch. 12

Question 124. C. This is a psychogenic seizure (also called nonepileptic seizure). Keys to a psychogenic seizure, or pseudoseizure, are lack of an aura, no cyanotic skin changes, no self injury, no incontinence, no postictal confusion, asynchronous body movements, absent EEG changes, and seizure activity being affected by the suggestion of the doctor.

K&S Ch. 10

Question 125. B. Internuclear ophthalmoplegia is a classic brainstem finding on neurologic examination of patients with demyelinating lesions of multiple sclerosis (MS). The lesion localizes to the medial longitudinal fasciculus (MLF) of the brainstem. The deficit involves abnormal horizontal ocular movements with absence or delayed adduction of the eye ipsilateral to the MLF lesion and coarse horizontal nystagmus in the abducting eye. Convergence is preserved. Bilateral internuclear ophthalmoplegia is highly suggestive of MS, but can also be seen with other brainstem lesions, particularly Arnold-Chiari malformation, Wernicke's encephalopathy, vascular lesions and brainstem gliomas.

B&D Ch. 60

Question 126. B. Paranoid schizophrenia is characterized by delusions of persecution or grandeur, as well as auditory hallucinations. Patients usually have their first break at a later age than other schizophrenic patients. They show more preservation of cognitive function than in other types of schizophrenia. Disorganized schizophrenia is marked by primitive, disinhibited, disorganized behavior. Patients have significant impairment in cognition.

Catatonic schizophrenia is characterized by stupor, negativism, rigidity and posturing. Mutism is common, and cognition and communication are impaired. Undifferentiated schizophrenic patients do not fit easily into one of the other categories. Residual schizophrenia consists of the continued presence of some symptoms of schizophrenia in a person who no longer meets full criteria for the disorder.
K&S Ch. 13

Question 127. E. Pathological gambling is categorized by the DSM as an impulse control disorder. Criteria for pathological gambling include preoccupation with gambling, gambling increased sums of money to obtain excitement, being unsuccessful at stopping or cutting back, gambling to escape dysphoric mood, lying to significant others about gambling, loss of important relationships over gambling, committing illegal acts in order to gamble, relying on others to pay the bills because of money lost gambling, and a desire to keep going back to break even.
K&S Ch. 25

Question 128. E. Asperger's disorder is characterized by the following clinical features. The patient has marked impairment in the use of nonverbal communication, failure to develop peer relationships, lack of desire to share experiences with others and restricted or stereotyped patterns of behavior. There can be preoccupation or obsessive focus on certain interests, rigid adherence to schedules, and stereotyped motor mannerisms. Unlike autism, there is not a delay in language or cognitive development. The child in this question clearly has Asperger's disorder. He is not breaking rules and violating social norms as one would expect with a conduct disorder. He is not fighting authority figures as one would expect of oppositional defiant disorder. He does not show irritability, impulsivity, and hyperactivity as one would find in attention deficit-hyperactivity disorder. His language and cognitive development are not delayed as would be expected in a case of autism.
K&S Ch. 42

Question 129. D. If you thought this was the same as question 128 you need to read more carefully! This is a case of autism. In autism there is marked impairment in the use of nonverbal communication, failure to develop peer relationships, lack of desire to share experiences with others, and restricted or stereotyped patterns of behavior. There can be preoccupation or obsessive focus on certain interests, rigid adherence to schedules, and stereotyped motor mannerisms. But very importantly, there is delay in, or total absence of spoken language. There is an inability to maintain conversation. There is stereotyped use of language. There is a lack of spontaneous or make believe play. Cognitive development is significantly impaired. There is a lack of social or emotional reciprocity.
K&S Ch. 42

Question 130. B. Derealization is a subjective feeling that the environment is strange or unreal. Depersonalization is a person's sense that they are unreal or unfamiliar. Fugue involves having amnesia for your identity and assuming a new identity. It usually also involves wandering to new places. Amnesia is the inability to recall past experiences. Anosognosia is an inability to recognize a neurological deficit that is occurring to oneself.
K&S Ch. 8

Question 131. E. Inhalants can cause a persisting dementia. It is irreversible except for the mildest cases. It may be the result of the neurotoxic effects of the inhalants, the metals they contain, or the effects of hypoxia. Inhalant use can also lead to delirium, psychosis, mood, and anxiety disorders. Signs of intoxication with inhalants include maladaptive behavior such

as assaultiveness, impaired judgment, as well as neurological signs such as dizziness, slurred speech, ataxia, tremor, blurred vision, stupor, and coma. The other answer choices have various effects, but do not cause a persisting dementia.
K&S Ch. 12

Question 132. E. Social skills training is an important part of psychiatric rehabilitation. Social skills are behaviors necessary for survival in the community. These are disrupted by severe illnesses such as schizophrenia. Social skills training has proven important in correcting deficits in patient's behaviors. Severely ill patients make slow progress, but can learn some necessary skills that enable them to engage in conversation and decrease social anxiety. Social skills training can be done both in a group and an individual format. The other answer choices in this question consist of unrelated pairs, some of which border on the ridiculous and are distracters.
K&S Ch. 35

Question 133. D. Multiple sclerosis (MS) is the most common inflammatory demyelinating disease. The classic onset of the disease is between the ages of 15 and 50 years. About two-thirds of patients have the relapsing-remitting form of the disease at onset, which is the most common form of the illness. Only about twenty percent of patients have primary progressive disease at onset. Optic neuritis (ON) is a common sign of multiple sclerosis and is frequently the cause of initial presenting symptoms. ON usually presents with eye pain that increases with eye movement followed by central visual loss (scotoma) in the affected eye. ON patients will have a relative afferent pupillary defect (Marcus Gunn pupil). This is tested by the swinging flashlight test which demonstrates that the abnormal pupil paradoxically dilates when a light is moved away from the normal to the affected eye. Internuclear ophthalmoplegia is a common sign of MS and involves a lesion in the medial longitudinal fasciculus of the brainstem that produces a characteristic eye movement abnormality. The eye ipsilateral to the lesions cannot adduct past the midline while the contralateral eye fully abducts and displays a coarse end-gaze nystagmus. The finding can sometimes be bilateral. Fatigue is a common complaint in patients with MS. It often has little to do with the amount of physical exertion carried out by the patient. It may occur upon waking despite a good night's sleep the night before. Heat sensitivity is a well-described phenomenon in MS. Increases in core body temperature can bring on symptoms or worsen already existing symptoms. This is known as Uhthoff's phenomenon. The condition occurs due to conduction block that occurs as body temperature rises. Lhermitte's sign is a transient neurologic sign described by patients as a sensation of an electric shock that descends down the spine or the extremities upon neck flexion. It is most often suggestive of MS, but can also be seen in other conditions involving the cervical spinal cord, such as disc herniations, trauma and tumors.
B&D Ch. 60

Question 134. C. Bulemia is categorized by a recurrent pattern of binge eating and self induced vomiting. Bulemic patients often develop a hypochloremic alkalosis, and are at risk for gastric and esophageal tears. Dehydration (hence low blood pressure) and electrolyte imbalances are likely. Many female bulimic patients have menstrual disturbances. Russell's sign is positive when cuts or scrapes to the backs of the hands are noted which are a result of sticking the fingers down the throat to induce vomiting.
K&S Ch 23

Question 135. D. Amphetamine intoxication presents with euphoria, anxiety, anger, hypervigilance, and impaired judgment and functioning. The effects are similar to those of cocaine. There is a risk for an amphetamine-induced

psychotic disorder as well, which is characterized by paranoia. One can also note visual hallucinations, hypersexuality, hyperactivity, confusion and incoherence.
K&S Ch. 12

Question 136. B. Acute stress disorder is characterized by similar symptoms to post-traumatic stress disorder, but with a different time frame. Symptoms occur for a minimum of two days, and a maximum of 4 weeks, and begin within 4 weeks of the traumatic event. The patient must have undergone a traumatic event. The patient then experiences emotional numbing, lack of awareness of surroundings, derealization, depersonalization, dissociative amnesia, flashbacks, avoidance of stimuli that remind them of the event, anxiety, irritability, increased arousal, or poor sleep.
K&S Ch. 16

Question 137. C. Children who are depressed can often present with irritability instead of, or in addition to depressed mood. Prepubertal children can report somatic complaints, psychomotor agitation, and mood-congruent hallucinations. Depressed children can also fail to make expected weight gains. Other signs of depression that children can present with include school phobia and excessive clinging to parents. Teens with depression often report poor school performance, substance abuse, promiscuity, antisocial behavior, truancy, and running away from home. They can withdraw from social activities and be grouchy and sulky.
K&S Ch. 49

Question 138. D. Schizoid personality disorder is characterized by a pervasive pattern of detachment from social relationships. The patient neither desires, nor enjoys close relationships. They choose solitary activities. They lack close friends or romantic relationships. They are indifferent to the opinions of others and are emotionally cold and detached. Some of the other choices in this question are references to schizotypal personality disorder. In the schizotypal patient, there are ideas of reference, magical thinking, paranoia, and excessive social anxiety which is fueled by paranoid thinking.
K&S Ch. 27

Question 139. A. Beneficence is the duty to do no harm to the patient. Autonomy is the duty to protect a patient's freedom to choose. Autonomy theory views the relationship between patient and doctor as between two adults, not as parent and child. Justice in this context means a fair distribution and application of services. Validity is a statistical word meaning that a test measures what it claims to measure.
K&S Ch. 58

Question 140. D. Tourette's disorder often involves both motor and vocal tics. The onset is usually around 7 years of age, but may come as early as 2 years. Motor tics usually start in the face and head, and progress down the body. Vocal tics are not done intentionally to provoke others, but are the result of sudden, intrusive thoughts and urges that the patient cannot control. These intrusive thoughts may involve socially unacceptable subject matter or obscenity.
K&S Ch. 46

Question 141. D. Substance abusers have the highest risk of becoming violent. Large doses of alcohol promote aggression, as do large doses of barbiturates. Paradoxical aggression can be observed with anxiolytics. Opioid dependence is associated with increased aggression. Stimulants, cocaine, hallucinogens, and sometimes cannabis can also lead to aggression. Aggressive behavior is more likely with those who have become acutely psychologically decompensated. More than half of people who commit homicide

and engage in assaultive behavior are under the influence of significant amounts of alcohol at the time the crime is committed. Although many major psychiatric disorders can lead to aggression, you are more likely to face substance-induced aggression simply because of the sheer number of cases of aggression and violence that are substance-induced.
K&S Ch. 4

Question 142. C. An ideal patient for psychodynamic psychotherapy should have the capacity for psychological mindedness, have at least one meaningful relationship, be able to tolerate affect, respond well to transference interpretation, be highly motivated, have flexible defenses and lack tendencies towards splitting, projection or denial. A useful screening tool for whether a patient has these characteristics is to understand the quality of their relationships, as the above-listed qualities often contribute to productive relationships.
K&S Ch. 35

Question 143. E. The clinical picture and scan are classic for multiple sclerosis (MS). The MRI scan reveals numerous subcortical white matter demyelinating lesions that are typical of MS. The lesions would be expected to enhance with gadolinium contrast early on during an attack and enhancement can persist up to eight weeks following an acute attack. The treatment of an acute attack is generally with intravenous corticosteroids. The protocol is usually with intravenous methylprednisolone 500–1000 mg daily in divided doses for three to seven days. This may or may not be followed with a one to two-week oral prednisone taper. Antibiotics such as ceftriaxone have no place in MS. Intravenous immunoglobulin therapy and plasmapheresis are treatments for myasthenia gravis and Guillain-Barré syndrome and not for MS. Aspirin and heparin therapies are generally instituted in the emergency room setting for acute ischemic stroke when recombinant tissue plasminogen activator cannot be given.
B&D Ch. 60

Question 144. A. Borderline patients often cut, self-mutilate, and make suicide attempts. The patient in question has made past suicide attempts and past attempts are the best predictor of future attempts. She is emotionally labile following an interpersonal conflict. She is already doing harm to herself through cutting and is becoming psychotic. All of these factors add up to one very important point: this patient is highly unpredictable and could very easily kill herself. The only reasonable answer choice is hospital admission where her impulsive, self-destructive, and self mutilating impulses can be limited and her behavior observed. The other answer choices do not take her unpredictability and self-destructiveness seriously enough. The choice for extended inpatient stay is wrong because you have no way of knowing how long she is going to need to stay based on the information given. She could potentially stabilize in a few days and be safe for discharge. She could also be in the hospital for several months. There is no way to predict length of stay based on the question stem.
K&S Ch. 27

Question 145. E. Research in recent years has found that depression following a heart attack increases the likelihood of another heart attack. There has been evidence to suggest that there are serotonin receptors on the surface of platelets which can modify and reduce platelet aggregation and thereby reduce heart attack risk. The prescription of a selective serotonin reuptake inhibitor antidepressant following a myocardial infarction has been shown to increase the amount of serotonin in the body as a whole. This in turn modulates platelet serotonin receptors, thus decreasing platelet aggregation and making a future heart attack less likely.
K&S Ch. 36

66

Question 146. B. Neurofibromatosus type 1 (NF1) is caused by a mutation in the 60 exon NF1 gene on chromosome 17q. NF1 is the most common of the neurocutaneous illnesses occurring in about 1 in 3000 individuals. NF2 is caused by a mutation in the NF2 gene on chromosome 22. It is less common than NF1 and appears in about 1 in 50 000 individuals. Patients with NF1 need to have any two of the following seven criteria to carry the diagnosis: six or more café au lait spots over 5 mm in diameter before puberty and over 15 mm if after puberty; axillary or inguinal freckling; optic glioma; two or more neurofibromas or one plexiform neurofibroma; a first-degree relative with NF1; two or more Lisch nodules (hamartomas of the iris); characteristic bony lesion such as thinning of long bones or sphenoid dysplasia. Patients with NF2 must have bilateral acoustic schwannomas in order to meet criteria for this condition. If the schwannoma is unilateral, the patient meets criteria only with a first-degree relative with NF2.
B&D Ch. 71

Question 147. E. Both delirium and dementia can present with sleep problems, disorientation to place, violent behavior and hallucinations. The hallmark of delirium however is alteration of consciousness. Criteria include disturbance of consciousness with reduced ability to sustain attention, changes in cognition (memory problems, language disturbance, disorientation), and perceptual disturbances. These develop over a short period of time and can fluctuate during the course of a day. Dementia on the other hand consists of multiple cognitive deficits including memory loss, aphasia, apraxia, agnosia, and disturbance of executive function.
K&S Ch. 10

Question 148. D. The first step in treating a sleep problem is to rule out any problems in the environment that could cause insomnia and to alter the environment to make it more conducive to sleep. This approach starts with the rule that the bed is to be used for sleep and sex only. Reading in bed or watching television in bed should not be permitted. If this should fail, then pharmacologic aids can be pursued. A sleep study is not warranted by a simple complaint of insomnia. That would be overkill. Of course, a detailed history is the best tool to determine whether or not a more serious sleep disturbance is present.
K&S Ch. 24

Question 149. E. The American Psychiatric Association does not see homosexuality as a disorder. As such, there is no therapy that is warranted to change it. It is seen as a normal variant of human sexuality. There is good data to suggest that therapy to change homosexuality can be damaging to the patient. There is no evidence that supports attempting to change a patient's sexual orientation. Such therapy should not be encouraged. Neither teens nor adults should be treated for being homosexual.
K&S Ch. 21

Question 150. D. Methylenedioxyamphetamine (MDMA) is also known as ecstasy. It is in the amphetamine family and is a common drug of abuse at clubs and raves. Symptoms of intoxication with amphetamines include euphoria, changes in sociability, hypervigilence, changes in interpersonal sensitivity, anxiety, anger and impaired judgment. Amphetamines can induce a psychosis which includes paranoia, hyperactivity and hypersexuality. Physical effects include fever, headache, cyanosis, vomiting (leading to dehydration), shortness of breath, ataxia, and tremor. More serious effects can include myocardial infarction, severe hypertension, and ischemic colitis. Cannabis intoxication presents as impaired coordination, euphoria or anxiety, sense of slowed time, social withdrawal and impaired judgment. Physical signs include conjunctival injection, increased appetite, tachycardia, and dry mouth. Ketamine is a relative of PCP. Intoxication presents as belligerence, impulsivity, psychomotor agitation, and impaired judgment. Physical signs include nystagmus, hypertension, ataxia, dysarthria, or muscle rigidity. Psychosis may be present and can persist for up to two weeks after intoxication. Diacetylmorphine is heroin. Intoxication results in euphoria followed by apathy, psychomotor agitation or retardation, impaired judgment, pupillary dilation, sedation, slurred speech and impaired attention or memory. Volatile inhalant intoxication presents as belligerence, assaultiveness, apathy, impaired judgment, dizziness, nystagmus, impaired coordination, unsteady gait, lethargy, tremor, psychomotor retardation, muscle weakness, euphoria or coma. Low doses of these substances can cause feelings of euphoria. High doses can cause paranoia, fearfulness and hallucinations.

K&S Ch. 12

Test Number **TWO**

1. All of the following are true, EXCEPT:
   A. Carl Jung focused on the growth of the personality and individuation
   B. Harry Stack Sullivan saw human development as a function of social interaction
   C. Erik Erikson developed a model of the life cycle that spanned from childhood to old age
   D. Jean Piaget developed a theory of cognitive development
   E. The work of Freud, Jung and Erikson was a function of carefully crafted psychological and neurodevelopmental studies

2. A 75 year-old woman presents to the emergency room with an acute onset of right hemisensory loss, mild right hemiparesis and a right-sided Babinski sign. On mental status examination, you note that she cannot repeat simple phrases, she can follow simple task instructions both verbal and on paper, she cannot write well, and she is having word-finding difficulties with multiple paraphasic errors. This clinical picture is consistent with a:
   A. Broca's aphasia
   B. Wernicke's aphasia
   C. Transcortical sensory aphasia
   D. Conduction aphasia
   E. Transcortical motor aphasia

3. All of the following statements regarding receptors are true, EXCEPT:
   A. Seven-transmembrane domain receptors require G proteins to open ion channels
   B. In the ligand-gated ion channel receptor, the channel is built into the complex that binds the ligand
   C. Seven-transmembrane domain receptors have an external NH$_2$ terminal end and an intracellular COOH terminal end
   D. Nerve growth factor (NGF) and brain-derived neurotropic factor (BDNF) bind to seven-transmembrane-domain receptors
   E. Hormones may diffuse into the cell and bind cytoplasmic receptors which leads to influence over gene expression

4. Correcting hyponatremia too rapidly with hypertonic saline replacement can result in:
   A. Guillain-Barré syndrome
   B. Acute thalamic hemorrhage
   C. Acute demyelinating encephalomyelitis (ADEM)
   D. Acute cerebellar syndrome
   E. Acute locked-in syndrome

5. A patient comes into your office and explains away why he beat his brother with a baseball bat. He gives several examples of how his brother had mistreated him in the past and says that if he had not gotten this beating the mistreatment would have continued. Which of the following defenses does this represent?
   A. Projection
   B. Blocking
   C. Externalization
   D. Rationalization
   E. Denial

6. A 34 year-old obese African-American woman presents to the emergency room with a complaint of six weeks of intermittent bifrontal headache and vague visual obscurations. She is on oral contraceptive medication and has a history of being on tetracycline therapy for a recent sexually transmitted disease. The immediate diagnostic test of choice in the emergency room is:
   A. Noncontrast head CT scan
   B. Lumbar puncture with cerebrospinal fluid opening pressure
   C. Brain MRI without gadolinium
   D. Serum sedimentation rate (ESR)
   E. Serum prolactin level

7. Which of the following organizations is made up of family members of the mentally ill?
   A. American Association for Mental Health
   B. National Mental Health Assembly
   C. National Alliance for the Mentally Ill
   D. Council for Mental Health Reform
   E. Association for the Advancement of Psychotherapy

8. All of the following are diagnostic criteria of migraine without aura, EXCEPT:
   A. Headache must last 4 to 72 hours
   B. Pulsatile quality
   C. Photophobia
   D. Nausea and vomiting
   E. Mild to moderate intensity

9. What is the lifetime prevalence of schizophrenia?
   A. 10%
   B. 5%
   C. 1%
   D. 0.5%
   E. 0.1%

10. All of the following are contraindications to the use of recombinant tissue plasminogen activator (r-TPA) in acute ischemic stroke, EXCEPT:
    A. Stroke occurrence 2 hours prior to r-TPA administration
    B. Major surgery within 2 weeks of r-TPA administration
    C. Uncontrolled hypertension
    D. Prothrombin time > 15
    E. Thrombocytopenia

11. Which of the following is based on active outreach to patients in the community?
    A. Traditional social work
    B. Assertive community treatment
    C. Day hospitals
    D. Psychiatric rehabilitation
    E. Electro-convulsive therapy

71

12. A 45 year-old woman presents to your office complaining of longstanding lower extremity discomfort, particularly at night prior to sleep onset. She reports shooting pains in the lower extremities that are relieved upon standing or walking. The discomfort is described as a "crawling" sensation. The treatment of choice for her condition is:

A. Sertraline

B. Cyproheptadine

C. Ropinirole

D. Levetiracetam

E. Ziprasidone

13. Which of the following is the best diagnostic procedure to determine if a 12 year-old boy is depressed?

A. MMPI

B. Scholastic achievement test

C. Dexamethasone suppression test

D. Face to face interview with the child

E. Interview the child's teacher by phone

14. A 65 year-old man presents to the emergency room with acute onset of vertigo, nausea, vomiting, dysarthria and nystagmus. On further examination, he is noted to have loss of pain and temperature sensation to the left-hand side of his face. He has right-sided loss of pain and temperature sensation to his trunk and leg. He has a left Horner's syndrome and falls to his left-hand side when you ask him to walk, and has left finger-to-nose dysmetria. You diagnose an acute stroke which is most likely localized to the:

A. Left hemisphere

B. Left lateral medulla

C. Left pons

D. Right pons

E. Right lateral medulla

15. Which of the following is associated with violence and aggression?

A. Blunted response to CRH stimulation test

B. Blunted growth hormone response to hypoglycemia

C. Decreased 5-HIAA in the CSF

D. Decreased dopamine in the CSF

E. Increased levels of norepinephrine in the CSF

16. Metachromatic leukodystrophy is inherited by _____ pattern of inheritance and results in a deficiency in _____:

A. Autosomal recessive; hexosaminidase A

B. Autosomal dominant; hexosaminidase A

C. Autosomal dominant; arylsufatase A

D. Autosomal recessive; arylsulfatase A

E. Autosomal recessive; galactocerebroside β-galactosidase

17. All of the following are true with respect to Seasonal Affective Disorders (SAD), EXCEPT:

    A. Patients are likely to respond well to light therapy

    B. The "with seasonal pattern" specifier can be applied to bipolar I, bipolar II, and major depressive disorders according to the DSM-IV

    C. It is not necessary to have full remissions of symptoms at other times of the year to make this diagnosis

    D. SAD involves a regular temporal relationship between the onset of symptoms and the time of year

    E. You must demonstrate at least two depressive episodes at the same time of year to make the diagnosis

18. All of the following primitive reflexes are generally expected to disappear by about 6 months of age, EXCEPT:

    A. Rooting

    B. Moro

    C. Palmar grasp

    D. Parachute response

    E. Tonic neck reflex

19. Which of the following would fall under the heading of somatoform disorder NOS?

    A. A patient with pain in one or more areas that is thought to be significantly mediated by psychological factors

    B. A patient with a persistent belief that she has cancer despite reassurance by her physician that nothing is wrong

    C. A patient who develops a motor deficit following significant psychological stressors

    D. A patient who feels that she is pregnant and presents with amenorrhea, enlarged abdomen, and breast engorgement, but a negative pregnancy test

    E. A patient with medical complaints involving pain, GI complaints, neurological complaints, and sexual complaints. No medical explanation can be found for these symptoms

20. An AIDS patient presents with decreased visual acuity. The most likely offending infectious agent responsible for this presentation is:

    A. Cytomegalovirus

    B. Toxoplasmosis

    C. Tuberculosis (mycobacterium)

    D. *Cryptococcus neoformans*

    E. JC virus

21. All of the following are true regarding schizophrenia, EXCEPT:
    A. The disorder is chronic and usually has a prodromal phase
    B. Eugen Bleuler coined the term schizophrenia
    C. The patient's overall functioning declines or fails to reach the expected level
    D. The most frequent hallucinations are olfactory
    E. Social withdrawal and emotional disengagement are common

22. All of the following are seen in narcolepsy EXCEPT:
    A. Cataplexy
    B. Nighttime awakening
    C. Excessive daytime sleepiness
    D. Sleep paralysis
    E. Hypnagogic hallucinations

23. Uncontrollable excessive talking, as seen in mania is also known as:
    A. Alexithymia
    B. Logorrhea
    C. Echolalia
    D. Flight of ideas
    E. Stilted speech

24. All of the following are appropriate therapies for status epilepticus, EXCEPT:
    A. Rectal diazepam
    B. Intravenous lorazepam
    C. Intramuscular phenytoin
    D. Intravenous valproic acid
    E. Oxygen by nasal cannula with airway protection

25. Which one of the following statements is true regarding atypical antipsychotics?
    A. Ziprasidone is an agonist at the 5-HT-1A receptor, and an inhibitor of reuptake of both serotonin and norepinephrine
    B. Risperidone is a significantly weaker antagonist of D2 than haloperidol
    C. Quetiapine is known for its high incidence of extrapyrimidal symptoms
    D. Olanzapine has been associated with weight loss in the majority of patients
    E. Clozapine has been shown to increase suicidality in chronically ill patients

26. Which of the following anticonvulsant agents is most appropriate for primary generalized seizures including tonic-clonic, absence, atonic and myoclonic seizure types?
    A. Divalproex sodium
    B. Phenytoin
    C. Oxcarbazepine
    D. Carbamazepine
    E. Ethosuximide

27. Which of the following is NOT a side effect of the tricyclic antidepressants?
    A. Tachycardia
    B. Prolonged PR interval
    C. Prolonged QRS interval
    D. Orthostatic hypotension
    E. Diarrhea

28. The L5 motor nerve root innervates the nerves responsible for:
    A. Foot extension
    B. Foot flexion
    C. Leg extension
    D. Hip flexion
    E. The ankle jerk reflex

29. Which one of the following antidepressants can be used as an antipruritic agent and for the treatment of gastric ulcer because of its potent histamine blockade?
    A. Trazodone
    B. Fluoxetine
    C. Citalopram
    D. Amitryptyline
    E. Amoxapine

30. A patient involved in a car accident is found on MRI to have a spinal fracture and a partial crush lesion to the cervical spinal cord that effectively causes a functional hemisection of the cord. His deficits would be expected to include:
    A. Contralateral loss of motor control and pain and temperature sensation with ipsilateral loss of proprioception and vibration sensation
    B. Ipsilateral loss of motor control and pain and temperature sensation with contralateral loss of proprioception and vibration sensation
    C. Ipsilateral loss of motor control and proprioception and vibration sensation with contralateral loss of pain and temperature sensation
    D. Contralateral loss of motor control and proprioception and vibration sensation with ipsilateral loss of pain and temperature sensation
    E. Ipsilateral loss of motor control and contralateral loss of proprioception, vibration, pain and temperature sensations

75

31. A child is able to use some symbols and language. Her reasoning is intuitive. She is unable to think logically or deductively. Which of Piaget's stages does this child fit into?

    A. Sensorimotor
    B. Preoperational thought
    C. Concrete operations
    D. Formal operations
    E. Trust vs mistrust

32. A 72 year-old man suffers a stroke with loss of motor functioning in the left leg and, to a lesser extent, the left arm. He has abulia and his eyes and head seem preferentially deviated to the right. His left arm is apraxic. His head CT is shown below. The arterial territory involved is that of the:

    A. Right middle cerebral artery
    B. Right posterior cerebral artery
    C. Right vertebral artery
    D. Right anterior cerebral artery
    E. Right posterior communicating artery

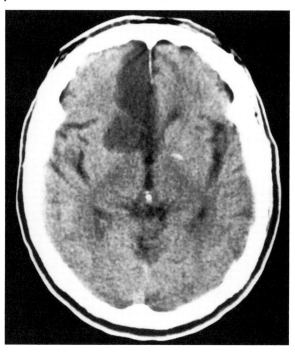

33. Which of the following is true regarding norepinephrine (NE) and/or the locus ceruleus?

    A. Norepinephrine is synthesized in the locus ceruleus
    B. Dopamine is synthesized in the locus ceruleus, NE in the dorsal raphe nuclei
    C. Acetylcholine is synthesized with NE in the substantia nigra
    D. 5-HT is synthesized in the locus ceruleus
    E. The locus ceruleus is the site of the formation of serotonin

34. Pure motor hemiparesis is most likely to result from a stroke localized to the:

    A. Midbrain
    B. Cerebellum
    C. Medulla
    D. Thalamus
    E. Internal capsule

35. Which one of the following receptor types is associated with weight gain and sedation?
    A. 5-HT-2A
    B. Alpha 1
    C. 5-HT-1A
    D. H1
    E. M1

36. The lesion causing a left-arm hemiballismus would most likely localize to the:
    A. Right subthalamic nucleus
    B. Left subthalamic nucleus
    C. Right putamen
    D. Left putamen
    E. Right globus pallidus interna

37. Which of the following is NOT a biogenic amine neurotransmitter?
    A. Dopamine
    B. GABA
    C. Epinephrine
    D. Acetylcholine
    E. Serotonin

38. The mechanism of action by which reserpine both improves the symptoms of adult-onset primary focal dystonia and can cause depression is:
    A. Direct postsynaptic dopamine antagonism
    B. Direct postsynaptic serotonin agonism
    C. Direct postsynaptic serotonin antagonism
    D. Presynaptic dopaminergic depletion
    E. Direct postsynaptic cholinergic antagonism

39. In the psychotic patient, the defense mechanism of projection takes the form of:
    A. Feelings of persecution
    B. Feelings of abandonment
    C. Feelings of sadness
    D. Feelings of gratification
    E. Feelings of isolation

40. The drainage of cerebrospinal fluid into the blood is a function of the:
    A. Choroid plexus
    B. Virchow-Robin spaces
    C. Dural mitochondria
    D. Ventricular ependymal cells
    E. Arachnoid granulations

41. Which one of the following is a method of making a prediction in order to compare the value of one variable to another?
    A. Probability
    B. Point prevalence
    C. Incidence
    D. Regression analysis
    E. Kappa

42. A 72 year-old woman with a history of smoking, diabetes, hypertension, hyperlipidemia and myocardial infarction presents to your emergency room by ambulance with an acute onset of obtundation with dense right hemiplegia, right hemisensory loss to light touch, pain and temperature, and mutism. You suspect a left lobar hemorrhage because of the acuity of onset of her symptoms and a blood pressure reading of 210/100 mmHg in the emergency room. Once stabilized, the best immediate diagnostic test of choice from the emergency room would be:
    A. Lumbar puncture with opening pressure and CSF assay for xanthochromia
    B. Brain MRI scan without gadolinium
    C. Blood work for coagulation panel (PT, PTT, INR)
    D. Noncontrast head CT scan
    E. Routine bedside electroencephalogram (EEG)

43. Which one of the following is most closely associated with prognostic outcome in psychodynamic therapy?
    A. Length of training
    B. Neutrality of the therapist
    C. Age of the therapist
    D. Gender of the therapist
    E. Empathy and warmth

44. Melatonin is a neuronal hormone that promotes sleep and is produced in the brain by the:
    A. Pineal gland
    B. Anterior pituitary gland
    C. Posterior pituitary gland
    D. Hypothalamus
    E. Thalamus

45. Which one of the following is an objective psychological test?
    A. Rorschach
    B. Sentence completion test
    C. Thematic apperception test
    D. MMPI
    E. Draw a person test

78

46. Subacute sclerosing panencephalitis is a rare late complication of which one of the following organisms:

    A. Measles virus
    B. Herpes simplex virus
    C. Epstein-Barr virus
    D. Mumps virus
    E. JC virus

47. All of the following could be descriptors of a patient with ADHD, EXCEPT:

    A. The patient fails to follow through on instructions and fails to finish schoolwork
    B. The patient often fidgets with hands or feet or squirms in his seat
    C. The patient often has difficulty awaiting his turn
    D. The patient often seems not to listen when spoken to directly
    E. The patient shows impairment from symptoms at school but not at home

48. A 13 year-old boy is brought to the emergency room from a group home because of acute agitation. On examination you note choreoathetotic movements, hyperreflexia, acute agitation, self-scratching and mutilating behavior, and a marked cognitive impairment. You peruse the group home chart and note that this young boy has an enzymatic deficiency in hypoxanthine-guanine phosphoribosyltransferase. Your keen memory brings you back to your pediatrics rotation in medical school and you realize the diagnosis is:

    A. Tay-Sachs disease
    B. Metachromatic leukodystrophy
    C. Krabbe disease
    D. Gaucher's disease
    E. Lesch-Nyhan syndrome

49. Which one of the following is NOT a DSM IV-TR criterion for schizophrenia?

    A. Delusions
    B. Presence of active phase symptoms for 6 months
    C. Hallucinations
    D. Disorganized speech
    E. Grossly disorganized or catatonic behavior

50. Botulinum toxin type A is the treatment of choice for all of the following disorders, EXCEPT:

    A. Hemifacial spasm
    B. Blepharospasm
    C. Cervical dystonia
    D. Restless legs syndrome
    E. Limb spasticity related to multiple sclerosis

51. A patient presents with a delusion about being poisoned that has been present for 5 months. The patient has no hallucinations or other psychotic symptoms. There has been no major impact on the patient's daily functioning. The patient has no mood symptoms. The most likely diagnosis is:

    A. Dementia
    B. Schizophrenia
    C. Schizoaffective disorder, bipolar type
    D. Delusional disorder
    E. Brief psychotic disorder

52. A young woman presents to the emergency room with a complaint of a band-like, bifrontal, squeezing headache that began six hours earlier. She denies nausea, vomiting, or any other associated symptoms. She describes the pain as waxing-and-waning in intensity throughout the six-hour period. Physical examination is unremarkable. She reports suffering from similar attacks in the past. The most likely diagnosis is:

    A. Tension-type headache
    B. Migraine without aura
    C. Migraine with aura
    D. Paroxysmal hemicrania
    E. Basilar migraine

53. All of the following are consistent with a major depressive episode, EXCEPT:

    A. Anhedonia
    B. Withdrawal from social situations
    C. Low frustration tolerance
    D. Weight loss
    E. Increased libido

54. The generator of migraine headache is thought to be the:

    A. Reticular activating system
    B. Trigeminal nucleus caudalis
    C. Dural and intracerebral blood vessels
    D. Suprachiasmatic nucleus
    E. Contraction of scalp and cranial muscles

55. A patient comes to your clinic with complaint of hypersomnia, hyperphagia, psychomotor slowing, and depressed mood. He states that this happens yearly usually around October or November. The treatment plan for this man should include:

    A. Risperidone
    B. Naloxone
    C. Exposure to bright artificial light for 2–6 hours per day.
    D. Flooding
    E. Alprazolam

56. What is the mechanism of action of carbidopa in the combination agent carbidopa-levodopa that is used for the treatment of Parkinson's disease?
    A. Post-synaptic dopamine receptor agonism
    B. Monoamine oxidase type B inhibition
    C. Dopa decarboxylase inhibition
    D. Catechol-O-methyltransferase inhibition
    E. Acetylcholine receptor antagonism

57. A young woman presents to the emergency room with complaints of palpitations, sweating, shortness of breath, chest pain and nausea. She thinks that she is having a heart attack. EKG reveals normal sinus rhythm with no ischemic changes. Cardiac enzymes are not elevated. Given her symptoms, an alternative diagnosis would be:
    A. Manic episode
    B. Myxedema madness
    C. Mad hatter's syndrome
    D. Psychotic disorder NOS
    E. Panic attack

58. The phenomenon of apoptosis refers to:
    A. Neuronal migration
    B. Neuronal maturation
    C. Neurogenesis
    D. Neuronal myelination
    E. Neuronal programmed cell death

59. Which of the following is not a tricyclic antidepressant?
    A. Amitriptyline
    B. Amoxapine
    C. Doxepin
    D. Desipramine
    E. Nortriptyline

60. A 2 year-old toddler is brought to the emergency room because of seizures, hemiparesis and apparent blindness. You immediately notice a marked reddish discoloration of the left side of the forehead and face. The parents tell you that their child has not met appropriate developmental milestones. Your most likely diagnosis is:
    A. Tuberous sclerosis
    B. Sturge-Weber syndrome
    C. Von Hippel-Lindau disease
    D. Ataxia-telangiectasia
    E. Fabry's disease

61. How is a doctor who agrees to take Medicare paid?
    A. He agrees to take only what Medicare pays for the service
    B. He is allowed to bill the patient for the difference between what Medicare pays and what he charges
    C. He is paid by a third party to make up the difference between his fee for service rate and the fee allowed by Medicare
    D. He can sue the government if his full fee is not paid
    E. He is not allowed to charge copays

62. The pain syndrome known as reflex sympathetic dystrophy can have all of the following characteristics, EXCEPT:
    A. Hypersensitivity to painful stimuli
    B. Myofascial trigger points
    C. Cyanosis of the extremities
    D. Sweating and shiny skin
    E. Warm or hot skin on the extremities

63. The police bring an acutely paranoid patient into the Emergency Room who was found wandering the streets. In your initial approach to this patient you should first:
    A. Sedate the patient with haloperidol and lorazepam
    B. Assess the dangerousness of the patient to self or others
    C. Obtain an EKG
    D. Contact the patient's family if possible
    E. Obtain any old charts from medical records

64. Carbamazepine can lower the levels and therefore the efficacy of all of the following agents, EXCEPT:
    A. Warfarin
    B. Clozapine
    C. Alprazolam
    D. Propranolol
    E. Citalopram

65. All of the following are true concerning the right to die and surrogate decision making, EXCEPT:
    A. Patients that believe that continuing treatment would lessen their quality of life have the right to demand that treatment be withheld or withdrawn
    B. Advanced directives or a living will are a way for patients to express their preferences before anything happens that would cause them to lose capacity
    C. If a patient leaves no clear instructions, the state will carry out a course of action to protect and preserve human life
    D. Surrogate decision makers can be appointed by the patient, or the courts
    E. The standard of substituted judgment means that the surrogate will do whatever is in the patient's best interests

66. Patients who smoke tobacco heavily can markedly reduce levels of psychotropic medications they are taking. Which one of the following medications is NOT affected by tobacco smoking in this way?

    A. Clozapine
    B. Olanzapine
    C. Haloperidol
    D. Risperidone
    E. Amitriptyline

67. A consultation-liaison psychiatrist is called to evaluate a patient who is in denial of a major illness. The most important obligation of the psychiatrist at the first evaluation is to:

    A. Confront the denial forcefully
    B. Tell the staff to "play along" with the patient's denial
    C. Obtain neuropsychological testing
    D. Meet with the patient's family
    E. Make sure the patient has been informed about the illness and treatment

68. A 38 year-old delivers twins by uncomplicated cesarean section at 37 weeks. The pregnancy, her first, was unremarkable. On day three following her delivery, she experiences an acute onset of what she describes as the worst headache of her life. The neurologist is called and discovers that she has a notable bitemporal hemianopsia, neck stiffness, a positive Kernig's sign, persistent hypotension and a right third nerve palsy. The most likely diagnosis is:

    A. Sheehan's syndrome
    B. Cushing's disease
    C. Subarachnoid hemorrhage
    D. Acute bacterial meningitis
    E. Familial hemiplegic migraine

69. A patient describes feeling anxious about being in places or situations from which escape may be difficult or in which help may not be available should the patient begin to panic. The patient avoids various situations because of these fears. The term that best describes this patient's symptoms is:

    A. Agonothete
    B. Agoniada
    C. Agoraphobia
    D. Agora
    E. Agouara

70. Normal-pressure hydrocephalus presents as the triad of:

    A. Dementia, parkinsonism, and visual hallucinations
    B. Dementia, ophthalmoplegia, and ataxia
    C. Dementia, incontinence, and gait disturbance
    D. Chorea, irritability, and obsessive-compulsive traits
    E. Dementia, axial rigidity, and vertical ophthalmoplegia

83

71. All of the following are true of cyclothymic disorder, EXCEPT:
    A. It is similar to bipolar disorder, but less severe
    B. Symptoms must be present for at least 2 years
    C. It is equally common in men and women
    D. Substance abuse is common in patients with cyclothymia
    E. There are often psychotic symptoms found in patients with cyclothymia

72. All of the following are potential risk factors for ischemic stroke, EXCEPT:
    A. Prior cardiac disease
    B. Depression
    C. Gender
    D. Family history
    E. Obesity

73. A patient enters your office. She is agitated, acts seductively, wears colorful clothes that are bizarre in appearance, has an excessive amount of makeup on, and vacillates between being entertaining, hyperexcited, and threatening. Based on this information, her most likely diagnosis is:
    A. Major depressive disorder
    B. Brief psychotic disorder
    C. Body dysmorphic disorder
    D. Bipolar disorder
    E. Delusional disorder

74. All of the following symptoms are suggestive of a carotid territory transient ischemic attack or stroke, EXCEPT:
    A. Ataxia with vertigo
    B. Aphasia
    C. Ipsilateral monocular blindness
    D. Contralateral body weakness
    E. Contralateral homonymous visual field defects

75. Which of the following is NOT commonly part of the thought process of the manic bipolar patient?
    A. Flight of ideas
    B. Clang associations
    C. Racing thoughts
    D. Tangentiality
    E. Suicidal ideation

76. All of the following agents are potentially useful for the treatment of essential tremor, EXCEPT:

    A. Lorazepam
    B. Primidone
    C. Propranolol
    D. Desipramine
    E. Botulinum toxin type A

77. To meet criteria for a major depressive disorder, a patient must have symptoms for:

    A. 1 week
    B. 2 weeks
    C. 1 month
    D. 2 months
    E. 6 weeks

78. Which one of the following tumors is associated with myasthenia gravis?

    A. Thyroid carcinoma
    B. Thymoma
    C. Glioblastoma multiforme
    D. Breast papilloma
    E. Non-Hodgkin's lymphoma

79. All of the following are true regarding schizophrenia, EXCEPT:

    A. Lifetime prevalence is about 1%
    B. Prevalence is greater in rural than in urban areas
    C. The male-to-female ratio is 1:1
    D. Onset is rare before age 10 years or after age 40 years
    E. There is a higher incidence of the disease in babies born in winter and early spring

80. All of the following genetically-inherited neurological disorders are acquired by autosomal dominant heredity, EXCEPT:

    A. Friedrich's ataxia
    B. Myotonic dystrophy
    C. Tuberous sclerosis
    D. Huntington's disease
    E. Neurofibromatosus

81. All of the following are characteristics of a major depressive episode, EXCEPT:
    A. Constipation
    B. Dry mouth
    C. Headache
    D. Disinhibited behavior
    E. Early morning awakening

82. Migraine is most likely a hereditary disorder that maps to which chromosome:
    A. Chromosome 14
    B. Chromosome 15
    C. Chromosome 17
    D. Chromosome 18
    E. Chromosome 19

83. Which one of the following would be listed under thought content in the mental status exam?
    A. Obsessions
    B. Word salad
    C. Flight of ideas
    D. Circumstantiality
    E. Tangentiality

84. CNS cysticercosis is caused by brain parenchymal invasion by which one of the following organisms:
    A. *L. major*
    B. *T. solium*
    C. *T. gondii*
    D. *E. granulosus*
    E. *T. spiralis*

85. Which of the following lab tests can be used to detect chronic alcohol abuse?
    A. RBC count
    B. WBC count
    C. GGT
    D. CPK
    E. Alkaline phosphatase

86. The most frequent neurological complication of chronic alcohol abuse is:
    A. Wernicke's encephalopathy
    B. Alcoholic cerebellar degeneration
    C. Alcoholic neuropathy
    D. Marchiafava-Bignami disease
    E. Alcoholic dementia

87. A study in which a group comes from a well-defined population and is followed over a long period of time is a:

   A. Case history study
   B. Cohort study
   C. Cross-sectional study
   D. Case-control study
   E. Retrospective study

88. The Miller-Fisher syndrome involves the classic symptom complex of:

   A. Dementia, parkinsonism, psychosis
   B. Gait ataxia, urinary incontinence and dementia
   C. Ataxia, areflexia, ophthalmoplegia
   D. Alexia without agraphia
   E. Right-left confusion, finger agnosia, acaculia

89. Konrad Lorenz, during his work with animals demonstrated which one of the following concepts which may be used to understand early human psychological development?

   A. Sensory deprivation
   B. Altruism
   C. Imprinting
   D. Stress syndromes
   E. Episodic dyscontrol

90. A 29 year-old woman presents to the ER by ambulance in a wheelchair. She was brought from home with a complaint of rapidly progressive bilateral leg weakness over the past two weeks. Her legs were also painful and she complained of numbness and tingling in the lower part of both legs. Just prior to the onset of symptoms she had a three-day bout of bad diarrhea with fever and chills that resolved spontaneously. All of the following would be likely findings on diagnostic testing and examination of this patient, EXCEPT:

   A. Diminished deep tendon reflexes
   B. High cell count with absent protein in CSF
   C. Conduction block and prolonged F-wave latencies on nerve conduction studies
   D. Positive *Campylobacter jejuni* antibody serology
   E. Complement fixing antibodies to peripheral nerve myelin on nerve biopsy

91. All of the following are second messengers, EXCEPT:

   A. Adenylyl cyclase
   B. cGMP
   C. Ca^{2+}
   D. cAMP
   E. IP_3

1:20

92. All of the following characteristics are more typical of a cortical dementia than of a subcortical dementia such as dementia of the Alzheimer type, EXCEPT:

    A. Apathy and depression
    B. Aphasia
    C. Dyspraxia
    D. Absence of motor abnormalities
    E. Gradual insidious progression of cognitive decline

93. A child is playing in his home, and at the same time that his dog barks the doorbell also rings. The child believes that the doorbell rang because the dog barked. This child would fit best into which of Piaget's stages?

    A. Sensorimotor
    B. Preoperational thought
    C. Concrete operations
    D. Formal operations
    E. Latency

94. The sensory dermatomes of the nipples and the umbilicus are respectively located at the level of:

    A. T2 and T8
    B. T3 and T9
    C. T4 and T10
    D. T5 and T11
    E. T6 and T12

95. Which one of the following receptor subtypes is associated with the neurotransmitter glutamate?

    A. Nicotinic
    B. Muscarinic
    C. Alpha 1
    D. AMPA
    E. GABA

96. Buspirone's mechanism of action is predominantly linked to which one of the following receptors:

    A. Serotonin 2A
    B. Serotonin 1A
    C. NMDA
    D. Dopamine 2
    E. Norepinephrine

97. Which one of the following statements is true regarding excitatory neurotransmitters?

   A. They open anion channels that depolarize the cell membrane and increase the likelihood of generating an action potential
   B. They open cation channels that hyperpolarize the cell membrane and increase the likelihood of generating an action potential
   C. They open cation channels that hyperpolarize the cell membrane and decrease the likelihood of generating an action potential
   D. They open anion channels that hyperpolarize the cell membrane and decrease the likelihood of generating an action potential
   E. They open cation channels that depolarize the cell membrane and increase the likelihood of generating an action potential

98. Phencyclidine (PCP) exerts its hallucinogenic effects primarily by mediation of which of the following receptors:

   A. Serotonin 2A
   B. Serotonin 1A
   C. NMDA
   D. Dopamine 2
   E. Norepinephrine

99. All of the following are immature defenses, EXCEPT:

   A. Hypochondriasis
   B. Introjection
   C. Sublimation
   D. Regression
   E. Passive aggression

100. Which one of the following agents is least likely to exacerbate the extra-pyramidal symptoms of Parkinson's disease?

   A. Amoxapine
   B. Perphenazine
   C. Thorazine
   D. Fluphenazine
   E. Phenelzine

101. Who was the author of *The Ego and Mechanisms of Defense,* and gave us the first comprehensive study of defense mechanisms?

   A. Sigmund Freud
   B. Kohut
   C. Erich Fromm
   D. Ana Freud
   E. Carl Jung

1:12

102. In order to be declared competent to stand trial, a patient must present with all of the following, EXCEPT:
    A. Understanding of the nature of the charges against him
    B. Not having a mental illness
    C. Having the ability to consult a lawyer
    D. Helping the lawyer in his defense
    E. Understanding of court procedure

103. Which one of the following is present in paranoid schizophrenia?
    A. Flat affect
    B. Catatonic behavior
    C. Incoherence
    D. Preoccupation with systematized delusions
    E. Grossly disorganized behavior

104. How long should a patient remain on antidepressant medication after having experienced four major depressive episodes in the last five years?
    A. 3 months
    B. 6 months
    C. 12 months
    D. 2 years
    E. Indefinitely

105. Which one of the following symptoms is NOT part of dysthymic disorder?
    A. Poor appetite
    B. Low self-esteem
    C. Feelings of hopelessness
    D. Hallucinations
    E. Fatigue

106. Which ruling determined that the physician-patient relationship imposes an obligation on the psychiatrist for care and safety of the patient and others?
    A. Wyatt vs Stickney
    B. Durham vs the United States
    C. O'Connor vs Donaldson
    D. Tarasoff vs regents of the University of California
    E. Clites vs State

107. Which one of the following tricyclic antidepressants is not considered a tertiary amine?

    A. Imipramine
    B. Amitriptyline
    C. Desipramine
    D. Clomipramine
    E. Trimipramine

108. All of the following surgical interventions can be used for the invasive treatment of idiopathic Parkinson's disease, EXCEPT:

    A. Thalamotomy
    B. Subthalamic nucleus deep brain stimulation
    C. Superior colliculus deep brain stimulation
    D. Pallidotomy
    E. Pallidal deep brain stimulation

109. The metabolite of which one of the following tricyclic antidepressants has potent dopamine blocking ability that can lead to antipsychotic-like side effects?

    A. Amoxapine
    B. Clomipramine
    C. Desipramine
    D. Trimipramine
    E. Imipramine

110. A patient presents with a non-dominant hemispheric stroke in the middle cerebral artery territory. All of the following symptoms and signs are possible to note on neurologic examination, EXCEPT:

    A. Hemi-inattention
    B. Anosognosia
    C. Right-left disorientation
    D. Impaired prosody of speech
    E. Visual and tactile extinction

111. Interaction with the enzyme CYP 2D6 has what bearing on the use of tricyclic antidepressants?

    A. None. Tricyclics do not interact with CYP 2D6
    B. Those with decreased CYP 2D6 activity will have lower than expected plasma drug concentrations
    C. Giving a patient on a tricyclic a CYP 2D6 inhibitor could cause a drop in the plasma concentration of the drug
    D. Cimetidine can cause an increase in tricyclic levels as a result of its interaction with CYP 2D6
    E. Concomitant use of drugs that inhibit CYP 2D6 with tricyclics may necessitate higher than usual prescribed doses of either drug to obtain the same levels

112. A 50 year-old man presents to the emergency room with a complaint of acute onset of right eye pain, ptosis, and diplopia. The symptoms began that morning immediately upon his awakening from sleep. Your examination reveals a normal-sized pupil that is fully reactive to light and a right eye that cannot adduct nasally with a ptotic right eyelid. The most likely cause of this condition is:

    A. Diabetes
    B. Stroke
    C. Posterior communicating artery aneurysm
    D. Multiple sclerosis
    E. Myasthenia gravis

113. Residual schizophrenia is characterized by:

    A. Absence of prominent hallucinations
    B. Delusions
    C. Incoherence
    D. Disorganized behavior
    E. Posturing

114. All of the following agents would be useful for the treatment of tics in Tourette's syndrome, EXCEPT:

    A. Fluphenazine
    B. Molindone
    C. Botulinum toxin type A
    D. Haloperidol
    E. Protryptiline

115. All of the following are characteristics of catatonic schizophrenia, EXCEPT:

    A. Mutism
    B. Negativism
    C. Rigidity
    D. Echolalia
    E. Grossly inappropriate affect

116. A right middle cerebral artery territory ischemic stroke posterior to the optic chiasm would be expected to cause:

    A. Bitemporal hemianopsia
    B. Left monocular blindness
    C. Left homonymous hemianopsia
    D. Right homonymous hemianopsia
    E. Right upper quadrantanopsia

117. All of the following statements are true regarding chemical signaling between neurons, EXCEPT?

    A. Neurotransmitter synthesis may be stimulated by influx of Ca^{2+}

    B. Norepinephrine-releasing neurons have presynaptic alpha receptors which are involved in a negative feedback system to stop NE release

    C. Once dopamine is released into the synaptic cleft it works until it diffuses away, or is removed by reuptake mechanisms

    D. Exocytosis is the process by which neurotransmitter storage vesicles release their contents into the synaptic cleft

    E. MAO type B metabolizes NE and serotonin

118. A 4 year-old boy presents to the ER in an acute state of agitation. Careful history-taking and examination reveal hypotonia, delayed developmental milestones, athetotic movements of the upper extremities and mental retardation. The parents explain that their son constantly bites his hands and lips to the point of bleeding. Lesch-Nyhan syndrome is the clinical diagnosis. This syndrome is caused by a deficiency of which of the following enzymes:

    A. Ornithine transcarbamylase

    B. Hypoxanthine-guanine phosphoribosyltransferase

    C. Adenylosuccinate deficiency

    D. Arginase

    E. Carbamoylphosphate synthase

119. A child is brought to your office for depression. During the course of your interview you see that the patient can think abstractly, reason deductively, and define abstract concepts. This child would fit into which of Piaget's developmental stages?

    A Sensorimotor

    B. Preoperational thought

    C. Concrete operations

    D. Formal operations

    E. Symbiosis

120. Predisposition for dementia pugilistica is increased in carriers with defects on which one of the following chromosomes:

    A. Chromosome 16

    B. Chromosome 17

    C. Chromosome 18

    D. Chromosome 19

    E. Chromosome 20

121. Which one of the tricyclic antidepressants has the most antihistaminic activity?
    A. Amoxipine
    B. Clomipramine
    C. Desipramine
    D. Nortriptyline
    E. Doxepin

122. All of the following are helpful in the treatment of obsessive-compulsive disorder, EXCEPT:
    A. Bupropion
    B. Fluvoxamine
    C. Clomipramine
    D. Sertraline
    E. Fluoxetine

123. Which one of the following is true regarding the tricyclic antidepressants?
    A. The down-regulation of β-adrenergic receptors correlates most closely with time needed for clinical improvement in patients
    B. Giving tricyclics leads to an increase in β-adrenergic receptors
    C. Giving tricyclics leads to an increase in 5-HT receptors
    D. Giving tricyclics leads to an increase in β-adrenergic receptors and a decrease in 5-HT receptors
    E. Giving tricyclics leads to a decrease in β-adrenergic receptors and an increase in 5-HT receptors

124. Enuresis in childhood can be treated effectively with all of the following, EXCEPT:
    A. Desmopressin
    B. Bell-and-pad conditioning
    C. Amitriptyline
    D. Imipramine
    E. Olanzapine

125. Which one of the following ions uses the second ion channel to open during an action potential, acts as a second messenger once in the neuron, activates the release of neurotransmitter, and activates ion channels that allow for influx of other ions that halt the action potential?
    A. Na^+
    B. K^+
    C. Cl^-
    D. Ca^{2+}
    E. IP_3

126. Patients with which one of the following disorders may have clinically significant side effects from tricyclic antidepressant drugs?
    A. Insomnia
    B. Benign prostatic hypertrophy
    C. Migraine
    D. Parkinson's disease
    E. Pituitary adenoma

127. Which one of the following statements is true regarding inhibitory neurotransmitters?
    A. They open chloride channels that depolarize the cell membrane and increase the likelihood of an action potential
    B. They open cation channels that depolarize the cell membrane and increase the likelihood of an action potential
    C. They open chloride channels that hyperpolarize the cell membrane and increase the likelihood of an action potential
    D. They open chloride channels that hyperpolarize the cell membrane and decrease the likelihood of an action potential
    E. They open potassium channels that depolarize the cell membrane and decrease the likelihood of an action potential

128. A patient with a fear of spiders is put in a room with many spiders, and immediately a live tarantula is placed on his hand for as long as necessary until the dissipation of his anxiety. This behavioral technique is called:
    A. Graded exposure
    B. Aversion therapy
    C. Flooding
    D. Assertiveness training
    E. Modeling

129. Which one of the following is true regarding psychoanalytic psychotherapy?
    A. All of the patient's remarks should be taken at face value
    B. Most of what the patient says is unimportant
    C. Disclaimers often precede emotionally charged material, and are important to note
    D. It's important to point out to the patient every instance in which they exhibit low self-esteem
    E. One should interpret the patient's resistance at each and every opportunity

130. An 82 year-old patient in a skilled nursing facility displays confusion, restlessness, agitation, and disorganized speech only during the evening hours. All of the following are appropriate treatment approaches, EXCEPT:

    A. Increased lighting in the room
    B. Low dose haloperidol at bedtime
    C. Having a calendar on the wall
    D. Flurazepam at bedtime for sleep
    E. Companionship and family support during the day

131. All of the following are techniques used in cognitive therapy, EXCEPT:

    A. Reattribution
    B. Role playing
    C. Thought recording
    D. Abreaction
    E. Developing alternatives

132. Heroin withdrawal can involve all of the following symptoms, EXCEPT:

    A. Pinpoint pupils
    B. Abdominal pain
    C. Piloerection
    D. Muscle twitching
    E. Dysphoria

133. Which one of the following is among the least sedating of the tricyclic anti-depressants?

    A. Desipramine
    B. Amitriptyline
    C. Trimipramine
    D. Doxepin
    E. Imipramine

134. All of the following are examples of secondary gain, EXCEPT:

    A. Getting money
    B. Getting medical help
    C. Getting out of having to work
    D. Getting out of family responsibilities
    E. Getting drugs of abuse

135. In hypothyroidism one would expect to find:

    A. Serum free T4 is increased
    B. Serum total T4 concentration is increased
    C. Serum thyroid stimulating hormone is increased
    D. Serum T3 uptake is increased
    E. Serum T3–T4 ratio is decreased

136. Which one of the following conditions involves increased risk in electro-convulsive shock therapy (ECT)?

    A. Pregnancy
    B. Hypopituitarism
    C. Uncontrolled epilepsy
    D. Neuroleptic malignant syndrome
    E. Cerebral aneurysm

137. Caution should be taken when prescribing which one of the following to a woman on oral contraception?

    A. Risperidone
    B. Valproic acid
    C. Gabapentin
    D. Lithium
    E. Carbamazepine

138. An 8 year-old child has a mental age of 6 years. For school placement purposes, the IQ should be reported as:

    A. 50
    B. 75
    C. 100
    D. 120
    E. 135

139. Psychiatrist: What's on your mind?

    Patient: I've been feeling depressed.
    Psychiatrist: Can you tell me more about what's been happening?
    Patient: I haven't been eating as much as I used to.
    Psychiatrist: Could you explain to me what you've been going through.
    The psychiatrist's approach is an example of:
    A. Closed-ended questions
    B. Open-ended questions
    C. Countertransference
    D. Detailed mini-mental status exam
    E. Negative reinforcement.

140. Violent or aggressive behavior is associated with:

    A. Decreased levels of 5-hydroxyindoleacetic acid in spinal fluid
    B. Decreased growth hormone response to insulin-induced hypoglycemia
    C. Abnormal dexamethasone suppression test
    D. Decreased response to corticotrophin releasing hormone stimulation test
    E. Decreased response to thyrotropin releasing hormone suppression test

141. All of the following are potential repercussions of lithium intoxication, EXCEPT:
    A. Seizure
    B. Renal toxicity
    C. Ataxia and coarse tremor
    D. Non-specific T-wave changes.
    E. Jaundice

142. Obsessive-compulsive disorder is associated with abnormality of which one of the following neurotransmitters?
    A. Norepinephrine
    B. Serotonin
    C. Melatonin
    D. Acetylcholine
    E. Dopamine

143. All of the following are true regarding use of the tricyclic antidepressants, EXCEPT:
    A. Due to their ability to prolong cardiac conduction time their use in patients with conduction defects is contraindicated
    B. These agents should be discontinued before elective surgery because they may cause hypertensive episodes during surgery
    C. Some patients who experience orthostatic hypotension may respond to the use of fludrocortisone
    D. Myoclonic twitches and tremors of the tongue and upper extremities are common in some patients on tricyclics
    E. Amoxapine is the least likely to cause parkinsonian symptoms of all the tricyclics

144. All of the following characteristics pertaining to vascular dementia are correct, EXCEPT:
    A. There is a step-wise decline in functioning
    B. Hypertension is a known risk factor
    C. There is abrupt onset of symptoms
    D. There is a good response to cholinergic therapies
    E. Smoking is a known risk factor

145. Which one of the following antidepressants is the most serotonin-selective of the tricyclics?
    A. Amoxapine
    B. Clomipramine
    C. Desipramine
    D. Nortriptyline
    E. Doxepin

146. A team comprised of a psychiatrist, psychologist, social worker, nurse, and medical student discharge a patient because the insurance will no longer pay for her stay. She kills herself. Who will be held legally responsible for the team's actions?
    A. The medical student
    B. The psychologist
    C. The social worker
    D. The nurse
    E. The psychiatrist

147. All of the following are side effects of treatment with tricyclic antidepressants, EXCEPT:
    A. Termination of ventricular fibrillation
    B. Increase collateral blood supply to ischemic heart muscle
    C. Decreased contractility
    D. Tachycardia
    E. Hypertension

148. The best indicator for future suicidal behavior is:
    A. Age
    B. Psychosis
    C. Past suicidal behavior
    D. Substance use
    E. Personality disorder

149. A patient presents to your office with obsessive-compulsive disorder (OCD). She has been tried on several SSRIs with little improvement. You decide to try a tricyclic. Which tricyclic has been shown to have significantly better efficacy in treating OCD than the others?
    A. Desipramine
    B. Doxepin
    C. Amitriptyline
    D. Clomipramine
    E. Nortriptyline

150. Which one of the tricyclic antidepressants is used to treat childhood enuresis?
    A. Desipramine
    B. Clomipramine
    C. Maprotiline
    D. Amoxapine
    E. Imipramine

Answers

Test Number **TWO**
ANSWER KEY

②

1	E	51	D	101	D		
N 2	D	N 52	A	102	B		
3	D	53	E	103	D		
N 4	E	N 54	B	104	E		
5	D	55	C	105	D		
N 6	B	N 56	C	106	D		
7	C	57	E	107	C		
N 8	E	58	E	N 108	C		
9	C	59	B	109	A		
10	A	N 60	B	N 110	C		
11	B	61	A	111	D		
N 12	C	N 62	E	N 112	A		
13	D	63	B	113	A		
14	B	64	B	114	E		
15	C	65	E	115	E		
N 16	D	66	D	N 116	C		
17	C	67	E	117	E		
N 18	D	N 68	A	N 118	B		
19	D	69	C	119	D		
N 20	A	N 70	C	N 120	D		
21	D	71	E	121	E		
22	B	N 72	B	122	A		
23	B	73	D	123	A		
N 24	C	N 74	A	124	E		
25	A	75	E	125	D		
N 26	A	N 76	D	N 126	B		
27	E	77	B	127	D		
N 28	A	N 78	B	128	C		
29	D	79	B	129	C		
N 30	A	N 80	A	130	D		
31	B	81	D	131	D		
N 32	D	N 82	E	132	A		
33	A	83	A	133	A		
N 34	E	N 84	B	134	B		
35	D	85	C	135	C		
N 36	A	86	C	136	E		
37	B	87	B	137	E		
38	D	N 88	C	138	B		
39	A	89	C	139	B		
N 40	E	N 90	B	140	A		
41	D	91	A	141	E		
N 42	D	N 92	A	142	B		
43	E	93	B	143	E		
N 44	A	N 94	C	N 144	D		
45	D	N 95	D	145	B		
N 46	A	96	B	146	E		
47	E	N 97	E	147	E		
N 48	E	98	C	148	C		
49	B	99	C	149	D		
N 50	D	N 100	E	150	E		

23   18   17

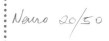

Neuro 20/50

ANSWER EXPLANATIONS

Question 1. E. There are several life-cycle theorists that are important to know. Freud's theory of development involving oral, anal, and phallic stages is important. Carl Jung felt that development of the personality occurs through experiences that teach a person who they intrinsically are. For him, libido included sexual energy, but also spiritual urges and a drive to understand the meaning of life. Harry Stack Sullivan focused on social interaction. In his theory he defined each stage of life through the need to interact with certain individuals. These interactions shaped the development of the personality. Erik Erikson developed a life cycle from childhood to adulthood. It consists of:

- Stage 1: Trust vs mistrust. Trust is shown by ease of feeding and depth of sleep, and depends on consistency of experience provided by the caretaker. If trust is strong, the child develops self-confidence. (Birth–1 year old)
- Stage 2: Autonomy vs shame and doubt. This stage includes the child learning to walk and feed himself. There is a need for outer control. Shame happens through excessive punishment, and self-doubt occurs if the child is made to feel ashamed of his actions. (Age 1–3)
- Stage 3: Initiative vs guilt. In this stage the child initiates both motor and intellectual activities. If reinforced, his intellectual curiosity is satisfied. If he is made to feel inadequate, he will develop guilt about self-initiated activities. (Age 3–5 years)
- Stage 4: Industry vs inferiority. In this stage the child is busy building, creating, and accomplishing. If he is inferior to his peers with use of tools and skills, he will have less status and develop a sense of inadequacy and inferiority. (Age 6–11 years)
- Stage 5: Ego identity vs role confusion. There is a struggle to develop a sense of inner sameness and continuity. The adolescent shows preoccupation with appearance, hero worship, and ideology. There are dangers of role confusion, and doubts about his sexual orientation and vocational identity. (Age 11 years–end of adolescence)
- Stage 6: Intimacy vs isolation. Intimacy is marked by formation of life-long attachments and self-abandonment. Separation occurs if the individual is isolates and views others as dangerous. (Age 21–40 years)
- Stage 7: Generativity vs stagnation. Generativity is marked by raising children, altruism, creativity, and guiding the next generation. Stagnation occurs if there is isolation, excessive self-concern, and an absence of intimacy. (Age 40–65 years)
- Stage 8: Ego identity vs despair. Integrity is a feeling of satisfaction that life has been worthwhile, along with an acceptance of one's place in life. Despair is the feeling of loss of hope, disgust, and fear of death. (Age 65+ years)

103

Piaget developed a theory of cognitive development. It consists of 4 stages: sensorimotor, preoperational thought, concrete operations, and formal operations. The work of Freud, Jung and Erikson was the result of observations of children, not of carefully crafted studies. Their theories are a framework to understand development, but are not intended to describe objective reality. Their work has been followed by more scientific longitudinal studies of development, and more neurobiological understandings of human behavior.

K&S Ch. 2

Question 2. D. The clinical picture given is that of a conduction aphasia. Conduction aphasia results from left hemispheric (dominant) lesions particularly in the inferior parietal or superior temporal regions. The area of predilection for this lesion is considered to be the arcuate fasciculus that connects Wernicke's and Broca's areas. Conduction aphasia is characterized by inability to repeat, relatively normal spontaneous speech, and the possibility of paraphasic errors and hesitancy. Naming may be impaired, but auditory comprehension is intact. Writing may or may not be impaired. Associated symptoms of a conduction aphasia may include right hemiparesis, right hemisensory loss, right hemianopsia, and limb apraxia. Broca's aphasia would involve a lesion of Broca's area in the left posterior inferior frontal gyrus. This results in broken, stuttering, staccato speech, with inability to repeat and phonemic and paraphasic errors. Reading is often impaired, although auditory comprehension is usually intact. Broca's aphasia is frequently associated with depression and right hemiparesis and hemisensory loss.

Wernicke's aphasia results from a lesion in the superior temporal gyrus in Wernicke's area. Speech is generally fluent, but comprehension is impaired. Speech may also be logorrheic, or overproductive. The speech displays paragrammatism, which involves neologisms, verbal paraphasic errors, and production of jargon. Repetition, naming, and auditory comprehension are impaired. Reading comprehension is impaired. Wernicke's aphasia is often accompanied by a right homonymous hemianopsia, with a marked absence of motor and sensory signs and symptoms.

Global aphasia results from large lesions involving the superior temporal, inferior frontal and parietal lobes. The region generally corresponds to the territory of the middle cerebral artery (MCA) and indeed a thrombus at the trifurcation of the MCA can produce a global aphasia. Speech is nonfluent or mute and comprehension is impaired. Naming, reading, repetition, and writing are all poor. Most patients present with a dense right hemiparesis, hemisensory loss and hemianopsia.

Transcortical aphasias involve the areas around and adjacent to Broca's and Wernicke's areas and essentially present with similar features to the two perisylvian aphasias, except that repetition is spared. Transcortical motor aphasia presents with similar features to Broca's aphasia, with telegraphic, stuttering speech, sparing of comprehension and fluent repetition. The area involved is usually anterior to Broca's area in the anterior cerebral artery territory. Transcortical sensory aphasia is the analogue of Wernicke's aphasia and presents with fluent paraphasic speech, paraphasic naming, impaired reading and auditory comprehension, and normal repetition. The lesion usually localizes to the temporo-occipital area. Transcortical mixed aphasia is a rare condition also known as isolation of the speech area. The classic presentation is that of a global aphasia with echolalic repetition only, and no propositional speech or comprehension. The patient can only repeat. The lesion localizes to large watershed areas in the left hemisphere, sparing the perisylvian areas.

B&D Ch. 12

Question 3. D. Major types of receptors found on neurons include the seven-transmembrane-domain receptor, which requires G proteins to open ion channels, and the ligand-gated ion channel receptor, which actually has an ion channel as part of its structure. The seven-transmembrane-domain receptor has a characteristic NH_2 terminal outside the cell, several intracytoplasmic loops, and an intracellular COOH terminal. It is the tyrosine kinase receptor which interacts with nerve growth factor (NGF) and brain derived neurotropic factor (BDNF). Through these interactions the tyrosine kinase receptor is thought to play a large role in neuronal plasticity and the remodeling of synaptic associations. It is also important to recall that hormones and steroids can diffuse into the neuron and bind to cytoplasmic receptors whose effects carry to the nucleus and regulate gene expression.

K&S Ch. 3

Question 4. E.   The classic complication of rapid sodium replacement in hyponatremia is central pontine myelinolysis. This can result in a clinical transection of the pons and a locked-in syndrome. Locked-in syndrome is the result of a pontine lesion that is clinically devastating and produces quadriplegia, mutism and a lower cranial nerve palsy with only the ability to move the eyes up and down and blink the eyelids being preserved. Only the upper brainstem function is preserved and patients usually need to be on a respirator. Cognition and comprehension are usually grossly intact and the patient is often quite aware of the predicament. Prognosis is very poor. The locked-in syndrome is most often the result of a ventral pontine infarct as a consequence of basilar artery thrombosis, but can in certain instances result from central pontine myelinolysis, which produces a more central pontine lesion. Other possible causes of locked-in syndrome are acute inflammatory demyelinating polyneuropathy (AIDP or Guillain-Barré syndrome), myasthenia gravis, and neuromuscular blocking agents.

B&D Ch. 57

Question 5. D.   This question contains an example of rationalization. Rationalization is characterized by offering rational explanations in an attempt to justify attitudes, beliefs or behaviors that may otherwise be unacceptable. Projection is perceiving and reacting to unacceptable inner impulses as if they are outside the self. Blocking is temporarily halting thinking. It often occurs in psychosis because of hallucinations and thought disorganization. Externalization is perceiving elements of your own personality in the external world or in external objects. It is a more general term than projection. Denial is avoiding awareness of some painful aspect of reality by negating sensory data. The most primitive of the defenses are the narcissistic defenses (denial, distortion, projection). The least primitive defenses are the mature defenses (altruism, anticipation, asceticism, humor, sublimation, suppression).

K&S Ch. 6

Question 6. B.   The clinical condition depicted in this question is that of pseudotumor cerebri, also called benign intracranial hypertension. Classically a problem seen in young obese African-American women, the exact etiology is unknown. Risk factors include hypervitaminosis A, high-dose corticosteroid therapy, tetracycline therapy, oral contraceptive use and head trauma. Patients typically present with a waxing and waning headache and intermittent visual obscurations. Neurologic examination can reveal papilledema on fundoscopic examination and enlargement of the blind spot on visual field testing. Brain imaging is usually normal, although some scans reveal slit-like ventricles. The diagnosis is established by lumbar puncture with measurement of the opening pressure which is elevated over $20\,cmH_2O$. The treatment modality of choice is pharmacologic, with acetazolamide 500 mg once or twice daily or with prednisone 20–40 mg daily. In certain cases patients opt for repeated lumbar

punctures to siphon off fluid to maintain normal cerebrospinal fluid pressure. Surgical options for treatment include ventriculoperitoneal shunting, or lumboperitoneal shunting if the ventricles are too small, and optic nerve sheath fenestration which can siphon off cerebrospinal fluid. ESR would be used as a diagnostic test for temporal arteritis. Serum prolactin level is sometimes drawn following a seizure to determine if it is epileptic or nonepileptic. The prolactin level would be expected to be elevated greater than twice normal within an hour after a true epileptic seizure.
B&D Ch. 52

Question 7. C. The National Alliance for the Mentally Ill (NAMI) is an advocacy group made up of families of the mentally ill that works at local, state, and federal levels to improve services for the mentally ill. They are involved with lawmakers, outreach and education. The other answer choices are distracters. The most important organization to know is NAMI.
K&S Ch. 4

Question 8. E. In 1988, the International Headache Society (IHS) established strict criteria for migraine with and without aura. The criteria for migraine without aura are as follows: at least five headache attacks lasting 4 to 72 hours (untreated or unsuccessfully treated), which have at least two out of four characteristics – unilateral location; pulsating quality; moderate or severe intensity; or aggravated by walking stairs or similar routine physical activity. During the headache at least one of the two following symptoms occur: phonophobia and photophobia; nausea and/or vomiting.
Migraine with aura involves at least two attacks with at least three of the following: one or more fully reversible aura symptoms indicating focal cerebral cortical and/or brainstem functions; At least one aura symptom develops gradually over more than four minutes, or two or more symptoms occur in succession; no aura symptom lasts more than 60 minutes; or headache follows aura with free interval of at least 60 minutes (it may also simultaneously begin with the aura). At least one of the following aura features establishes a diagnosis of migraine with typical aura: homonymous visual disturbance; unilateral paresthesias and/or numbness; unilateral weakness; or aphasia or unclassifiable speech difficulty.
B&D Ch. 75

Question 9. C. The lifetime prevalence of schizophrenia is 1%. It is estimated that there are somewhere in the vicinity of 2 million patients with schizophrenia in the United States. The other answer choices are distracters.
K&S Ch. 4

Question 10. A. Recombinant tissue plasminogen activator (r-TPA) is FDA-approved for acute thrombolysis of ischemic cerebrovascular accident within three hours of the occurrence of the event. Inclusion criteria for intravenous r-TPA administration include acute ischemic stroke with a clear time of onset less than or equal to three hours prior to desired r-TPA administration, neurologic deficit measurable on the NIH stroke scale and CT scan of the head demonstrating an absence of intracranial hemorrhage. Exclusion criteria are: rapidly improving or minor stroke symptoms or deficits, seizure at the onset of stroke, prior intracranial hemorrhage, pretreatment blood pressure greater than 185/110 mmHg, major surgery within the previous 14 days, a prior stroke or head injury within the last three months, intestinal or urinary bleeding within three weeks prior to the stroke, subarachnoid hemorrhage, blood glucose level <50 mg/dL or >400 mg/dL, recent myocardial infarction, current use of oral anticoagulants (PT > 15 or INR > 1.7) or heparin use within the last 48 hours, a platelet count of < 100 000 per µL, or arterial puncture at a noncompressible site within the last seven days.

B&D Ch. 57

Question 11. B. Assertive community treatment is based on the model whereby teams of psychiatrists and other mental health workers go out into the community to patients' homes to maintain contact with them, monitor their status, and encourage medication compliance. The goal is to prevent decompensation of severely mentally ill patients and catch them before they severely decompensate and require hospitalization.

K&S Ch. 4

Question 12. C. The condition described in this question is that of restless legs syndrome (RLS). The only FDA-approved treatment is ropinorole (Requip), a dopamine agonist, which can improve symptoms at low doses starting at 0.5 mg prior to bedtime. Other dopamine agonists, pergolide, pramipexole and bromocriptine can be useful, but are not specifically FDA approved. Other helpful agents include benzodiazepines, opiate analgesics, gabapentin and levodopa/carbidopa. Restless legs syndrome has a prevalence rate of about 5% and is most often seen in middle to older-aged patients. It is usually idiopathic, but has been associated with polyneuropathy, uremia, and iron deficiency. The classic symptoms of RLS are crawling or creeping sensations (paresthesias or dysesthesias) of the lower extremities that are worse when lying down or in bed and occur most often at the onset of sleep. There is an urge to move the legs during rest, or when lying down or sitting. The urge to move is generally relieved by movement, like walking or stretching. Symptoms are worse at night or only occur in the evening or at night. Family history can be positive in 40–50% of patients, which suggests an autosomal dominant pattern of inheritance.

B&D Ch. 74

Question 13. D. The best method to diagnose depression is the standard psychiatric interview. Psychiatric interviews serve two functions: to find and classify symptoms, and to find psychological determinants of behavior. Interviews can either be insight or symptom oriented. The other answer choices all have major flaws. The MMPI is a self-report inventory used to assess personality traits, and as such is not appropriate to the task. The scholastic achievement test is completely unrelated to symptom identification for depression. The dexamethasone suppression test is used to demonstrate abnormal activity of the hypothalamic–pituitary–adrenal axis which can be found in 50% of major depression patients. However, the test has limited clinical usefulness because of the frequency of false positive and negative test results. Interviewing the patient's teacher is a good idea, but in no way can it replace a face-to-face meeting with the child or be the sole basis for diagnosing depression.

K&S Chs 1&15

Question 14. B. This question describes a left lateral medullary syndrome (also called a Wallenberg's syndrome). The Wallenberg syndrome is a brainstem stroke syndrome usually caused by occlusion of one of the vertebral arteries, or less commonly, one of the posterior inferior cerebellar arteries. The area of infarction is the lateral medulla. The clinical syndrome involves an ipsilateral Horner's syndrome, ipsilateral loss of pain and temperature sensation in the face, cerebellar ataxia and weakness of the vocal cords, pharynx and palate. There is contralateral loss of pain and temperature sensation to the hemibody. The visual system is not affected with this syndrome.

B&D Ch. 57

Question 15. C. Decreased levels of serotonin in the cerebrospinal fluid (CSF) have been shown to be linked to higher levels of aggression in patients. In general,

dopamine seems to promote aggression, whereas norepinephrine and serotonin seem to inhibit it, as does GABA. Rapid declines in serotonin levels have been linked to irritability and aggression, and low CSF serotonin has been linked to increased frequency of suicide. Corticotropin-releasing hormone (CRH) is a hormone that may increase in major depression, anorexia, and anxiety disorders. It is produced by the hypothalamus. It has no relation to aggression. Growth hormone is also unrelated to aggression.
K&S Ch. 4

Question 16. D. Metachromatic leukodystrophy (MLD) is an autosomal recessive metabolic disorder of myelin that results in a deficiency in arylsulfatase A (ASA). The result is an abnormal accumulation of sulfatides in the brain and peripheral nerves. High sulfatide levels lead to progressive demyelination. The ASA gene is located on chromosome 22q13. Gait disorder with hypotonia and lower limb areflexia are early manifestations of the disease and often precedes central nervous system involvement in infantile and juvenile forms of the disease. Adult-onset MLD tends to present with progressive dementia and behavioral problems. Nerve conduction velocities (NCV) are slowed in both juvenile and adult patients. Delayed visual and somatosensory evoked potential latencies are noted more often in adult cases. The classic neuropathologic findings are segmental nerve demyelination on nerve biopsy and metachromatic inclusions within Schwann cells and macrophages. Although nerve biopsy is diagnostic of MLD, MRI of the brain combined with urine assay for increased sulfatide excretion and abnormal ASA enzyme assay in leukocytes is less invasive and the preferred diagnostic method today. Treatment by bone marrow transplantation may increase brain ASA levels sufficiently to slow or stop disease progression.
Tay-Sachs disease is the severe infantile form of the autosomal recessive gangliosidosis that results in hexosaminidase A deficiency. Hexosaminidase A codes to chromosome 15q23-q24. The classic infantile picture is that of developmental retardation, paralysis, dementia, and blindness with death in the second or third year of life. The classic finding is a "cherry-red spot" on fundoscopic examination. Babies with Tay-Sachs disease have a persistent hypersensitivity to loud noise with a marked hyperreactivity of startle response.
Krabbe's disease, also called globoid cell leukodystrophy, is an autosomal recessive disease caused by a deficiency in lysosomal enzyme galactocerebrosidase β-galactosidase. The gene has been localized to chromosome 14q31. Multinucleated macrophages in central white matter are accompanied by extensive central and peripheral demyelination. Infants present with rapid deterioration in motor and intellectual development, hypertonicity, optic atrophy, opisthotonic posture, and seizures. Stem cell transplantation can improve central nervous system manifestations by providing a source of missing enzyme.
B&D Ch. 82

Question 17. C. Seasonal affective disorder is a non-DSM term used to describe a seasonal specifier added to the diagnoses of bipolar I & II disorders, and major depressive disorder. It is associated with depressive symptoms that occur at a certain time of year, with complete remission of symptoms at other times of the year. One must show a pattern of two episodes during the same season of the previous two years to make the diagnosis. In addition, the seasonal depressive episodes must substantially outnumber any non-seasonally related depressive episodes during the patient's lifetime. The treatment is light therapy.
K&S Ch. 15

Question 18. D. The parachute response can persist far longer than 6 months. The Moro reflex is elicited by startle and is usually present in the normal infant up to 6 months of age. The child extends the arms symmetrically when the head is rapidly but gently dropped a few centimeters into the examiner's hand with the baby in a supine position. The tonic neck reflex is normally present from birth to about 3 months of age. Grasp and rooting reflexes usually disappear at or about the 6 month of age mark. Any persistence of these reflexes beyond this period or recurrence later in life, would be considered abnormal. Positive grasp and rooting reflexes in the adult would be considered frontal release signs and would signal extensive frontal white matter damage or disease.

B&D Ch. 30

Question 19. D. Answer choice D describes pseudocyesis, which is listed in the DSM under somatoform disorders NOS. It involves a false belief that one is pregnant, and can involve physical signs associated with pregnancy, such as those described. However, the patient is not pregnant and there is no endocrine disorder present to explain the findings. Other patients that fall under the heading of somatoform disorder NOS include those with other somatic symptoms that do not meet the time criteria for other diagnoses. Answer choice A describes pain disorder, in which a patient experiences pain that can not be explained by a medical condition and is thought to be significantly mediated by psychological factors. Answer choice B describes hypochondriasis, in which a patient is convinced that he has a serious disease, based on misinterpretation of bodily symptoms, and despite the reassurance of doctors. Choice C describes conversion disorder, in which the patient develops neurological symptoms with no medical explanation that are thought to be mediated by psychological factors. Choice E describes somatization disorder, in which the patient has physical complaints spanning several organ systems that have no medical explanation and are thought to be associated with psychological factors. To make the diagnosis of somatization disorder, the patient must exhibit at any time during the disturbance, four pain symptoms, two gastro-intestinal symptoms, one sexual symptom, and one pseudoneurological symptom.

K&S Ch. 17

Question 20. A. Cytomegalovirus (CMV) is the most common offending infectious agent in AIDS-related retinopathy. It accounts for 30% of cases of HIV-related retinopathy. Toxoplasmosis is less common, likely involved in about 5% of retinitis cases. Tuberculosis is a rare cause of AIDS-related retinitis. *Crypto coccus neoformans* is usually responsible for a fungal meningitis and not a retinitis in AIDS patients with low CD4 counts. JC virus is the offending agent in progressive multifocal leukoencephalopathy in AIDS patients.

B&D Ch. 59

Question 21. D. The most common hallucinations in schizophrenia are auditory. Visual, olfactory and tactile hallucinations are also possible. Schizophrenia was first discovered by Morel who called it "démence precoce". Later Kraepelin used "dementia praecox" to describe a group of illnesses that started in adolescence and ended in dementia. Bleuler coined the term "schizophrenia." The disorder is chronic and has a prodromal, active, and residual phase.

K&S Ch 13

Question 22. B. Nighttime awakening is not considered to be part of the clinical picture of narcolepsy. Narcolepsy is a lifelong sleep disorder that is believed to have a hereditary component. In the United States, the prevalence is about 3 to 6 in 10 000. One to two per cent of first-degree relatives of narcoleptic patients manifest the illness compared to 0.02–0.18% of the population at large. Narcolepsy is linked to the dysfunction of the hypocretin (orexin) peptide system.

The hallmark of the disease is excessive daytime sleepiness and sleep attacks. Sleep attacks manifest as the irresistible desire to fall asleep. Attacks can occur at any waking moment and last for a few minutes up to thirty minutes' duration. Performance at school, work, and in social situations usually suffers.

The second major manifestation of narcolepsy is cataplexy. Cataplexy is the sudden loss of muscle tone in the voluntary muscles, with sparing of the respiratory and ocular muscles. Attacks of cataplexy involve the patient falling to the ground following rapid complete loss of muscle tone. Consciousness is preserved during cataplexic attacks. Anywhere from 60–100% of narcoleptic patients suffer from cataplexy.

Sleep paralysis is the third major symptom of narcolepsy. It can be noted in one-quarter to one-half of narcoleptic patients. These attacks are characterized by hypnagogic or hypnopompic sudden bilateral or unilateral limb paralysis. Consciousness is preserved during these attacks, but the patient cannot move or speak.

Hypnagogic hallucination is the fourth major symptom of narcolepsy. These can occur at onset of sleep or during early morning awakening. About 20–40% of narcoleptic patients experience these hallucinations. Other major symptoms of narcolepsy include disturbance of night sleep in about 70–80% of patients and automatic behavior that can resemble a fugue-like state, which can occur in 20–40% of narcoleptic patients.

The only medications FDA-approved for narcolepsy are modafinil and sodium oxybate. Modafinil, which can be given in a single dose of 100–200 mg daily, modulates the hypocretin (orexin) neurons in the brainstem and is a non-amphetamine stimulant. Sodium oxybate (Xyrem) is a drug that was initially FDA-approved specifically for cataplexy, but now has an approval for narcolepsy as well.

B&D Ch. 74

Question 23. B. Logorrhea is uncontrollable, excessive talking. Alexithymia is a difficulty in recognizing and describing one's emotions. Echolalia is the imitative repetition of the speech of another. Flight of ideas is rapid shifting from one topic to another. Stilted speech is a formal stiff speech pattern.

K&S Ch. 8

Question 24. C. Intramuscular phenytoin is a poor choice for treatment of status epilepticus because of its erratic rate of absorption. Useful status epilepticus treatments include rectal or intravenous diazepam, intravenous lorazepam, intravenous phenytoin or phosphenytoin, intravenous valproic acid, oxygen by nasal cannula and airway protection, and intravenous phenobarbital. Phenobarbital is acceptable treatment, but not the best choice because of the narrow therapeutic window and possibility of overdose leading to respiratory depression and possible death.

B&D Ch. 73

Question 25. A. Of the statements listed, the only correct one is answer choice A. Ziprasidone is an agonist at 5-HT-1A and does inhibit reuptake of serotonin and norepinephrine. It is also an antagonist at 5-HT-1D, 2A, and 2C, as well as D2 and D3. It has low affinity for histaminic, muscarinic and alpha-2 receptors. Because of its action on serotonin and norepinephrine, it has been postulated to be of benefit not only in psychosis, but also in anxiety and depression. Risperidone is a similar blocker of D2 when compared to haldol, and as such carries one of the highest risks for EPS among the atypicals. Quetiapine is known for its low incidence of EPS, as it has only a moderate affinity for the D2 receptor. It has a high affinity for 5-HT types 2 and 6, H1, and alpha 1 and 2. It has low affinity for muscarinic receptors. Olanzapine has been associated with weight gain in many patients. It is very anticholinergic and carries with it the corresponding side effects. Clozapine has been shown to be associated with a decreased risk of suicide in schizophrenic patients. Major side effects of clozapine include seizures and agranulocytosis, among others. And while we're on the topic of anticholinergic side effects, the treatment of choice for urinary retention is urecholine (Bethanechol).

K&S Ch. 35

Question 26. A. Divalproex sodium (valproic acid) has the broadest spectrum of coverage and indication of all the anticonvulsant medications. It has proven efficacy in primary-generalized tonic-clonic seizures, absence seizures, and myoclonic seizures. Its likely mechanism of action is by blockade of voltage-dependent sodium channels and GABA enhancement. Phenytoin is not indicated for absence seizures and has no place in their treatment. It is indicated for treatment of partial and generalized tonic-clonic seizures. Its mechanism of action is by blockade of voltage-dependent sodium channels. Oxcarbazepine and carbamazepine are indicated for partial complex and secondary generalized seizures, but both can worsen absence seizures. Oxcarbazepine does not produce autoinduction of its own metabolism in the way that carbamazepine does. Ethosuximide is indicated only in uncomplicated absence seizures and has no place in the treatment of partial complex or secondary generalized tonic-clonic seizures. Its mechanism of action is by lowering voltage-dependent calcium conductance in thalamic neurons.

B&D Ch. 73

Question 27. E. Constipation is a common side effect of the tricyclic antidepressants as a result of the anticholinergic activity of these drugs. Other tricyclic side effects include dry mouth, blurry vision, sweating, orthostatic hypotension, sedation, lethargy, agitation, tremor, slowed cardiac conduction (as evidenced by prolonged PR and QRS intervals), and tachycardia.

K&S Ch. 36

Question 28. A. Foot flexion (also called dorsiflexion; the bending of the foot upwards) involves the tibialis anterior muscle innervated by nerves that emanate from the L5 motor nerve root. L5 also controls the extension (bending upwards) of the big toe (extensor hallucis longus). A lesion at L5 often causes a foot drop from dorsiflexor muscle weakness. Foot extension (pushing down on the gas pedal) involves the gastrocnemius (calf) and soleus muscles innervated by nerves that emanate from the S1 nerve root predominantly. Leg extension is a function of the quadriceps muscles (anterior thigh) which are innervated by nerves emanating from the L3 and L4 nerve roots. Hip flexion (raising of the knee in the air) is a function of the iliopsoas muscles which are innervated by the L1, L2 and L3 nerve roots. The Achilles or ankle jerk motor reflex is a function of the S1 motor nerve root.

B&D Ch. 26

Question 29. D. Amitriptyline can be used for gastric ulcer because of its strong histamine blockade. Other drugs that can also be used for this purpose include doxepin and trimipramine.

K&S Ch. 36

Question 30. A. The condition noted in this question is that of the classic Brown-Séquard syndrome due to a hemisection of the spinal cord. The correct combination of deficits is that of loss of motor control and posterior column function ipsilateral to and below the level of the lesion coupled with contralateral loss of pain and temperature sensation one to two dermatomal levels below the level of the lesion. Frequent causes include disc herniation, penetrating trauma, spinal fracture and radiation injury. The cervical spinal cord is most commonly affected.

B&D Ch. 27

Question 31. B. This question focuses on Piaget's stages of cognitive development. In the sensorimotor stage children respond to stimuli in the environment, learning during the process. They eventually develop object permanence (objects exist independent of the child's awareness of their existence), and begin to understand symbols (as in the use of words to express thoughts). During the preoperational stage there is a sense that punishment for bad deeds is unavoidable (immanent justice). There is a sense of egocentrism, and phenomenalistic causality (the thought that events that occur together cause one another). Animistic thinking (inanimate objects are given thoughts and feelings) is also seen.

In the concrete operations stage, egocentric thought changes to operational thought where another's point of view can be taken into consideration. In concrete operations children can put things in order and group objects according to common characteristics. They develop the understanding of conservation (a tall cup and a wide cup can both hold equal volumes of water) and reversibility (ice can change to water and back to ice again).

During formal operations children can think abstractly, reason deductively, and define abstract concepts. Trust vs mistrust is one of Erik Erikson's stages and is a distracter in this question.
K&S Ch. 2

Question 32. D. The anterior cerebral artery (ACA) territory is the area affected by this stroke. The ACA irrigates the medial frontal lobes and therefore when affected causes preferential leg greater than arm and face weakness contralateral to the side of the lesion. The destruction of the nearby frontal eye fields causes loss of tonic opposition of the gaze to the opposite side so the eyes will often be noted to look toward the side of the lesion. Sphincteric incontinence is sometimes seen if the cortical bowel and bladder areas are affected. Patients often suffer from abulia, a loss of will power or the lack of ability to do things independently. Bilateral ACA territory damage can result in akinetic mutism.
B&D Ch. 57

Question 33. A. Norepinephrine is made in the locus ceruleus. Serotonin is made in the dorsal raphe nuclei. Dopamine is made in the substantia nigra. Acetylcholine is made in the nucleus basalis of Meynert.
K&S Ch. 3

112

Question 34. E. Pure motor hemiparesis is one of the classic lacunar stroke syndromes and would be expected from an infarct in the area of the internal capsule, the basis pontis, or the corona radiata. Lacunar strokes are characterized as ischemic strokes resulting from small vessel lipohyalinosis that is caused by hypertension and diabetes as the two major risk factors. Lacunar infarcts by definition are small and range from 0.5 mm to 1.5 cm in diameter. Microembolism may also be a mechanism of lacunar strokes.

Other lacunar syndromes include pure sensory stroke, usually from a small lesion in the venteroposterolateral nucleus of the thalamus; sensory-motor stroke, from a stroke to the internal capsule and thalamus, or the posterior limb of the internal capsule; ataxic hemiparesis, which results from a lacunar infarct to either the basis pontis or posterior limb of the internal capsule; and the dysarthria-clumsy hand syndrome, resulting from a stroke to the deep areas of the basis pontis.
B&D Ch. 57

Question 35. D. Of the receptors listed, it is the histamine receptor that is associated with weight gain and sedation. The M1 receptor is associated with constipation, blurred vision, dry mouth, and drowsiness. Alpha 1 receptors are associated with dizziness and decreased blood pressure. The 5-HT-1A

receptor is a presynaptic autoreceptor involved in the response of neurons to the SSRIs. The 5-HT-2A receptor is one of the post-synaptic serotonin receptors involved in the neuron's response to the SSRIs. The serotonin receptors are associated with modulation of depression and anxiety, but not with weight gain or sedation.
K&S Ch. 3

Question 36. A. The contralateral subthalamic nucleus of Luys is most often the area where a lesion will produce hemiballismus. Hemiballismus is a dramatic, flinging movement of the proximal extremities. It can affect both the upper and lower limbs and is most often unilateral. Most frequently, the cause of hemiballismus is an acute stroke.
B&D Ch. 77

Question 37. B. The six biogenic amine neurotransmitters are dopamine, epinephrine, norepinephrine, acetylcholine, histamine, and serotonin. Of these, dopamine, norepinephrine, and epinephrine are all synthesized from the precursor tyrosine, and are known as a group as the catecholamines. GABA is an amino acid neurotransmitter, not a biogenic amine. Of note is that cocaine works by blocking the reuptake of the biogenic amines, more specifically serotonin, norepinephrine, and dopamine.
K&S Ch. 3

Question 38. D. Reserpine interferes with the magnesium and ATP-dependent uptake of biogenic amines which results in the depletion of dopamine, norepinephrine and serotonin neurotransmitters. In this way, it can relieve symptoms of dystonia and can also cause depression, sedation, and a Parkinson's like syndrome.
B&D Ch.77

Question 39. A. Projection is perceiving and reacting to unacceptable inner impulses as though they were outside the self. On a psychotic level it takes the form of delusions about external realities that are usually persecutory in nature. One's own impulses and hostilities are projected onto another who is now assumed to have intentions to persecute you. The other answer choices are distracters which have nothing to do with projection.
K&S Ch. 6

Question 40. E. The arachnoid (pacchionian) granulations are the major sites for drainage of cerebrospinal fluid (CSF) into the blood. These granulations protrude through the dura into the superior sagittal sinus and act as one way valves or siphons for the CSF. Equilibrium is maintained by the arachnoid granulations, for if CSF pressure drops below a certain level, absorption stops. If the CSF pressure increases, more fluid is absorbed. The choroid plexuses that protrude into the ventricles are responsible for the majority of CSF production in humans. In humans, the rate of CSF production is about 0.35 mL/minute. Drugs that can temporarily reduce production of CSF and ease increased intracranial pressure include acetazolamide and mannitol. States of hypothermia, hypocarbia, hypoxia and hyperosmolality can also temporarily decrease CSF production. Virchow-Robin spaces act as a duct for substances in the subarachnoid space to enter the brain. The other answer choices are distracters.
B&D Ch. 65

Question 41. D. Regression analysis is a method of predicting the value of one variable in relation to another variable based on observed data. Probability is the likelihood that an event will occur. A probability of 0 means it will not occur. A probability of 1 means it will definitely occur. Point prevalence is the number of people with a disorder at a specific point in time divided by the total population at that point in time. Incidence is the number of

new cases of a disease over a given time divided by the total number of people at risk during that time. Central tendency is a central value in a distribution around which other values are arranged. Examples of central tendency are the mean, median, and mode. The mean is the average. The median is the middle value in a series of values. The mode is the value that appears most frequently in a series of measurements. Kappa is a variable used to indicate a constant value that does not change. Sensitivity is the ability of a test to detect that which is being tested for.
K&S Ch. 4

Question 42. D. Noncontrast head CT is the best immediate test of choice in the emergency room if a lobar hemorrhage is suspected. MRI of the brain can add precision, but in the hyperacute stage may not be able to reveal acute bleeding as well as the CT scan. The most common location of intracranial hemorrhage is from the putamen, which accounts for about 35% of cases. Lobar hemorrhage is second to putaminal hemorrhage in frequency and accounts for about one-quarter of cases. Hypertension remains the most frequent cause of intracranial hemorrhage, but arteriovenous malformations, cerebral amyloid angiopathy and sympathomimetic agents can also account for quite a number of cases.

Emergency room management of suspected intracranial hemorrhage begins with stabilization of vital signs and airway protection. Intubation is indicated if the level of consciousness drops to a Glasgow Coma Scale score of 8 or less. CT scan of the head must next be done to determine the location and size of the hemorrhage. Neurosurgical consultation may be indicated if the hemorrhage is large and increased intracranial pressure is suspected.

Blood work checking the coagulation panel is very important. If the patient is on oral or parenteral anticoagulation therapy, it is imperative to consider reversing anticoagulation by protamine sulfate for those on heparin or with parenteral vitamin K or fresh frozen plasma for those patients on warfarin therapy.

Bedside EEG is not indicated unless there is pervasive coma or seizures. Lumbar puncture is usually contraindicated if intracranial or lobar hemorrhage is suspected, because it can trigger uncal herniation and eventual death if the patient is already in a state of increased intracranial pressure. The lumbar puncture with CSF xanthochromia assay is useful only if a subarachnoid hemorrhage is suspected.
B&D Ch. 57

Question 43. E. Outcomes in psychodynamic therapy have been found to be closely associated with the empathy provided by the therapist. The goal is for the therapist to be in tune with the patient's internal state in an empathic way. When patients feel that therapists understand their internal world they are more likely to accept interpretations made by the therapist. The other answer choices, while important are not the most important. Some of these distracters may have impacts on the therapeutic relationship, but will not be the universally most important factor in the outcome of therapy.
K&S Ch. 35

Question 44. A. Melatonin is believed to be released principally by the pineal gland and there is a feedback loop between the pineal gland and the suprachiasmatic nucleus in the hypothalamus that helps with sleep regulation. Melatonin is secreted predominantly at night and levels peak between 3:00 am and 5:00 am, and decrease to lower levels during the day. Melatonin is a modulator of human circadian rhythm for entrainment by the light-dark cycle.
B&D Ch. 74

Question 45. D. The Minnesota Multiphasic Personality Inventory (MMPI) is an objective psychological test. It is a self report inventory used to find areas of pathological personality structure. The other tests listed are projective tests. In projective tests the patient is given a picture or incomplete piece of information and asked to fill in the details or complete the unfinished task. The answers that the patient gives reveal aspects of his personality, thought content, thought structure, and psychological makeup. In the Rorschach test the patient is shown ink blots and asked to share what he thinks the ink blots look like. In the sentence completion test the patient is asked to finish incomplete sentences. In the thematic apperception test the patient is shown a series of pictures and asked to make up stories based on the pictures. In the draw a person test the patient is asked to draw a person of the same and opposite sex. The person of the same sex is thought to represent the patient. Interpretations are made based on the details the patient puts into the drawings.

K&S Ch. 5

Question 46. A. Subacute sclerosing panencephalitis (SSPE) is the result of a persistent and nonproductive viral infection of the neurons and glia that is caused by the measles virus. It is a late complication of the measles. Children 5 to 10 years of age are affected most often. Clinical manifestations include personality and cognitive changes, myoclonic seizures, spasticity, choreoathetoid movements, difficulty swallowing, eventually leading to coma and death. The three tests of choice are lumbar puncture for cerebrospinal fluid (CSF) assay, electroencephalogram (EEG) and brain biopsy. CSF reveals an elevated measles antibody titer, oligoclonal bands, absence of pleocytosis, normal glucose and normal to elevated protein. Brain biopsy may reveal neuronal and glial nuclear and cytoplasmic viral inclusion bodies. EEG reveals a characteristic pattern of periodic bursts of generalized slow-wave complexes. There is no specific accepted treatment, but studies have revealed that intraventricular interferon-α combined with oral isoprinosine can be helpful. Prognosis is generally poor and often death can be expected within twelve months if response to treatment is poor. There is no evidence that SSPE results from measles vaccination in children.

B&D Ch. 59

Question 47. E. Attention deficit hyperactivity disorder (ADHD) is diagnosed by six or more symptoms of inattention or six or more symptoms of hyperactivity-impulsivity that persist for 6 months or more. Some symptoms that cause impairment should be present before age 7 years. Impairment must be present in more than one setting to make the diagnosis. Symptoms of inattention involve failure to pay close attention to tasks, failure to sustain attention, not listening, not following through on tasks, problems organizing tasks, forgetfulness, and being easily distracted by extraneous stimuli. Symptoms of hyperactivity-impulsivity include fidgeting, inability to remain seated when expected, running or climbing excessively, difficulty playing quietly, acting as if driven by a motor, talking excessively, blurting out answers, difficulty awaiting turn, and interrupting others.

K&S Ch. 42

Question 48. E. Lesch-Nyhan syndrome is an X-linked recessive hereditary disorder of purine and pyrimidine metabolism. Hyperuricemia results from a deficiency in hypoxanthine-guanine phosphoribosyltransferase (HGPRT). Clinical symptoms and signs of the syndrome include choreoathetosis, hyperreflexia, hypertonia, dysarthria, behavioral disturbances, cognitive impairment and self-mutilatory behavior. Neurologic signs and symptoms are likely a result of diminished dopamine concentrations in the cerebrospinal fluid and basal ganglia.
Metachromatic leukodystrophy is an autosomal recessive disorder which is caused by arylsulfatase-A (ASA) deficiency. There is an accumulation of excess sulfatides in the nervous system which leads to progressive demyelination. The disorder localizes to chromosome 22q13.

Tay-Sachs is a recessive disorder localizing to chromosome 15q23-24. It is caused by a deficiency in hexosaminidase A. The adult form presents as progressive weakness in the proximal muscles of the upper and lower extremities. Associated symptoms may involve spasticity, dysarthria, cognitive and psychiatric impairment.

Krabbe disease, also called globoid cell leukodystrophy, is an autosomal recessive disease that localizes to chromosome 14q31. It is a result of a deficiency in lysosomal enzyme galactocerebroside β-galactosidase. Generalized central and peripheral demyelination is the hallmark of the disorder, as well as the presence of multinucleated macrophages (globoid cells) in cerebral white matter. Infantile arrest of motor and cognitive development is noted, with seizures, hypertonicity, optic atrophy and opisthotonic posturing. Stem cell transplantation may reverse the neurologic deficits by providing the missing enzyme.

Gaucher's disease is an autosomal recessive disorder resulting from β-glucosidase deficiency. It localizes to chromosome 1q21. There are three identified types. Type I presents with the characteristic findings of hematologic anomalies, hypersplenism, bone lesions, skin pigmentation and ocular pingueculae.

B&D Chs 68&82

Question 49. B. In order to diagnose schizophrenia, active phase symptoms must be present for a 1 month period only. It may be diagnosed if other symptoms (i.e., negative) are present over a 6 month period, but at least one month of that 6 months must have contained active symptoms. All other answer choices are part of the characteristic active phase symptoms for schizophrenia. Social isolation is a bad prognostic sign for schizophrenia. Good prognostic signs include late age of onset, acute onset, and the presence of an affective component.

K&S Ch. 13

Question 50. D. Botulinum toxin type A is FDA-approved for the treatment of cervical dystonia, blepharospasm, hemifacial spasm, strabismus, and axillary hyperhydrosis, and cosmetically for hyperactive glabellar lines of the procerus muscles of the forehead. Although not FDA-approved for spasticity related to multiple sclerosis, it is an excellent treatment for that particular disorder. Botulinum toxin type A is also used off-label for the treatment of migraine. The mechanism of action of botulinum toxin type A is through blockade of neuromuscular transmission via blockade of presynaptic acetylcholine release. Botulinum toxin type A has no place in the treatment of restless legs syndrome.

B&D Ch. 54

Question 51. D. This question is a clear description of a delusional disorder. In a delusional disorder, the patient usually presents with a nonbizarre delusion (i.e., something that could happen in real life). There are no other psychotic symptoms present. His ability to function in his daily life is preserved. There is not a significant mood component to the disease. The question says nothing about memory impairment, therefore dementia is not correct. The patient does not meet criteria for active phase schizophrenic symptoms, therefore schizophrenia and schizoaffective disorder are ruled out. Brief psychotic disorder lasts less than a month, and this patient has had symptoms for 5 months, so this answer choice is incorrect.

K&S Ch.14

Question 52. A. The clinical presentation described in this question is that of classic tension-type or muscle contraction headache. These headaches can result from both muscular and emotional tension and stress. These headaches are not well understood and muscle tension may not fully explain their pathogenesis. The hypothalamic-mamillothalamic tract may be implicated in the generation of the pain, but studies have yet to investigate this thoroughly. Often treatment with rest, sleep, or simple analgesics is sufficient to bring relief. These headaches can begin at any age, are most often bilateral and are described as band-like around the head. Patients describe squeezing, pressure or burning types of pain. The pain can wax and wane throughout the day and can be present, if left untreated, from a period of hours to days. This headache type is usually free of any associated or autonomic symptoms, which helps to differentiate it from migraine. Treatment of tension-type headache usually begins with aspirin or acetaminophen. If headaches are more severe, combination drugs like acetaminophen-butalbital-caffeine (Fioricet) may be helpful, or non-steroidal anti-inflammatory agents such as naproxen or ibuprofen. Migraine is differentiated from tension-type headache mainly by its stereotyped features and associated autonomic symptoms. Migraine is generally unilateral, pulsatile and is accompanied by photophobia, phonophobia, or osmophobia. Other features can include nausea and vomiting, anorexia, blurred vision, and lightheadedness. The aura that can precede a migraine involves transient visual, motor, or focal neurologic deficits or symptoms. The scintillating scotoma is the most common visual manifestation of aura. The patient can perceive a shimmering arc or zigzag pattern of light in the peripheral visual field that can gradually enlarge. Sensory aura can involve transient numbness and tingling in the extremities that can last from seconds up to a half an hour's duration. Motor aura is rare and can manifest as a transient motor weakness or hemiparesis, in much the same way as the sensory deficits. The patient may therefore misinterpret these symptoms as the onset of a stroke. Basilar migraine usually presents with occipital headache and neurologic symptoms attributable to the brainstem. The aura can involve visual and sensory phenomena, but these are often accompanied by vertigo, dysarthria, tinnitus and speech deficits. Loss of consciousness may occur if the reticular activating system of the pons is involved. The patient will often experience severe occipital pain after awakening from the aura. These attacks resemble stroke-like symptoms in the vertebrobasilar territory. Paroxysmal hemicrania is a special headache entity that falls into the category of indomethacine-responsive headache syndromes. This headache type begins early in life and is more common in women than in men (2:1 ratio). The hemicrania can be episodic or chronic. Pain is unilateral and brief, occurring generally in the periorbital or temporal areas. Attacks are frequent, usually five or more daily and each lasts about 20 minutes. Each attack is accompanied by autonomic features such as conjunctival injection, lacrimation, ptosis, rhinorrhea, ipsilateral to the side of the headache. Response to indomethacin 25 mg–100 mg daily in divided doses is usually dramatic. The mechanism of indomethacin's efficacy in this headache variety is not well understood.

B&D Ch. 75

Question 53. E. In major depressive disorder libido is decreased. Increased libido is often found in mania.

K&S Ch. 15

Question 54. B. The best answer to this question is the trigeminal nucleus caudalis (TNC). Many theories exist to try to explain the pathogenesis of migraine, and unfortunately there is no perfect unified theory. It is generally believed that abnormal intracranial and extracranial vascular reactivity accounts for the pulsatile nature of migraine by the abnormal dilatation of these vessels. It is believed that the aura of migraine is caused by a phenomenon called spreading oligemia or spreading depression. This refers to a phase of oligemia that spreads over the occipital cortex at a rate of about 2–3 mm/minute and causes the scintillating scotoma noted during aura. This was described by Lashley in 1941, by

117

his analysis of his own aura. Abnormal neuronal impulses from the tri-geminal nucleus caudalis in the pons send messages along the trigeminal ophthalmic branches to nerve terminals that release substance P, neuroki-nin A and calcitonin gene-related peptide (CGRP). These polypeptides in turn activate a cascade of sterile neurogenic perivascular inflammation in the brain. Vessels then dilate and by vascular endothelial activation, there is an extravasation of plasma proteins that triggers an inflammatory response. Ergot alkaloid medications and triptan medication effectively block neuronal firing in the TNC and can abort an attack. The reticular activating system (RAS) refers to the ascending tracts in the pons that are responsible for maintenance of wakefulness. Bilateral pontine le-sions affecting the RAS can result in impairment of consciousness. The suprachiasmatic nuclei (SCN) in the hypothalamus are thought to be the generator of the human biological clock that regulates circadian rhythms. Melatonin is the neurohormone produced by the pineal gland that acts at melatonin receptor sites in the SCN by a feedback loop. The SCN has no known role in migraine. Muscular contraction of the scalp and cranial musculature is not believed to be associated with migraine, but may play a role in the manifestation of tension-type headache.

B&D Ch. 67 & 75

Question 55. C. This is a case of seasonal affective disorder, which is a depression that sets in during the fall and winter and resolves during the spring and summer. It is often characterized by hypersomnia, hyperphagia, and psychomotor slowing. Treatment involves exposure to bright artificial light for 2–6 hours each day during the fall and winter months. It is thought to be related to abnormal melatonin metabolism. All other answer choices given are distracters and are unrelated to the patient's primary problem.

K&S Ch. 15

Question 56. C. Carbidopa serves a simple function: it inhibits dopa decarboxylase and thereby prevents the peripheral metabolism of levodopa to dopamine before it can cross the blood–brain barrier. The dopamine agonists such as ropinirole, pramipexole, pergolide and bromocriptine are direct post-synaptic dopamine receptor agonists indicated for Parkinson's disease treatment. Selegeline is the selective monamine oxidase type B (MAO-B) inhibitor that blocks dopamine degradation by MAO-B and can potenti-ate the action of levodopa in the central nervous system. Catechol-O-methyltransferase (COMT) inhibitors such as tolcapone and entacapone prevent peripheral degradation of levodopa and central metabolism of levodopa and dopamine, thereby increasing central levodopa and dopamine levels. COMT inhibitors are usually taken simultaneously with doses of levodopa-carbidopa. Anticholinergic agents such as tri-hexyphenidyl and benztropine can reduce tremor in Parkinson's disease by blockade of postsynaptic muscarinic receptors. These agents carry the danger of toxic side effects that include confusion, blurred vision, urinary retention, constipation and dry mouth.

B&D Ch. 77

Question 57. E. This question includes common symptoms found in a panic attack. Others include trembling, choking sensations, dizziness, fear of losing control, fear of death, paresthesias, chills, or hot flushes. The patient in question does not present with the characteristic signs and symptoms of a manic episode. Myxedema madness is a depressed and psychotic state found in some patients with hypothyroidism. Mad Hatter's syndrome presents as manic symptoms resulting from chronic mercury intoxica-tion. The patient describes no psychotic symptoms, so psychotic disorder NOS is clearly the wrong choice.

K&S Ch. 16

Question 58. E. Apoptosis refers to programmed neuronal cell death. This concept is believed to account for the pathophysiology of several neurodegenerative diseases. These diseases include spinal muscular atrophy, Parkinson's disease, amyotrophic lateral sclerosis, and Alzheimer's dementia.
B&D Ch. 45

Question 59. B. Amoxapine and maprotiline are tetracyclic, not tricyclic antidepressants. Amoxapine has significant dopamine blocking activity, and can produce side effects similar to those found with many antipsychotics, such as tardive dyskinesia and dystonia. Maprotiline is one of the most selective inhibitors of norepinephrine reuptake. It has mild sedative and anticholinergic side effects. Notably there is an increased incidence of seizure associated with its use. It has a long half life of 43 hours.
K&S Ch. 36

Question 60. B. Sturge-Weber syndrome is a neurocutaneous disorder that is sporadic and not genetically inherited. The hallmark is the presence of a facial cutaneous angioma (port-wine nevus) usually with a brain angioma ipsilateral to the skin lesion. Other characteristics can include contralateral hemiparesis, mental retardation and homonymous hemianopia. Glaucoma is common and if untreated can lead to blindness. Seizures develop in over 70% of Sturge-Weber patients and present most often as motor seizures or generalized tonic-clonic seizures. Treatment of seizures is achieved with anticonvulsant medication, which if proven ineffective, may lead to the consideration of surgical intervention such as hemispherectomy to excise the offending brain tissue.
Von Hippel-Lindau syndrome (VHL) is a heritable neurocutaneous disorder that is transmitted by autosomal dominant pattern of inheritance. The VHL gene is a tumor-suppressor gene on chromosome 3. Prevalence is about 1 in 40 000 to 100 000. The predominant clinical presentation is characterized by retinal and CNS hemangioblastomas and visceral cysts and tumors. Hemangioblastomas are slow-growing vascular tumors that are benign but can bleed and cause local mass effect. The most common CNS sight of this tumor type is the cerebellum in about 50% of cases. Renal cysts occur in about half of patients with VHL. Pheochromocytoma occurs in about 10–20% of patients. Frequent follow-up and screening for tumors is the management of choice for patients with VHL.
Ataxia-telangiectasia is a neurodegenerative neurocutaneous disorder that is inherited by autosomal recessive pattern of inheritance. Prevalence is about 1 in 40 000 to 100 000. The hallmark of the disorder is the development of early-onset ataxia in childhood. Ataxia tends to develop at around 12 months of age, when the child begins to walk. Children typically are wheelchair-bound by 12 years of age. Telangiectases (small dilated blood vessels) tend to develop later, from about age 3–6 years, and often affect the earlobes, nose and sclerae. There is also a higher risk of lymphoma and leukemia in patients with the disorder than in the general population at large. Abnormal eye movements are common in children with the disorder. These include nystagmus, ocular motility impairment and gaze apraxia.
Fabry's disease is an X-linked lysosomal storage disease resulting from deficiency in α-galactosidase A. Stigmata of the disease include the development of asymptomatic red or purple papules that occur around the umbilicus, hips, thighs and scrotum area. Other characteristics include corneal deposits, painful dysesthesias of the distal extremities, cerebral thrombosis or hemorrhage, and eventual vascular narrowing from deposition of glycolipids in the arterial endothelium. Renal failure is a common cause of death due to renal vascular compromise. Treatments are disappointing in Fabry's disease. Enzyme repletion does not help the clinical problems. Plasmapheresis is also not particularly effective. Renal

119

transplantation can delay systemic complications and alleviate renal failure, but is not curative.

Tuberous sclerosis is discussed elsewhere in this volume in great detail.

B&D Ch. 71

Question 61. A. The doctor who takes Medicare must accept Medicare's maximum fee. This fee includes any appropriate copays set forth in the patient's policy. The physician can not bill the patient or another party for the difference between what Medicare allows and what you want to charge.

K&S Ch. 4.

Question 62. E. Reflex sympathetic dystrophy is one of the so-called complex regional pain syndromes. It is the result of regional pain and sensory changes following trauma or a noxious event. There may or may not be a diagnosable underlying nerve lesion to the problem. Soft tissue injury is the trigger in about 40% of cases and bony fracture in about 25% of cases.

There are three stages to the disorder. Stage one (acute) is associated with pain that is out of proportion to the initial injury. There is usually hypersensitivity to painful stimuli or physical contact with the extremity. Stage two (dystrophic) is associated with tissue edema and skin that is cool, cyanotic, hyperhidrotic, with livedo reticularis. Pain is constant and increases with any physical contact to the affected extremity. Stage three (atrophic) is associated with paroxysmal pain and irreversible tissue damage. The skin can become thin and shiny and the fascia can become thickened or contractured. Treatments begin with intense physical therapy which can be helpful by improving mobility of the affected extremity. Steroids may be helpful in certain cases. Phenoxybenzamine, which is a sympathetic blocking agent, can also be useful, if tolerated. Some patients require invasive anesthesia by regional block, which can be helpful in certain patients.

B&D Ch. 33

Question 63. B. In the situation where you are presented with an unknown psychotic or paranoid patient, the first step is to make sure that patient and staff are safe. All other options are valid, but would be taken after an initial assessment of the patient's safety has been made. When given a question such as this on an examination, maintenance of safety comes first, and diagnosis and treatment come later. You would not automatically give sedation to the patient if they were not agitated or dangerous, so answer choice A is not the correct first move. Remember that past violence is the best predictor of future violence.

K&S Ch. 33

Question 64. B. Carbamazepine is an inducer of cytochrome P450 2C19 and 3A4. It can therefore induce the metabolism of any substrate of the 2C19 and 3A4 systems. The 3A4 substrates that can be induced by carbamazepine include erythromycin, clarithromycin, alprazolam, diazepam, midazolam, cyclosporine, indinavir, ritonavir, saquinavir, diltiazem, nifedipine, amlodipine, verapamil, atorvastatin, simvastatin, aripiprazole, buspirone, haloperidol, tamoxifen, trazodone, propranolol, zolpidem, zaleplon, methadone, estradiol (oral contraceptives), progesterone, testosterone, and fentanyl, to name but a few. The 2C19 substrates that can be induced by carbamazepine include amitriptyline, citalopram, clomipramine, imipramine, R-warfarin, propranolol, and primidone. Carbamazepine can lower lamotrigine levels by induction of glucuronidation enzyme 1A4. Clozapine is a substrate of cytochrome P450 1A2 and is not affected by carbamazepine.

B&D Ch. 36

Question 65. E. The standard of substituted judgment holds that a surrogate decision maker will make decisions based on what the patient would have wanted, and implies that the decision maker be familiar with the patient's values and attitudes. The best interest principle, which was the past, but not current standard, states that a decision maker will decide which option would be in the patient's best interests. Patients do have the right to refuse treatment that they feel would lessen their quality of life. Advanced directives and the living will are ways for patients to preserve their wishes in writing such that the correct decisions are made for them should they become incapacitated. The state will follow the course that preserves human life should a suitable surrogate decision maker not be present. Surrogate decision makers can be appointed by the patient, courts, or the hospital. In many cases this person is the patient's next of kin.

K&S Ch. 56

Question 66. D. Tobacco smoking is a potent inducer of cytochrome P450 1A2. As such it can significantly lower levels of amitriptyline, fluvoxamine, clozapine, olanzapine, haloperidol, and imipramine. Risperidone is a substrate of cytochrome P450 2D6 and its levels can be lowered by 2D6 inducers such as dexamethasone and rifampin. Risperidone levels can be significantly increased by 2D6 inhibitors such as bupropion, citalopram, clomipramine, doxepin, duloxetine, escitalopram, fluoxetine, paroxetine, sertraline, and perphenazine. Risperidone levels are not affected by tobacco smoking.

B&D Ch. 36

Question 67. E. One cannot treat what is assumed to be denial before actually knowing that it is denial. Often in medical settings things are not clearly explained to patients in language they can understand. As such it is first necessary to explain what is going on to the patient clearly and in language they can follow. Confronting the patient's denial forcefully, and aggressively removing his defenses against overwhelming emotion, is potentially more harmful than helpful. Playing along with the denial can lead to noncompliance and failed treatment outcomes and is a bad idea. Neuropsychological testing is not necessary if a patient is in denial. If he had a neurocognitive deficit that precluded his understanding of the material presented to him it could be considered, but those were not the circumstances described in this question. Meeting the family is important, but not more important than making sure the patient has had the situation explained properly. The patient is the primary person who has to understand. Informing the family while the patient is left in the dark is not the best approach.

K&S Ch. 28

Question 68. A. This is a classic case of Sheehan's syndrome, which is essentially a postpartum pituitary infarction or apoplexy. The classic symptoms are those similar to a pituitary hemorrhage. The pituitary infarction can cause chiasmal compression that can lead to bitemporal hemianopsia from bilateral medial optic nerve compression. Hypotension can occur due to pre-existing adrenocorticotropic hormone deficiency. The clinical picture can resemble a subarachnoid hemorrhage due to the rupture of a berry aneurysm or an arteriovenous malformation. This would account for the severe acute headache and cranial nerve palsy. The syndrome can also result in meningeal irritation with positive Kernig's and Brudzinski's signs and a stiff neck. The diagnosis can often be confirmed by a CT or MRI scan of the brain. Treatment is generally supportive and only in certain cases is it necessary to provide corticosteroid replacement or conduct a surgical decompression.

Cushing's disease is caused by endogenous overproduction of adrenocorticotropic hormone from the anterior pituitary gland. Cushing's syndrome is the result of exposure to either excessive exogenous or endogenous corticosteroids. The clinical picture is that of hypertension, truncal obesity, impaired glucose tolerance or diabetes mellitus, menstrual irregularities, hirsutism, acne, purplish abdominal striae, osteoporosis, thin skin with excessive bruising, and proximal myopathy. The diagnostic test of choice is the dexamethasone suppression test. Subarachnoid hemorrhage is most often the result of an intracranial arterial aneurysmal rupture. The acute presentation very often consists of a sudden explosive headache ("the worst headache of my life"), meningeal signs, nausea, vomiting, photophobia, and obtundation. Head CT scan is the imaging test of choice as it reveals acute blood better than MRI. CT scans can only reveal subarachnoid blood in about 90–95% of patients within 24 hours of the hemorrhage. This sensitivity drops to about 80% after 72 hours. A negative CT scan should therefore be followed by a lumbar puncture with centrifuging of CSF looking for characteristic xanthochromia (from lysed red blood cells). If either CT or lumbar puncture is positive for subarachnoid hemorrhage, then cerebral angiography should be performed as soon as possible to determine the location of the aneurysm and best method of intervening. The most popular interventions for intracranial aneurysms are endovascular coiling, microsurgical clipping, and balloon embolization. Saccular or berry aneurysms are the most common kind of intracranial aneurysms. Between 80% and 85% of aneurysms stem from the anterior cerebral circulation, most often arising from the anterior communicating artery, posterior communicating artery, or the trifurcation of the middle cerebral artery. Between 15% and 20% of aneurysms originate in the posterior circulation, most often from the origin of the posterior inferior cerebellar artery or at the bifurcation of the basilar artery.

Bacterial meningitis presents in adults as a febrile illness involving headache, stiff neck, and signs of cerebral dysfunction, which are present in over 85% of patients. Associated signs and symptoms include nausea, vomiting, photophobia, and myalgia. Often Kernig's and Brudzinski's signs can be elicited. Cerebral dysfunction can involve delirium, confusion, and decreased level of consciousness that ranges from lethargy to coma. Seizures can occur in about 40% of cases. Cranial nerve palsies can be seen in 10–20% of patients. Increased intracranial pressure may result in the appearance of bilateral VI nerve palsies. Lumbar puncture and blood cultures clinch the diagnosis. Cerebrospinal fluid (CSF) opening pressure is high (200–500 mmH$_2$O) and protein is also high (100–500 mg/dL, normal = 15–45 mg/dL), with decreased glucose and marked pleocytosis (100–10000 WBC/μL, normal = <5), with 60% or more polymorphonuclear leukocytes. CSF cultures are positive in about 75% of cases. In the United States, the predominant causative organism in children ages 2 to 18 years is *N. meningitidis* and in adults, *S. pneumoniae*. Intravenous ampicillin, penicillin-G and third-generation cephalosporins (ceftriaxone, cefotaxime, ceftazidime) are the usual agents of first-line treatment.

Familial hemiplegic migraine (FHM) is a rare autosomal dominant migraine subtype in which the aura is accompanied by hemiplegia. FHM has been mapped to chromosome 19p13 that codes for the α1-subunit of brain-specific voltage-gated P/Q-type calcium channel. There is some notion that because FHM has similar symptoms to traditional migraine with aura that this implies that migraine with aura may also be genetically linked to chromosome 19.

B&D Ch. 47 & 59

Question 69. C. The question stem accurately describes agoraphobia. The other answer choices are distracters. Agonothete is the judge of games in ancient Greece. Agoniada is the bark of a South American shrub. Agora is the market place in ancient Greece. Agouara is a South American wild dog or a crab eating raccoon. Needless to say, the only one that will show up on the boards is agoraphobia.

K&S Ch. 16

Question 70. C. Normal-pressure hydrocephalus (NPH) presents with the triad of dementia, incontinence, and gait disturbance. The cause, in up to one-third of cases, is undetermined. NPH can be caused by trauma, infection, or subarachnoid hemorrhage. Brain CT scan or MRI reveal enlargement of the third, fourth, and lateral ventricles. NPH causes an apraxic, or magnetic gait, making it difficult for the patient to raise the legs off the ground. The dementia is considered to be subcortical, and results in slowing of verbal and motor functioning while the cortical functions remain intact. Abulia, apathy and depression are common in NPH. Urinary incontinence occurs early in the course of the illness, particularly when there is prominent gait disturbance. Lumbar puncture reveals a normal opening pressure. Serial lumbar punctures with drainage of cerebrospinal fluid can improve the symptoms and support the diagnosis of NPH. Ventriculoperitoneal shunting is the treatment of choice and is successful in up to 80% of cases. Shunts fail about one-third of the time and complications of shunting include subdural hematoma and infection.

Diffuse Lewy-body disease, or dementia with Lewy bodies is the second-most prevalent dementia after Alzheimer's disease. The symptomatic triad is that of dementia, parkinsonism, and visual hallucinations. A hallmark of the disease is extreme sensitivity to dopamine receptor antagonists which can result in severe parkinsonism when treatment with neuroleptics is undertaken. Dopaminergic therapy is generally not that helpful. Hallucinations are ideally treated with the newer antipsychotics, particularly quetiapine, clozapine, and ziprasidone. Rivastigmine and donepizil may be useful cholinergic therapy to try to improve cognition.

Wernicke's encephalopathy presents with the acute triad of mental confusion, ophthalmoplegia and gait ataxia, predominantly in alcoholic patients. On autopsy, the neuropathologic hallmark is multiple small hemorrhages in the periventricular gray matter, mainly around the aqueduct and the third and fourth ventricles. MRI of the brain often reveals abnormalities in the periaqueductal regions, bilateral mamillary bodies, and medial thalami.

Sydenham's chorea (SC) is a result of rheumatic fever. It is extremely rare these days because of the widespread availability of antistreptococcal therapy. The disorder is more frequent in girls, generally between 5 and 15 years of age. Chorea begins insidiously over a period of weeks and can last up to 6 months. Behavioral manifestations can include irritability, obsessive-compulsive traits and restlessness. Enlargement of the basal ganglia can be noted on MRI. Symptoms are generally self-limited, lasting up to about 6 months. Anti-basal ganglia antibodies can be detected by Western blot testing and these antibodies seem to account for the mechanism of the disorder. Valproic acid is a useful therapy for the chorea.

B&D Chs 72&77

123

Question 71. E. Cyclothymic disorder does not involve psychotic symptoms, although these symptoms may be found in bipolar disorder. Cyclothymia is a less severe form of bipolar with alternation between hypomania and moderate depression. Symptoms must exist for two years to make the diagnosis. It is equally common in men and women. Substance use often co-exists. The onset is usually insidious and occurs in late adolescence or early adulthood.

K&S Ch. 15

Question 72. B. Depression is not considered a stroke risk factor. Common risk factors for stroke include older age, male gender, low socioeconomic status, diabetes mellitus, obesity, cigarette smoking, excessive alcohol consumption, and family history. Other important risk factors are arterial hypertension, prior stroke or transient ischemic attack, asymptomatic carotid bruit, dyslipidemia, hyperhomocysteinemia and oral contraceptive use.

Hereditary blood dyscrasias also elevate stroke risk, such as protein C or S deficiency, antithrombin III deficiency and factor V leiden deficiency.
B&D Ch. 57

Question 73. D. This question gives a classic description of the appearance of a patient in the manic phase of bipolar disorder. They are often very bizarre, colorful, seductive and erratically behaved. A depressed patient would be apathetic and psychomotor retarded, not hyperexcited. There was no mention made in the question of psychosis or delusions so brief psychotic disorder and delusional disorder are incorrect. There is also no mention of abnormally perceived body image so body dysmorphic disorder is incorrect as well. There is an equal prevalence of bipolar disorder in women versus men. Bipolar I disorder in women most often starts with depression.
K&S Ch. 15

Question 74. A. Ataxia is indicative of a cerebellar lesion and the cerebellum is perfused by the vertebrobasilar arterial system. Symptoms indicative of a carotid territory transient ischemic attack or stroke would be: transient ipsilateral monocular blindness (amaurosis fugax), contralateral body weakness or sensory loss, aphasia with dominant hemisphere involvement, contralateral homonymous visual field deficits. Symptoms that suggest a vertebrobasilar territory stroke or transient ischemic attack include: bilateral, shifting, or crossed weakness or sensory loss (ipsilateral face with contralateral body), bilateral or contralateral homonymous visual field defects or binocular visual loss, two or more of vertigo, diplopia, dysphagia, dysarthria and ataxia.
B&D Ch. 57

Question 75. E. Suicidal ideation is part of the thought content of the depressed patient. It is possible to find it in the manic bipolar patient, but is more likely during the depressed phase of the illness and is not part of the thought process.
K&S Ch. 15

Question 76. D. Essential tremor (ET) is one of the most common movement disorders. It has been noted in up to 5% of patients over 60 years of age. It is defined as a postural and kinetic tremor of the forearms and hands (sometimes with other body parts) that gradually increases in amplitude over time. ET is believed to be a monosymptomatic illness, without other neurologic deficits. As many as two-thirds of patients have a positive family history of ET. The disease is likely heterogeneous with an autosomal dominant pattern of inheritance.

The mainstay of treatment is the use of β-adrenergic blocking agents and primidone. Propranolol is the β-blocker of choice and can be given in doses of 120–320 mg daily in divided doses. This helps reduce tremor amplitude in roughly half of patients. Primidone can be given as a single nighttime dose of 25 mg and subsequently titrated to a therapeutic dose of 50–350 mg daily. Benzodiazepine sedative-hypnotic agents, like clonazepam and lorazepam are also frequently used and can be helpful. Botulinum toxin type A can be injected intramuscularly for head and hand tremor and can be effective in certain cases. Desipramine and the tricyclic antidepressants are not useful in ET and may in fact worsen tremor. If oral therapy fails, surgical intervention can be contemplated if symptoms are serious. Stereotactic thalamotomy has been shown to reduce contralateral tremor by 75% in as many as 90% of cases. Thalamic deep brain stimulation has also been demonstrated to be effective in treating ET and can improve symptoms in up to 80% of cases.
B&D Ch. 77

Question 77. B. To qualify for a diagnosis of major depressive disorder, symptoms must be present for at least two weeks. Symptoms can include depressed mood, diminished interest in activities, weight loss or gain, insomnia or hypersomnia, psychomotor retardation, fatigue, feelings of worthlessness, decreased concentration, recurrent thoughts of death, and recurrent suicidal ideation.

K&S Ch. 15

Question 78. B. The thymus gland is believed to play a role in the pathogenesis of myasthenia gravis (MG). MG is an autoimmune disorder and the thymus gland is involved in tolerance to self-antigens. Ten per cent of patients with MG have a thymic tumor and 70% have cellular hyperplasia of the thymus indicative of an active immune response. About 20% of patients with MG who develop symptoms between ages 30 and 60 years have a thymoma. The thymus contains myoid cells that express the AChR (acetylcholine receptor) antigen, antigen presenting cells and immunocompetent T cells. The thymus is believed to produce AChR subunits that act as autoantigens in the sensitization of the patient against the AChR. Most thymomas in MG patients are benign and are amenable to easy surgical resection which may in certain cases improve symptomatology. The other tumor types mentioned above are not typically associated with MG.

B&D Ch. 84

Question 79. B. Prevalence for schizophrenia is higher in urban than in rural areas, as are morbidity and severity of presentation. The lifetime prevalence is about 1%. The male to female ratio is 1:1. Onset is usually between 15 and 35 years, with onset before 10 years and after 40 years being rare. There is a higher incidence of cases in babies born in the winter and early spring.

K&S Ch. 13

Question 80. A. Friedrich's ataxia (FA) is an autosomal recessive disease that localizes to chromosome 9q13-21.1. It is the result of an unstable expansion of a trinucleotide repeat (GAA). Onset is typically noted in adolescence with gait ataxia, loss of lower extremity proprioception, and absence of deep tendon reflexes, more often in the lower extremities. There is also predominant central nervous system involvement with noted dysarthria, presence of Babinski signs and eye movement anomalies. The natural progression of the disease is towards a complete loss of ambulation ability and ultimately death due to hypertrophic cardiomyopathy in about 50% of cases. Death occurs on average by late in the fourth decade. Myotonic dystrophy (MD) type I is an autosomal dominantly inherited disease with trinucleotide repeat expansion of CTG that codes to chromosome 19q13.3. The incidence is 1 in 8000 live births. Classic symptoms and signs include ptosis, bifacial weakness, frontal baldness, triangular drooping facies. Motor weakness is greater distally than proximally. Myotonia is a classic sign, which is the inability to relax a contracted muscle or group of muscles. For example, a patient is unable to let go after shaking hands. Percussion myotonia can also be demonstrated, particularly in the thenar and hypothenar hand muscles. This is involuntary contraction of muscles after percussion with a reflex hammer. Fibrotic or infiltrative cardiomyopathy is a frequent associated problem in myotonic dystrophy. DNA testing by serum polymerase chain reaction is the diagnostic modality of choice for MD. Electromyography reveals myopathic features and myotonic discharges ("dive-bomber" sound after muscular relaxation). Perifascicular muscle fiber atrophy is the classic histopathologic finding on muscle biopsy. Please note that the other three answer choices are explained in questions elsewhere in this volume and are all diseases inherited by autosomal dominant transmission.

B&D Chs 78&85

Question 81. D. Disinhibited behavior is more characteristic of mania than it is of depression. All of the other symptoms are somatic or sleep complaints that are

frequently associated with depression. Patients with depression have disrupted REM sleep, including shortened REM latency, increased percentage of REM sleep, and a shift in REM distribution from the last half to the first half of the night. Acetylcholine is associated with the production of REM sleep.
K&S Ch. 15

Question 82. E. It is believed that migraine maps to several regions on chromosome 19, because of the entity FHM (familial hemiplegic migraine) that has been associated with this gene locus. FHM is thought to be a channelopathy involving a brain-specific calcium channel α-1 subunit gene that has been mapped to chromosome 19p13. Given the similarity between FHM and typical migraine, researchers believe that chromosome 19 may well be the locus that links both disorders.
B&D Ch. 75

Question 83. A. Obsessions are part of thought content, as are delusions, ideas of reference, phobias, suicidal or homicidal thought, depersonalization, derealization, and neologisms, to name a few. Thought process would include word salad, flight of ideas, circumstantiality, tangentiality, clang associations, perseveration, and goal directed ideas.
K&S Ch. 7

Question 84. B. CNS cysticercosis involves parenchymal invasion of the brain by the larval stage pork tapeworm *T. solium.* Cysticercosis occurs by ingestion of undercooked pork containing cysticerci. The infection occurs most frequently in Central and South America where poor hygiene and sanitation lead to unsanitary conditions. After ingestion of tainted pork, the tapeworm eggs hatch in the gastric tract, develop to larval stage and eventually penetrate the bowel to migrate to host tissue, most often in the CNS. Clinical presentation ranges from epilepsy, focal neurological deficits, hydrocephalus, cognitive decline, meningitis, or myelopathy. Diagnosis is confirmed by brain MRI demonstrating the parasites in the brain and from confirmatory serology and/or CSF ELISA tests. ELISA on CSF is more sensitive and specific than serologic tests. Treatment is with albendazole or praziquantel oral therapy, coupled with parenteral steroids. *T. spiralis* infection causes trichinosis which is also caused by ingestion of poorly cooked pork or other game meats in endemic areas. *E. granulosus* are the larval tapeworms that cause CNS echinococcosis. Humans generally acquire echinococci through contact with dogs that are infected. *E. granulosus* tends to cause solitary CNS spherical cysts without edema. Treatment can involve surgical resection of the cyst or conservative medical management with albendazole if the cysts are not resectable. *L. major* is a protozoan that causes leishmaniasis. The vector is a sandfly bite. Visceral disease can be accompanied by inflammatory neuropathies that resemble Guillain-Barré syndrome. Treatment is by parenteral administration of antimony or amphotericin B. *T. gondii* is the intracellular protozoan responsible for toxoplasmosis infection. Vectors include migratory birds and cats and so the infection can be found worldwide. Toxoplasmosis rarely occurs in immunocompetent patients, but is more often seen in AIDS patients with low CD4 counts. CNS lesions present as ring enhancing on both CT and MRI. CSF titers may contain *T. gondii* DNA detectable by PCR. Treatment is usually a combined regimen of pyrimethamine and sulfadiazine with folinic acid. Ventricular shunting may be required if lesions are space-occupying and cause hydrocephalus.
B&D Ch. 59

Question 85. C. The effects of alcohol can be seen in several lab tests. The GGT will be elevated in 80% of alcoholic patients, while MCV is increased in 60% of alcoholic patients. Uric acid, triglycerides, AST and ALT can also be elevated. The other lab values given in the question are unrelated to alcohol abuse.

K&S Ch. 12

Question 86. C. Alcoholic neuropathy is the most common neurologic manifestation of chronic alcoholism. Up to 75% of alcoholic patients are diagnosed with this disorder. Most patients are chronic alcohol abusers between 40 and 60 years of age. This type of neuropathy is a mixed motor and sensory disorder. Symptoms usually begin gradually, symmetrically in the feet. Alcoholic dementia refers to older patients with a lifelong history of heavy alcohol use, who experience an insidious decline in their cognitive functioning. Nearly 20% of older alcoholics have some form of dementia, but this is complicated by the presence of other comorbidities such as liver abnormalities, head trauma, malnutrition and stroke. Alcoholic dementia results in more of a predominance of fine motor control and verbal fluency deficits than is seen in patients with dementia of the Alzheimer type.

Marchiafava-Bignami disease is a rare demyelinating disease preferentially affecting the corpus callosum in chronic alcoholics. The exact etiology of the disorder is not well-understood. It may be related to nutritional factors or direct toxic effects of alcohol on the cerebral white matter, but this is unclear. The most common neurologic manifestation is that of frontal lobe damage and dementia noted on neurologic examination. The central portion of the corpus callosum is more often affected than the anterior or posterior portions. Treatment is directed at nutritional support and alcoholic rehabilitation.

Alcoholic-nutritional cerebellar degeneration is seen more often in men than in women. The disorder presents in longstanding alcoholics as unsteadiness in walking evolving over weeks to months. The most common presentation on examination is truncal ataxia, with a wide-based gait and difficulty with tandem walking. Pathologically, the disorder results from preferential atrophy of the superior and anterior cerebellar vermis, with lesser involvement of the cerebellar hemispheres. Wernicke's encephalopathy is explained extensively elsewhere in this volume.

B&D Chs 63&82

Question 87. B. A cohort study is when a group from a well-known population is chosen and followed over a long period of time. These studies give us estimates of risk based on suspected causative factors for a given disease. Case history studies look back on people with a given disease. Cross-sectional studies give information on prevalence of a disease in a population at a given point in time. Retrospective studies are based on past data, as opposed to prospective studies which are based on observing things as they occur.

K&S Ch. 4

Question 88. C. The Miller-Fisher syndrome is a variant of Guillain-Barré syndrome (GBS, acute inflammatory demyelinating polyneuropathy). The classic triad of symptoms is gait ataxia, areflexia and ophthalmoplegia. This accounts for about 5% of GBS cases. Motor strength is usually intact. Serum IgG antibodies to the ganglioside GQ1b can be detected in serum early in the course of the Miller-Fisher variant of GBS. F-wave latencies may be intact on EMG with reduced or absent SNAP amplitudes. CSF protein is elevated without pleocytosis about one week into the course of the illness. Dementia, parkinsonism and psychosis make up the triad of dementia with Lewy bodies. The clinical picture is that of dementia, extrapyramidal symptoms, fluctuations and visual hallucinations. Visual hallucinations occur in as many as 80% of cases. Neuroleptic sensitivity is another diagnostic characteristic. The classic pathologic finding is the Lewy bodies which are diffuse throughout the cortex and are eosinophilic inclusions with a core halo on hematoxylin and eosin stain. Treatment

127

with newer atypical antipsychotics, particularly clozapine, is usually best and cholinesterase inhibitors such as donepizil may also be helpful. The triad of gait ataxia, urinary incontinence and dementia is classic for normal pressure hydrocephalus.

B&D Ch. 82

Question 89. C. Konrad Lorenz is known best for his work with imprinting. Imprinting is the phenomenon whereby during a critical period of early development a young animal will attach to their parent, or whatever surrogate is in the parent's place. From then on the presence of that parent or surrogate will elicit a specific behavior pattern even when the animal is much older. In Lorenz's case newborn goslings imprinted on him instead of their mother and followed him around as if he were their mother. This has correlates in psychiatry because it is evidence of the link between early experiences and later behaviors. Lorenz also studied aggression in animals and worked on the need for aggression in humans given the pressures of natural selection. All the other answer choices in this question are distracters which have nothing to do with the work of Lorenz.

K&S Ch. 4

Question 90. B. This case depicts a classic case of acute inflammatory demyelinating polyneuropathy (Guillain-Barré syndrome or GBS). The annual incidence is 1.8 in 100 000. About 65% of patients report a prior "insult" before the onset of symptoms. This often takes the form of a gastrointestinal infection, an upper respiratory infection, surgery, or immunization a few weeks before symptoms appear. The most commonly identified organism responsible for prodromal infection is *Campylobacter jejuni*. *C. jejuni* can be detected in stool cultures and serologic studies. The clinical presentation of GBS can vary from case to case. Typically patients present with symmetrical lower extremity weakness, with paresthesias and possibly with sensory symptoms. The paralysis is usually an ascending paralysis and the most worrisome outcome is paralysis of the muscles of respiration which can prove fatal in some cases. Deep tendon reflexes are usually greatly diminished or absent. Diagnostic testing reveals the classic nerve conduction abnormalities of conduction block and prolonged F-wave latencies, which are pathognomonic of GBS. CSF studies reveal cytoalbuminergic dissociation: elevated protein with an acellular fluid. In certain cases, nerve biopsy can reveal complement fixing antibodies to peripheral nerve myelin. Treatment should take place in the hospital and in an intensive care unit setting if respiratory compromise is imminent. Two treatments of choice are high dose intravenous immunoglobulin administration and plasmapheresis. These have been proven to be equally efficacious in numerous recent studies.

B&D Ch. 82

Question 91. A. Second messengers are molecules that work within the cell to carry on the message delivered by the neurotransmitter on the cell surface. IP_3, cGMP, Ca^{2+}, cAMP, DAG, NO, and CO are all common second messenger molecules. Adenylyl cyclase is not a second messenger itself, but rather is the enzyme that makes cAMP from ATP. Adenylyl cyclase is turned on or off by G proteins depending on the need for cAMP. Binding cAMP to transcription factors regulates gene transcription, including the machinery to make certain neurotransmitters. Calcium plays a number of roles within the cell, and excess Ca^{2+} is linked to production of NO and cell death through excitotoxicity. One of the major functions of IP3 is to cause the release of intracellular Ca^{2+} from the endoplasmic reticulum.

K&S Ch. 3

Question 92. A. The cortical dementias such as Alzheimer's disease generally produce a gradual decline in cognitive function, with normal speed of cognition and the presence of aphasia, dyspraxia, and agnosia. Depression is less common in cortical dementia than in subcortical disease. Motor abnormalities are typically absent in cortical dementia, unless the disease is in the terminal stages. Subcortical dementia, as exemplified in Parkinson's disease, typically presents with dysarthria and extrapyramidal motor abnormalities. Apathy and depression are often present. Frontal memory impairment, with recall aided by cues, is often noted. Speed of cognition in subcortical dementia is slow.

B&D Ch. 72

Question 93. B. This question focuses on Piaget's stages of cognitive development. In the sensorimotor stage children respond to stimuli in the environment, and learn during this process. They eventually develop object permanence (objects exist independent of the child's awareness of their existence), and begin to understand symbols (as in the use of words to express thoughts). During the preoperational stage there is a sense that punishment for bad deeds is unavoidable (immanent justice). There is a sense of egocentrism, and phenomenalistic causality (the thought that events that occur together cause one another). Phenomenalistic causality is the subject of this question. Animistic thinking (inanimate objects are given thoughts and feelings) is also seen.

In the concrete operations stage, egocentric thought changes to operational thought where another's point of view can be taken into consideration. In concrete operations children can put things in order and group objects according to common characteristics. They develop the understanding of conservation (a tall cup and a wide cup can both hold equal volumes of water) and reversibility (ice can change to water and back to ice again).

During formal operations children can think abstractly, reason deductively, and define abstract concepts. Latency is a distracter. It occurs in Freud's model after the genital phase and before puberty.

K&S Ch. 2

Question 94. C. T4 is the dermatome at the level of the nipples. T10 is the dermatome at the level of the umbilicus. Other important dermatomes to remember include: C2 – back of head, C4 – above collar bone, C6 – thumb, C7 – middle fingers, C8 – little finger, L1 – groin, L2 – lateral thigh, L3 – medial thigh, L4 – medial leg, L5 – lateral leg, big toe, S1 – little toe, sole of foot, S5 – perianal area.

B&D Ch. 27

Question 95. D. The three receptor types associated with glutamate are AMPA, kainate, and NMDA. Acetylcholine is associated with the nicotinic and muscarinic receptors. Norepinephrine is associated with the alpha 1, alpha 2, and beta receptors. Serotonin is associated with the various 5-HT receptors. GABA is associated with the GABA receptor. Opioids are associated with the mu and delta receptors. Dopamine is associated with the D1, D2 etc. receptors.

K&S Ch. 3

Question 96. B. Buspirone is a serotonin 1A agonist or partial agonist. It is indicated for the treatment of anxiety disorders, in particular, generalized anxiety disorder. It does have activity at the serotonin 2 and dopamine 2 receptor sites, but its significance at those sites is not well understood. It may have mild dopamine 2 agonistic and antagonistic effects, but this is not its predominant mechanism of action. Buspirone takes two to three weeks to exert therapeutic effects. The initial dose is 15 mg daily in two or three divided doses. Therapeutic effects are usually not seen until a dose of 30 mg or above is reached. The maximum approved daily dose is 60 mg. Buspirone can increase blood levels of haloperidol. Buspirone cannot be used with monoamine oxidase inhibitors (MAOI) and a two-week wash-out needs to happen after an MAOI is stopped before buspirone can be started. Buspirone levels can be increased by nefazodone, erythromycin, itraconazole and grapefruit juice by their inhibition of cytochrome P450 3A4 in the liver.

K&S Ch. 36

Question 97. E. Excitatory neurotransmitters open cation channels that depolarize the cell membrane and increase the likelihood of generating an action potential. These neurotransmitters elicit excitatory postsynaptic potentials or EPSPs.

K&S Ch. 3

Question 98. C. Phencyclidine (PCP) is a potent N-methyl-D-aspartate (NMDA) receptor antagonist. The NMDA receptor is a subtype of the glutamate receptor. PCP has calcium channel binding properties and prevents the influx of calcium into neurons. PCP also has dopaminergic properties that would seem to explain the reinforcing effects of the drug.

Tolerance can occur with PCP, but it is generally held that PCP does not cause a physical dependence. There is psychological dependence to the agent and users can become dependent to its euphoric effects in this way. PCP intoxication is characterized by maladaptive behavioral changes, such as violence, impulsivity, belligerence, agitation, impaired judgment. Symptoms of intoxication include nystagmus, hypertension, decreased pain responsiveness, ataxia, dysarthria, muscle rigidity, seizures, coma, and hyperacusis. PCP can induce a delirium with agitated, bizarre, or violent behavior. It can also cause an acute psychotic disorder with delusions and hallucinations that can persist for several weeks following ingestion of the drug. PCP can remain in the blood and urine for more than a week. Treatment of the behavioral abnormalities related to PCP is best undertaken with benzodiazepines and dopamine antagonists.

K&S Ch. 12

Question 99. C. Sublimation is one of the mature defenses. It is characterized by obtaining gratification by transforming a socially unacceptable aim or object into an acceptable one. Sublimation allows instincts to be channeled in an acceptable direction rather than blocked. All other choices are immature defenses. Hypochondriasis is exemplified by exaggerating an illness for the purpose of evasion or regression. Introjection is demonstrated by internalizing the qualities of an outside object. It is an important part of development but can also be used as an unproductive defense. The classic example is identification with an aggressor. Regression is characterized by attempting to return to an earlier libidinal phase of functioning to avoid the tension and conflict of the current level of development. Passive aggression takes the form of expressing anger towards others through passivity, masochism, and turning against the self. Manifestations can include failure and procrastination.

K&S Ch. 6

Question 100. E. Phenelzine is a monoamine oxidase inhibitor and is not likely to worsen the movement disorder symptoms of Parkinson's disease. The other four agents are antagonists of dopamine D2 receptors and can of course worsen symptoms of Parkinson's disease and cause drug-induced parkinsonism. The pathophysiology involves D2 receptor antagonism in the caudate. Patients who are elderly and female are at greatest risk for neuroleptic-induced parkinsonism. More than half of patients exposed to neuroleptics on a long-term basis have been noted to develop this unwanted adverse effect. Amoxapine (Asendin) is a dibenzoxazepine tetracyclic antidepressant that has strong D2 antagonistic properties because it is a chemical derivative of the neuroleptic loxapine (Loxitane). Because of its unique

structure and chemical properties, amoxapine can also cause akathisia, dyskinesia and infrequently, neuroleptic malignant syndrome.
K&S Ch. 36

Question 101. D. Ana Freud wrote *The Ego and Mechanisms of Defense* and was the first to give a comprehensive study of the defense mechanisms. She maintained that all people, healthy or neurotic, use a number of defense mechanisms. Freud was the father of psychoanalysis whose work focused on the importance of libido, aggression, and the oedipal complex, among other concepts. Kohut was the father of self psychology. Fromm defined five character types common to western culture. Jung went beyond Freud's work and founded the school of analytic psychology. It focused on the growth of the personality through one's experiences.
K&S Ch. 6

Question 102. B. In the case of Dusky vs United States, the US Supreme Court determined that, in order to have the competence to stand trial, a criminal defendant must be able to have the ability to consult his lawyer with a reasonable degree of rational understanding and he must have a reasonable and rational understanding of the proceedings against him. The McGarry instrument is a clinical guide that identifies thirteen areas of functioning that must be demonstrated by a criminal defendant in order to be declared competent to stand trial. Answer choices A, C, D, and E are included in these thirteen areas, as well as the ability to plan legal strategy, the ability to appraise the roles of participants in courtroom procedure, capacity to challenge prosecution witnesses realistically, capacity to testify relevantly, ability to appraise the likely outcome, and understanding the possible penalties, among several others.
K&S Ch. 57

Question 103. D. Paranoid schizophrenia is characterized by systematized delusions or frequent auditory hallucinations related to a single theme. None of the other answer choices are characteristic of paranoid schizophrenia, but may be found in other types of schizophrenia.
K&S Ch 13

Question 104. E. Studies have indicated that depression tends to be a chronic, relapsing disorder. The percentage of patients who recover following repeated episodes diminishes over time. About one-quarter of patients have a recurrence within the first six months after initial treatment. This figure rises to about 30–50% in the first two years and even higher to about 50–75% within five years. It has been proven than ongoing antidepressant prophylaxis helps to lower relapse rates. As a patient experiences more depressive episodes over time, the time between episodes decreases and the severity of the episodes worsens.
K&S Ch. 15

131

Question 105. D. Dysthymic disorder is characterized by decreased mood over a period of two years with poor appetite or over eating, sleep problems, fatigue, low self esteem, poor concentration, and feelings of hopelessness. Hallucinations are not considered part of dysthymia, although it is possible to have hallucinations as part of a major depressive episode.
K&S Ch. 15

Question 106. D. Tarasoff vs regents of the University of California is the landmark case from 1976 in which the California Supreme Court ruled that any psychotherapist who believes that a patient could injure or kill someone must notify the potential victim, the victim's relatives or friends, or the authorities. In 1982, the same court issued a second ruling that broadened Tarasoff to include the duty to protect, not only to warn the intended victim.

The Durham Rule was determined by the ruling in the case of Durham vs the United States in 1954 by Judge Bazelon. This rule stipulates that a defendant cannot be found criminally responsible if the criminal act was the product of a mental illness or defect. In 1972 the District of Columbia Court of Appeals in the ruling United States vs Brawner, discarded the Durham Rule.

In 1976 in the ruling of O'Connor vs Donaldson, the United States Supreme Court ruled that harmless mentally ill patients cannot be confined involuntarily without treatment if they can survive outside an institution. Clites vs State was a landmark case pertaining to a ruling in favor of a patient and his family who sued for damages resulting from chronic neuroleptic exposure that resulted in tardive dyskinesia. The appellate court ruled that the defendants deviated from the usual standards of care by failing to conduct physical examinations and routine laboratory tests and failed to intervene at the first signs of tardive dyskinesia.

K&S Ch. 57

Question 107. C. All of the drugs listed are tertiary amines except desipramine, which is a secondary amine. The other tertiary amine is doxepin. The secondary amines include desipramine, nortryptyline, and protryptyline. During metabolism the tertiary amines are converted into secondary amines.

K&S Ch. 35

Question 108. C. Surgical approaches to Parkinson's disease include deep brain stimulation, surgical stereotactic ablation of overactive brain areas and cellular implantation of dopaminergic neuronal cells. Stereotactic thalamotomy can reduce tremor and rigidity contralaterally in about 75–85% of patients. There is little effect on bradykinesia. Bilateral thalamotomy can cause cognitive and speech deficits. Thalamic deep brain stimulation is better tolerated and results are similar to thalamotomy without the risks involved with the ablative procedure. Stereotactic posteroventral pallidotomy can improve dopa-induced dyskinesia and akinesia in about 70% of patients. Pallidal deep brain stimulation has also been shown to be almost as effective as pallidotomy. Subthalamic deep brain stimulation is the most preferred of the surgical procedures and has demonstrated 40–50% improvement in the motor fluctuations of Parkinson's disease. Human fetal substantia nigra transplantation into the putamen has been shown to be modestly effective on an experimental basis. Injection of glial-derived neurotrophic factor (GDNF) into brain parenchyma may be of future utility, but up until recently has only been studied in animal models. The superior colliculus is not an area that is targeted in neurosurgical intervention for Parkinson's disease.

B&D Ch. 77

Question 109. A. Amoxapine has a 7-hydroxymetabolite that has potent dopamine blocking activity. This can lead to antipsychotic-like side effects that result from the drug's use.

K&S Ch. 35

Question 110. C. Right-left disorientation is a result of a lesion to the dominant angular gyrus and is one of the symptoms of Gerstmann's syndrome. A large stroke in the right middle cerebral artery territory can result in hemi-neglect, visual and tactile extinction, impaired speech prosody (loss of musical and emotional inflection), anosognosia (not knowing that you have a deficit or problem), and behavioral problems such as delirium and confusion. The patient may not recognize that the affected left arm and/or hand is his own and may have limb apraxia. A contralateral homonymous hemianopia or inferior quadrantanopia can also be noted in nondominant hemispheric strokes.

B&D Ch. 57

Question 111. D. The metabolism of tricyclic antidepressants by CYP2D6 is an important topic that has led to an FDA recommended precaution. Tricyclics are metabolized by CYP 2D6, and as such anything that decreases the activity of CYP 2D6 will increase the plasma level of the tricyclic, even into the toxic range. Some people are naturally "poor metabolizers" who have decreased CYP 2D6 activity, and as such, higher plasma levels. Cimetidine inhibits CYP 2D6 and as such will increase tricyclic levels. The same holds true for quinidine. Several drugs are substrates for CYP 2D6 and will decrease its ability to clear tricyclics when present. These include fluoxetine, sertraline, paroxetine, carbamazepine, phenothiazines, propafenone, and flecainide.
K&S Ch. 35

Question 112. A. This question depicts a classic diabetic third nerve palsy. The differential diagnosis of greatest importance with an isolated third nerve palsy is diabetes (benign) versus that of an internal carotid artery (ICA) aneurysm (potentially fatal). Aneurysms that most commonly affect third nerve functioning are those originating at the ICA near the origin of the posterior communicating artery. A third nerve palsy resulting from an aneurysm is usually associated with a dilated pupil and eyelid ptosis, as contrasted with a diabetic third nerve palsy that usually spares the pupillary function.
B&D Ch. 57

Question 113. A. Residual schizophrenia is characterized by the absence of prominent hallucinations, delusions, incoherence, and disorganized behavior. Two or more of the residual symptoms may be present (i.e., negative symptoms or active phase symptoms present in a clearly attenuated form). Posturing is a characteristic symptom of catatonic schizophrenia.
K&S Ch. 13

Question 114. E. Severe motor tics in Tourette's syndrome are best treated by neuroleptics, in particular haloperidol and pimozide. Recently the atypical neuroleptics have come to be used more readily because of their superior safety profiles, in particular risperidone, quetiapine, olanzapine, ziprasidone and clozapine. Fluphenazine, molindone, and other conventional antipsychotics are also acceptable treatment choices. Clonidine is also a frequently used and effective treatment of tics and is particularly favored by pediatric neurologists for its excellent safety profile. Botulinum toxin type A can be effective for blepharospasm, eyelid motor tics, and is in fact FDA-approved for this indication. Protryptiline and the other antidepressants may be effective for associated obsessive-compulsive symptoms, but these agents are not useful for treatment of tics.
B&D Ch. 77

Question 115. E. Grossly inappropriate affect is a characteristic of disorganized schizophrenia, along with disorganized behavior, incoherence, and loosening of associations. In addition to the symptoms listed in the question, catatonic schizophrenia can also present with stupor, purposeless excitement, posturing, and echopraxia.
K&S Ch. 13

Question 116. C. The middle cerebral artery territory includes the optic radiations. A lesion of these tracts results in either a contralateral homonymous hemianopsia or a contralateral inferior quadrantanopsia ("pie on the floor"). Bitemporal hemianopsia is of course caused by invasion of the optic chiasm, often by a sellar lesion such as a pituitary macroadenoma. Left monocular blindness would result from an ipsilateral central retinal artery occlusion.
B&D Ch. 57

Question 117. E. The process by which neurotransmitter is released into the synaptic cleft is called exocytosis. Neurotransmitters are synthesized in the presynaptic neuron, and both their synthesis and release are mediated by Ca^{2+} influx into the cell. Feedback receptors exist on the presynaptic membranes of many cells, a good example being the alpha 2 receptor on the noradrenergic neuron which participates in a negative feedback loop to stop the release of norepinephrine. Neurotransmitters such as dopamine, norepinephrine, and serotonin will remain active until they diffuse out of the cleft or are removed by reuptake mechanisms. Degradation of recycled neurotransmitters is done via monoamine oxidases (MAOs), with MAO type A degrading NE and serotonin and MAO type B degrading dopamine.
K&S Ch. 3

Question 118. B Lesch-Nyhan syndrome is an X-linked recessive disorder. Hyperuricemia results from a deficit in hypoxanthine-guanine phosphoribosyltransferase. Clinical hallmarks of the disorder include cognitive impairment, self-mutilatory behavior, hypertonia, hyperreflexia, dysarthria, developmental delay and choreoathetotic movements. Low dopamine concentrations in the basal ganglia and cerebrospinal fluid may be a cause of the movement disorder noted in Lesch-Nyhan syndrome.
Ornithine transcarbamylase deficiency is an X-linked inborn error of metabolism of the urea cycle that causes hyperammonemia, encephalopathy and respiratory alkalosis. Treatment with low-protein diet and dietary arginine supplementation can be effective.
Carbamoylphosphate synthase deficiency is an autosomal recessive inborn error of metabolism of the urea cycle that causes hyperammonemia, encephalopathy and respiratory alkalosis. There are two forms of the disorder, type I an early fatal form and type II a delayed-onset form which may only present later in childhood or early adulthood. Treatment with dietary arginine repletion may be helpful in certain cases.
Arginase deficiency results in hyperammonemia as well. The disorder is usually caused by a point-mutation or deletion on chromosome 6q23 that codes for the ARG1 gene. The incidence of the disorder is less than 1 in 100 000.
Adenylosuccinase deficiency results in autism, growth retardation, and psychomotor delay. It is believed to be an autosomal recessive cause of autism. Seizures may also arise as a result of this disorder.
B&D Ch. 68

Question 119. D. This question focuses on Piaget's stages of cognitive development. In the sensorimotor stage children respond to stimuli in the environment, and learn during this process. They eventually develop object permanence (objects exist independent of the child's awareness of their existence), and begin to understand symbols (as in the use of words to express thoughts). During the preoperational stage there is a sense that punishment for bad deeds is unavoidable (immanent justice). There is a sense of egocentrism, and phenomenalistic causality (the thought that events that occur together cause one another). Animistic thinking (inanimate objects are given thoughts and feelings) is also seen.
In the concrete operations stage, egocentric thought changes to operational thought where another's point of view can be taken into consideration. In concrete operations children can put things in order and group objects according to common characteristics. They develop the understanding of conservation (a tall cup and a wide cup can both hold equal volumes of water) and reversibility (ice can change to water and back to ice again.) During formal operations children can think abstractly, reason deductively, and define abstract concepts. Symbiosis is one of Mahler's stages of separation-individuation. It is unrelated to Piaget.
K&S Ch. 2

Question 120. D. Post-traumatic dementia most often results in frontotemporal cognitive dysfunction from diffuse subcortical axonal shear that disrupts cortical and subcortical circuitry. Slowing of mental processing and difficulty with executive functioning, set-shifting, organization and planning, are the most frequent cognitive deficits noted. Dementia pugilistica can occur in patients with repeated head trauma and is not simply limited to boxers. Clinical features include severe memory and attentional deficits and extrapyramidal signs. ApoE4 carriers (which resides on chromosome 19) are at increased risk of post-traumatic dementia as well as Alzheimer's disease.
B&D Ch. 72

Question 121. E. Doxepin is the tricyclic with the most antihistaminic activity.
K&S Ch. 35

Question 122. A. Bupropion is neither indicated nor effective in the treatment of obsessive-compulsive disorder (OCD). The selective serotonin reuptake inhibitors (SSRIs) have demonstrated proven efficacy in treating OCD. Trials of four to six weeks' duration are usually needed to produce results, but often trials need to be extended to eight to sixteen weeks to achieve maximal therapeutic benefit. The standard of care is to start either an SSRI or clomipramine which generally generate a response in 50–70% of cases. Four of the SSRIs have been FDA-approved for OCD, fluoxetine, fluvoxamine, paroxetine and sertraline. Higher doses may be needed in order to achieve a response. Clomipramine (Anafranil) is the most serotonergic of the tricyclic and tetracyclic antidepressant agents, which are more noradrenergic in their nature. Clomipramine was the first agent specifically FDA-approved for OCD. It needs to be titrated upwards gradually over several weeks in order to minimize gastrointestinal and anticholinergic side effects. The best results are achieved with a combination of drug and cognitive behavioral therapy.
K&S Ch. 16

Question 123. A. Giving tricyclic antidepressants leads to a decrease in the number of β-adrenergic and 5-HT receptors. This downregulation of receptors is what correlates most closely with the time to clinical improvement in patients.
K&S Ch. 35

Question 124. E Enuresis should first be treated with the bell-and-pad behavioral conditioning method before pharmacotherapy is instituted. The principle is simple: a bell awakens the child when the mattress becomes wet. Tricyclic antidepressants, such as amitriptyline and imipramine can reduce the frequency of enuresis in about 60% of patients. Desmopressin (DDAVP) is effective in about half of patients. Tricyclic antidepressants are to be given about one hour before bedtime. The response to therapy can be as rapid as a few days. Desmopressin is administered intranasally in doses of 10–40 mg daily. Children who respond completely to any of these pharmacological agents should continue the therapy for several months to prevent relapse. Olanzapine and the antipsychotic medications are not generally used in the treatment of enuresis.
K&S Ch. 53

Question 125. D. This question stem is referring to Ca^{2+}. During an action potential, the first ion channel to open is the Na^+ channel. This lets Na^+ flow into the neuron. Next Ca^{2+} channels open allowing more positively charged ions to enter and contribute to the action potential. Once inside, Ca^{2+} ions act as second messengers involved in protein–protein interactions and gene regulation. Calcium ions are critical to the release of neurotransmitter and also activate the opening of potassium ion channels that then put a stop to the action potential through the after-hyperpolarization of the

membrane. With regard to receptors, also keep in mind that the GABA receptor is a chloride ion channel.
K&S Ch. 3

Question 126. B. The most worrisome side effects of the tricyclic antidepressant agents are cardiac conduction abnormalities, because of course these side effects can lead to fatal cardiac arrhythmias if the medication is taken in overdose. These agents can cause flattened T waves, tachycardia, prolonged QT intervals and depressed ST segments on electrocardiograms. The tricyclics are also noted for causing orthostatic hypotension by alpha-1 adrenergic blockade and they can of course cause sedation and the lowering of the seizure threshold. The tricyclics can also cause anticholinergic side effects, which consist of dry mouth, constipation, blurred vision and urinary retention. In the male patient suffering from benign prostatic hypertrophy, the anticholinergic load can lead to severe urinary retention and even anuria, which can be very problematic. Bethanecol 25–50 mg three to four times daily can reduce urinary hesitancy and retention. Tricyclic antidepressants can actually help with migraine and neuropathic pain prophylaxis, particularly at lower dosages. These are off-label uses for these agents.
K&S Ch. 36

Question 127. D. Inhibitory neurotransmitters open chloride channels that hyperpolarize the membrane and decrease the likelihood of an action potential being generated. They cause inhibitory postsynaptic potentials or IPSPs.
K&S Ch. 3

Question 128. C. This question addresses different types of behavior therapy for a simple phobia of spiders (arachnophobia). Flooding (implosion) involves exposing the patient to the feared stimulus in vivo immediately, without a gradual buildup, as would be expected in therapeutic graded exposure. The goal of flooding is immediate exposure and response prevention until the patient can tolerate the anxiety and gain a sense of mastery of the anxiety. Therapeutic graded exposure is similar to systematic desensitization, except that relaxation techniques are not involved and the technique is carried out in real situations. Progress is graded and at first the patient may be exposed to pictures of the spiders only, and then later exposed to the real spiders themselves. Participant modeling involves the patient learning a new behavior by observation first, then eventually by doing it, often accompanied by the therapist. This model can work particularly well with agoraphobia. Aversion therapy is the use of a noxious stimulus or punishment to suppress an undesired behavior. Using a bad-tasting nail polish to prevent nail-biting, or taking disulfiram to prevent alcohol use would be excellent examples of aversion therapy. Assertiveness training teaches the patient to develop social and interpersonal skills through responding appropriately in social or occupational situations, expressing opinions acceptably, and achieving personal goals. Techniques such as role modeling, positive reinforcement and desensitization can be used to develop assertiveness.
K&S Ch. 35

Question 129. C. Disclaimers such as "I know you don't agree with this but ..." or "I don't know why I think this but..." often precede emotionally charged material. They serve to soften the delivery of such material and relieve anxiety on the part of the person making them. Whenever a disclaimer is made by the patient in therapy the therapist should listen closely to the material that follows as that material is often a window into how the patient truly feels. The other answer choices in this question border on the ridiculous.
K&S Ch. 35

Question 130. D. This question depicts a patient with an acute delirium. The mainstay of treatment of delirium is to treat the underlying cause if it is identifiable. The other goal of treatment is to give the patient environmental, sensory and physical support. Environmental support can be given by increasing the lighting level in the room, providing a clock and calendar in the room showing the correct time and date, and by dimming the lights and closing the blinds only at night. Physical support can be provided to patients by the presence of friends and relatives in the room, or a constant caregiver figure. This can help prevent falls and other physical accidents. Low-dose haloperidol in either oral or intramuscular form can be helpful to treat psychotic symptoms or agitation. Benzodiazepines, particularly those of high potency and short duration of action like flurazepam (Dalmane) should be avoided, as they can paradoxically agitate and further confuse the delirious patient.

K&S Ch. 10

Question 131. D. Abreaction is an emotional release after recalling a painful event. It is part of psychodynamic therapy and is a large part of what Freud thought brought about cure during psychoanalysis of conversion disorder patients during his early work. The other answer choices are part of cognitive behavioral therapy (CBT). In CBT the false belief systems that underlie maladaptive behaviors and mood disturbance are examined through techniques such as those listed in the question. Underlying assumptions that feed false belief systems are also examined. The goal of therapy is to correct the underlying thoughts and assumptions, and in so doing, change the mood and behavior.

K&S Ch. 35

Question 132. A. Pinpoint pupils are a feature of opioid intoxication or usage and not withdrawal. Opioid withdrawal consists of dysphoric mood, nausea or vomiting, muscle aches or twitches, lacrimation or rhinorrhea, papillary dilatation, piloerection, sweating, diarrhea, yawning, fever and insomnia. Associated symptoms can include hypertension, tachycardia, and temperature dysregulation such as hypothermia or hyperthermia. Other possible symptoms can include depression, irritability, weakness and tremor.

K&S Ch. 12

Question 133. A. The least sedating tricyclic antidepressants are desipramine and protriptyline. Moderately sedating tricyclics include imipramine, amoxapine, nortriptyline and maprotiline. The most sedating include amitriptyline, trimipramine, and doxepin.

K&S Ch. 35

Question 134. B. Secondary gain refers to tangible advantages that a patient may get as a result of being unwell. Examples of secondary gain include getting out of responsibility, getting money, drugs, or other financial entitlements, or controlling other people's behavior. Getting or seeking medical help, or enjoying playing the sick role for its own sake, would be considered a form of primary gain.

K&S Ch. 17.

Question 135. C. In hypothyroidism, one would expect to find an increased TSH and a low free T4 level. Sub-clinical cases of hypothyroidism will present with a high TSH and a normal T4 level. Other answer choices are distracters, and are not the most important lab values to look for when trying to diagnose hypothyroidism.

K&S Ch. 7

Question 136. E. There are no absolute contraindications to electroconvulsive shock therapy (ECT). Pregnancy is not a contraindication for ECT. Fetal monitoring is only considered important if the pregnancy is high risk or complicated. Brain tumors increase the risk of ECT, especially of brain edema and herniation after ECT. If the tumor is small, complications can be minimized by administration of dexamethasone prior to ECT and close monitoring of blood pressure during the treatment. Patients with aneurysms, vascular malformations or increased intracranial pressure are at greater risk during ECT because of increased blood flow during the induction of the seizure. This risk can be decreased by careful control of blood pressure during the seizure. Epilepsy and prior neuroleptic malignant syndrome are not problematic with the administration of ECT. Recent myocardial infarction is another risk factor, but the risk decreases markedly 2 weeks after the infarction and even further 3 months after the infarction. Hypertension, if controlled and stabilized with antihypertensive medication, does not pose an increased risk during ECT.

K&S Ch. 36

Question 137. E. Carbamazepine has many drug–drug interactions because of its effects on the cytochrome P450 system. Of importance is the fact that it lowers concentrations of oral contraceptives, leading to breakthrough bleeding and uncertain protection against pregnancy. It has a long list of other drugs with which it interacts including lithium, some antipsychotics, and certain cardiac medications. It should not be combined with MAOIs. Combining clozapine with carbamazepine will increase the risk of bone marrow suppression.

K&S Ch. 36

Question 138. B. Alfred Binet developed the idea of mental age in 1905 as the average intellectual level of a particular age. Intelligence quotient (IQ) is simply the quotient of mental age divided by chronological age multiplied by 100. An IQ of 100 is therefore considered to be the average, that is, when mental age and chronological age are equal. An IQ of 100 represents the 50th percentile in intellectual ability for the general population.

K&S Ch. 5

Question 139. B. Open-ended questions are those that allow the patient to express what he is thinking and do not direct the patient to speak about a specific topic that the doctor chooses. Ideally an interview should begin with open ended questions and become more specific and close-ended as it continues. Closed-ended questions can often be answered in one or few words. Open-ended questions often require the patient to explain and provide information.

K&S Ch. 1

Question 140. A. The Karolinska Institute has shown in numerous studies that diminished central serotonin plays a role in suicidal behavior. This group was the first to demonstrate that low levels of cerebrospinal fluid (CSF) 5-hydroxyindoleacetic acid (5-HIAA) is associated with suicidal behavior. It has also been shown that low 5-HIAA levels predict future suicidal behavior and that low 5-HIAA levels have been shown in the CSF of adolescents who kill themselves.

K&S Ch. 34

Question 141. E. Symptoms of lithium toxicity include ataxia, tremor, nausea, vomiting, nephrotoxicity, muscle weakness, convulsions, coma, lethargy, confusion, hyperreflexia, and nystagmus. Non-specific T-wave changes can also be seen at high lithium concentrations. Jaundice is a result of hepatic dysfunction. Lithium damages the kidneys, not the liver. Lithium induced polyuria is the result of lithium antagonism to the effects of ADH (anti-diuretic hormone).

K&S Ch. 36

Question 142. B. Obsessive-compulsive disorder (OCD) is believed to be a result of an imbalance in the serotonin system. Data show that serotonergic drugs are more effective in relieving symptoms of OCD than drugs that work on other neurotransmitter systems. Studies are unclear as to whether serotonin actually is involved in the cause of OCD. Cerebrospinal fluid (CSF) assays of 5-hydroxyindoleacetic acid (5-HIAA) have reported variable findings in patients with OCD. In one study CSF levels of 5-HIAA decreased after treatment with clomipramine, leading researchers to the conclusion that the serotonin system is involved in OCD symptom genesis.
K&S Ch. 16

Question 143. E. Amoxapine is the most likely of the tricyclic antidepressants to cause parkinsonian symptoms. It can also cause akathisia or dyskinesia. This is because its metabolites have dopamine blocking activity. It can even cause NMS in rare cases. Tricyclics are contraindicated in patients with cardiac conduction deficits. They should be stopped before elective surgery because of the risk of hypertension when tricyclics are given concomitantly with anesthetics. Fludrocortisone can help some patients with orthostatic hypotension. Myoclonic twitches and tremors can be seen in patients on desipramine and protriptyline.
K&S Ch. 35

Question 144. D. Vascular dementia, formerly known as multi-infarct dementia, is generally the result of one or more cerebrovascular accidents that are the consequence of ischemic or embolic risk factors for cerebrovascular events. Vascular dementia occurs more frequently in men, particularly those with known cerebrovascular risk factors, which include smoking, hypertension and diabetes. Symptoms are generally abrupt in onset and a pattern of step-wise decline in cognition and functioning can often be noted. There is often a presence of demonstrable focal neurologic deficits. Vascular dementia is generally poorly responsive to cholinergic repletion therapy by acetylcholinesterase inhibitors.
K&S Ch. 10

Question 145. B. Clomipramine is the most serotonin-selective of the tricyclic antidepressants.
K&S Ch. 35

Question 146. E. The psychiatrist is the member of the team who is held legally responsible for the team's decisions. It stems from the concept that the highest person in the hierarchy is responsible for the actions of those he or she supervises. The psychiatrist is considered the head of this team. As such, the attending psychiatrist is responsible for the actions of the residents he or she supervises, and is responsible for the actions of the team.
K&S Ch. 57

Question 147. E. The tricyclic antidepressants have many cardiac side effects that are worsened in overdose. They act as type 1A antiarrhythmics. As such they can terminate ventricular fibrillation, and increase collateral blood supply to ischemic heart tissue. In overdose they can be highly cardiotoxic and will cause decreased myocardial contractility, tachycardia, hypotension, and increased myocardial irritability. Also important to note is that nortriptyline is unique in that it has a therapeutic window. Blood levels should be obtained and the therapeutic range is 50–150 ng/mL. Levels above 150 ng/mL may reduce its efficacy.
K&S Ch. 35

Question 148. C. Past suicidal behavior is the best predictor of future suicidal behavior. It is a better predictor than any of the other answer choices given in this question. As such, one of the most important questions to ask a patient who has suicidal thoughts is about their history of past suicide attempts.

Other risk factors for suicide are as follows: men are more likely than women, divorced or single more likely than married, elderly are less likely to attempt, but more likely to succeed when they do, whites are more likely than other ethnic groups, and the higher the social status the higher the risk.

K&S Ch. 34

Question 149. D. Clomipramine has been shown to be particularly useful in treating obsessive-compulsive disorder in comparison to the other tricyclics. Its efficacy when compared to the SSRIs for OCD is equal or better, depending on the study.

K&S Ch 35

Question 150. E. Imipramine is often used to treat childhood enuresis. Desmopressin is also useful in 50% of patients. Improvement can range from cessation of enuresis to leaking less urine. Drugs should be given one hour before bedtime and results are usually evident within days. Patients who achieve full dryness should take the medication for several months to prevent relapse.

K&S Ch. 35

THREE

Test Number **THREE**

1. During which one of Piaget's stages of development will a child be able to understand that a tall glass and a short wide glass can contain the same volume of water despite their different shapes?

    A. Sensorimotor stage
    B. Preoperational thought stage
    C. Concrete operations stage
    D. Formal thought stage
    E. Anal stage

2. Transient global amnesia presents with all of the following characteristics, EXCEPT:

    A. Loss of personal information and identity
    B. Reversible anterograde and retrograde memory loss
    C. Inability to learn newly acquired information
    D. Preservation of alertness without motor or sensory deficits
    E. Men are affected more commonly than women

3. All of the following answer choices are true regarding GABA, EXCEPT:

    A. GABA is thought to suppress seizure activity
    B. GABA is thought to exacerbate mania
    C. GABA is thought to decrease anxiety
    D. GABA-A activity is potentiated by topiramate
    E. Gabapentin has no activity at the GABA receptors or transporter

4. An 8 year-old boy has been at sleep-away summer camp for two weeks and presents with a sudden onset of facial diplegia. The most likely infectious organism that might have caused this symptom is:

A. *T. pallidum*

B. *B. burgdorferi*

C. *L. interrogans*

D. *R. rickettsii*

E. *Y. pestis*

5. A middle aged man has been referred to your office by a plastic surgeon. The man is seeking a face lift for his "excessively large cheeks". The surgeon has not been able to find anything abnormal about the man's face or skin, and when he comes to see you, you fail to see anything wrong either. The patient insists that his cheeks are grotesque and ruining his whole appearance. When pressed, he admits that others may not consider his cheeks to be as bad as he does. His most likely diagnosis is:

A. Malingering

B. Schizophrenia

C. Somatization disorder

D. Conversion disorder

E. Body dysmorphic disorder

6. Tourette's syndrome often involves which one of the following psychiatric manifestations?

A. Generalized anxiety disorder

B. Social anxiety disorder

C. Panic disorder

D. Obsessive-compulsive disorder

E. Psychotic disorder

7. A young woman comes to the emergency room with a one week history of pressured speech, decreased sleep, grandiosity, and loosening of associations. The patient feels that she is being monitored by a satellite and she is seen talking to herself when no one else is in the room. Which one of the following criteria must be met to diagnose this patient with schizoaffective disorder instead of bipolar disorder?

A. Presence of mania

B. Psychotic symptoms in the absence of mood symptoms for a 1 week period

C. At least one prior episode of depression

D. Presence of psychotic symptoms during a manic episode

E. Psychotic symptoms in the absence of mood symptoms for a 2 week period

8. Which one of the following therapies would be best-suited to a bipolar patient in a manic episode during pregnancy?

   A. Haloperidol

   B. Lithium

   C. Aripiprazole

   D. Divalproex sodium

   E. Electroconvulsive shock therapy

9. You are called to evaluate a 60 year-old man with a history of depression. His family reports that he has not been himself for the past 5 days. On examination he makes poor eye contact, is inattentive, mutters incoherently, keeps rearranging pieces of paper on his bed tray with no apparent logic, and drifts off to sleep while you are talking to him. What is his most likely diagnosis?

   A. Depression

   B. Dementia

   C. Delusional disorder

   D. Delirium

   E. Obsessive compulsive disorder

10. Which one of the following pharmacologic agents would be most likely to cause extrapyramidal side effects and possible tardive dyskinesia?

   A. Hydroxyzine

   B. Diphenhydramine

   C. Metoclopramide

   D. Ondansetron

   E. Tizanidine

11. The most common symptom seen in patients with narcolepsy is:

   A. Hypnopompic hallucinations

   B. Sleep paralysis

   C. Hypnagogic hallucinations

   D. Sleep attacks

   E. Cataplexy

12. The primary auditory cortex localizes to which one of the following brain regions?

   A. Temporal lobe

   B. Parietal lobe

   C. Frontal lobe

   D. Occipital lobe

   E. Thalamus

13. Which one of the following neurotransmitters works as an adjunctive neurotransmitter for glutamate as well as an independent neurotransmitter with its own receptors?

    A. GABA
    B. Norepinephrine
    C. Serotonin
    D. Dopamine
    E. Glycine

14. All of the following agents are acceptable and useful for the treatment of postherpetic neuralagia, EXCEPT:

    A. Gabapentin
    B. Lidoderm
    C. Pregabalin
    D. Carbamazepine
    E. Phenytoin

15. A construction worker is brought to the emergency room immediately after an accident on a job site. He was standing very near a three story scaffold that fell and missed crushing him by inches. He reports feeling anxiety, a sense of numbing, detachment, difficulty remembering the accident, and states that he feels like he is in a daze. The most likely diagnosis is:

    A. Generalized anxiety disorder
    B. Major depression
    C. Delirium
    D. Dissociative amnesia
    E. Acute stress disorder

16. Trauma to which one of the following vessels or groups of vessels commonly causes epidural hematoma?

    A. Middle meningeal artery
    B. Meningeal bridging veins
    C. Cavernous sinus
    D. Basilar artery
    E. Transverse sinus

17. A 26 year-old woman comes into the emergency room. She reports that she has been having mood swings that go from depressed to elated to rageful in minutes to hours. She has been having paranoid feelings and vague auditory hallucinations over the past week since breaking up with her boyfriend. On this past Monday she cut her arms with a razor, but only superficially. Her history reveals promiscuity, unstable relationships, and cocaine use. She now reports suicidal ideation. Her most likely diagnosis is:

   A. Bipolar disorder
   B. Depression with psychotic features
   C. Schizoid personality disorder
   D. Borderline personality disorder
   E. Schizotypal personality disorder

18. What is the characteristic electroencephalographic pattern noted in Creutzfeldt-Jakob disease?

   A. Three-per-second spike and wave
   B. Periodic high-amplitude sharp wave complexes
   C. Temporal spikes
   D. Generalized background slowing
   E. Periodic lateralizing epileptiform discharges (PLEDS)

19. To be diagnosed with polysubstance dependence, how many substances must a patient be found dependent on?

   A. Six substances, including caffeine
   B. Two groups of substances, where dependence criteria were met for one of the groups
   C. Four substances, including nicotine, but excluding caffeine
   D. Five specific substances
   E. Three or more groups of substances where dependence criteria were met for the groups, but not necessarily for any one particular substance

20. Which one of the following cerebrospinal fluid findings is indicative of aseptic meningitis?

   A. Variably increased lymphocytes, slightly decreased glucose, very high protein
   B. Moderately increased lymphocytes, decreased glucose, mildly elevated protein
   C. Highly increased neutrophils, decreased glucose, very high protein
   D. Slightly increased lymphocytes, normal glucose, mildly elevated protein
   E. Absent or few lymphocytes, normal glucose, very high protein

21. A small child is in the park with her mother. As the two interact, the child goes off to play for a brief time, then returns to her mother, then goes off to play, then returns to her mother. The child continues this pattern, regularly checking to see that the mother is still there. She would best fit into which one of Mahler's stages of separation-individuation?

    A. Normal autism
    B. Symbiosis
    C. Rapprochement
    D. Practicing
    E. Object constancy

22. What type of systemic poisoning results in the development of characteristic Mees' lines of the fingernails as in the photograph below?

    A. Mercury
    B. Arsenic
    C. Lead
    D. Organophosphates
    E. Ionizing radiation

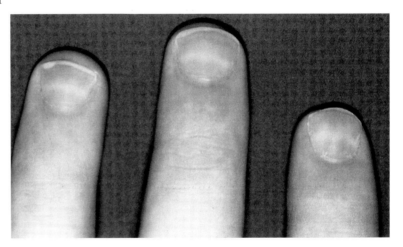

23. The assumption that there is no significant difference between two random samples of a population is called:

    A. Correlation coefficient
    B. Control group
    C. Analysis of variance (ANOVA)
    D. Regression analysis
    E. Null hypothesis

24. Organophosphate poisoning by pesticide exposure causes neurologic deficits by which one of the following mechanisms?

    A. Anticholinergic toxicity
    B. Cholinergic toxicity
    C. Gamma-aminobutyric acid blockade
    D. Serotonergic toxicity
    E. Dopaminergic toxicity

25. Emil Kraepelin used which one of the following terms in reference to schizophrenia?

    A. ~~Language delay~~
    B. Dementia praecox
    C. ~~Split-personality~~
    D. Rebound hyperactivity
    E. ~~Downward drift~~

26. Which one of the following agents causes poisoning in humans that can result in a blue line at the gingival margin?

    A. Manganese
    B. Thallium
    C. Arsenic
    D. Mercury
    E. Lead

27. The police bring a man into the hospital who has been stealing satellite dishes off of houses and setting them up in his own yard because he feels that he has a chip in his head that allows him to talk directly to God. He states that God has instructed him to do this as preparation for the second coming. When his wife is questioned about her husband's behavior she responds that indeed God has been directly communicating with her husband, and that she has helped him steal some of the larger satellite dishes. The wife's condition can best be described as:

    A. Schizoid personality disorder
    B. Delusional disorder
    C. Shared psychotic disorder
    D. Bipolar disorder
    E. Substance-induced psychotic disorder

28. Truncal ataxia or instability can result most specifically from a lesion to the:

    A. Cerebellar hemispheres
    B. Cerebellar vermis
    C. Cerebellopontine angle
    D. ~~Thalamus~~
    E. ~~Midbrain~~

29. Which one of the following neurotransmitters has large numbers of receptors in the spinal cord, is synthesized primarily from serine, and has been the subject of research involving negative symptom reduction in schizophrenia?

    A. GABA
    B. Glycine
    C. ~~Serotonin~~
    D. ~~Dopamine~~
    E. ~~Glutamate~~

147

30. All of the following are contraindications to lumbar puncture, EXCEPT:
    A. Thrombocytopenia
    B. Cerebral mass lesion
    C. Suspected meningitis with obtundation
    D. Recent head trauma
    E. Papilledema

31. What is the difference between posttraumatic stress disorder and acute stress disorder?
    A. The nature of the trauma
    B. The symptoms that follow the trauma
    C. The impairment resulting from the symptoms
    D. The duration of the symptoms
    E. The age of the patient

32. Which chromosomal abnormality is the most common cause of mental retardation?
    A. Trisomy 21
    B. Trisomy 18
    C. Cri-du-chat syndrome
    D. Fragile X syndrome
    E. Prader-Willi syndrome

33. Ending up in strange places with no recollection of how one got there, or finding objects in one's possession that one doesn't recall acquiring is most characteristic of:
    A. Anxiety
    B. Psychosis
    C. Histrionic personality
    D. Dissociation
    E. Depression

34. Which one of the following child abuse injuries is the most likely to result in death or long term sequelae?
    A. Embolic stroke from multiple bone fractures
    B. Subdural hematoma from head trauma
    C. Skull fracture from head trauma
    D. Cerebral hypoxia from choking
    E. Seizures from head and brain trauma

35. A 59 year-old man comes into your office complaining of depression. His wife of 25 years died unexpectedly five weeks ago. Since then he has been crying, has had little appetite but has lost no weight, and reports difficulty sleeping. He has been going out to dinner once each week with friends and says that it helps get his mind off of his wife's death. He is not suicidal. This is the first time in his life that he has had symptoms such as these. His most likely diagnosis is:
    A. Bipolar disorder
    B. Major depressive disorder
    C. Acute stress disorder
    D. Bereavement
    E. Dysthymic disorder

36. All of the following are considered lower motor neuron signs, EXCEPT:
    A. Hypotonia
    B. Muscle atrophy
    C. Fasciculations
    D. Babinski's sign
    E. Hyporeflexia

37. Mahler's stage that is characterized by a baby considering himself a fused entity with his mother, but developing increased ability to differentiate between the inner and outer world is called:
    A. Normal autism
    B. Symbiosis
    C. Differentiation
    D. Rapprochement
    E. Object constancy

38. Which one of the following therapeutics can eliminate benign paroxysmal positional vertigo?
    A. Diazepam
    B. Brandt-Daroff exercises
    C. Meclizine
    D. Metoclopramide
    E. Gabapentin

39. All of the following are diagnostic criteria for kleptomania, EXCEPT:
    A. Recurrent failure to resist stealing objects
    B. Decreased sense of tension immediately preceding the theft
    C. Pleasure at the time of committing the theft
    D. The theft is not done to express anger
    E. The act is not in the context of an antisocial personality disorder

40. The persistent vegetative state is characterized by all of the following, EXCEPT:
    A. Preserved eye opening
    B. Preserved response to noxious stimuli
    C. Preserved eye tracking
    D. Preserved swallowing
    E. Preserved sleep-wake cycles

41. An Hispanic man comes into the emergency room complaining of headache, insomnia, fear, anger, and despair. Your differential diagnosis is most likely to include which one of the following?
    A. Schizophrenia
    B. Schizoaffective disorder
    C. Panic disorder
    D. Attaque de nervios
    E. Myoclonic sleep disorder

42. What is the most typical effect of depression on nocturnal sleep?
    A. Decreased total sleep time
    B. Initial insomnia
    C. Middle insomnia
    D. Early morning awakening
    E. Sleep-wake cycle reversal

43. All of the following are symptoms that would be expected in a patient with pyromania, EXCEPT:
    A. Deliberate and purposeful fire setting
    B. Tension before the act
    C. Fascination with fire
    D. Pleasure when setting fires
    E. Setting fires for monetary gain or as an expression of political ideology

44. Apoptosis mediated by the *N*-methyl-D-aspartate (NMDA) receptor complex is most likely caused by elevated intracellular levels of which one of the following ions?
    A. Calcium
    B. Magnesium
    C. Sodium
    D. Potassium
    E. Chloride

45. A patient is brought into the emergency room following a fight with police. Upon examination the psychiatrist finds that the patient has a history of several discrete assaultive acts. His aggression in these situations was out of proportion to what one would consider normal. The patient has no other psychiatric disorder and no history of substance abuse. He has no significant medical history. What is his most likely diagnosis?

A. Impulse control disorder NOS
B. Pyromania
C. Mania
D. Temporal lobe epilepsy
E. Intermittent explosive disorder

46. A 45 year-old woman comes to the emergency room by ambulance unconscious and barely breathing. Paramedics found an empty bottle of 90 tablets of 2 mg clonazepam on her dresser that was filled at the pharmacy the day before. One of the first agents to administer to this patient in the acute setting is:

A. Naloxone
B. Flumazenil
C. Dimercaprol
D. Atropine
E. Epinephrine

47. All of the following should be considered in the differential diagnosis for intermittent explosive disorder, EXCEPT:

A. Delirium
B. Dementia
C. Temporal lobe epilepsy
D. Obsessive compulsive disorder
E. Substance intoxication

48. The electroencephalographic pattern that most often characterizes infantile spasms is:

A. Three-per-second spike and wave
B. Hypsarrhythmia
C. Periodic lateralizing epileptiform discharges (PLEDS)
D. Triphasic sharp waves
E. Burst-suppression pattern

49. Psychiatric symptoms which can be found with AIDS include all of the following, EXCEPT:

A. Progressive dementia
B. Personality changes
C. Heat intolerance
D. Depression
E. Loss of libido

50. Which one of the following structures is NOT considered part of Papez' circuit?

    A. Amygdala
    B. Mamillary body
    C. Fornix
    D. Cingulate gyrus
    E. Hippocampus

51. A child is in the doctor's office for an evaluation. His mother is waiting outside in the waiting area. The child is aware that his mother still exists even though she is not present in the room. For this to be true, the child must have reached which one of Mahler's stages of separation-individuation?

    A. Normal autism
    B. Practicing
    C. Differentiation
    D. Symbiosis
    E. Object constancy

52. All of the following neurologic disorders are believed to be caused by defects in the calcium channel system, EXCEPT:

    A. Lambert-Eaton myasthenic syndrome
    B. Malignant hyperthermia
    C. Hypokalemic periodic paralysis
    D. Familial hemiplegic migraine
    E. Benign familial neonatal convulsions

53. A young woman comes to her psychiatrist's office for help. She feels that others are exploiting her, but has no hard evidence. She is preoccupied with the lack of loyalty that she feels all of her friends have. She reads hidden demeaning connotations into the psychiatrist's comments. She bears grudges and is unforgiving of slights. Her most likely diagnosis is:

    A. Schizophrenia
    B. Schizotypal personality disorder
    C. Paranoid personality disorder
    D. Schizoid personality disorder
    E. Dementia

54. All of the following are clinical features of phenylketonuria, EXCEPT:

    A. Sensorineural deafness
    B. Infantile spasms
    C. Microcephaly
    D. A characteristic 'mousy' odor
    E. Light hair and skin pigmentation

55. Which one of the following dopaminergic tracts or areas is responsible for the parkinsonian side effects of antipsychotic medications?

    A. Mesolimbic-mesocortical tract
    B. Tuberoinfundibular tract
    C. Nigrostriatal tract
    D. Caudate neurons
    E. Ventral striatum

56. Which one of the following disorders is correctly depicted in the photomicrograph below?

    A. Lissencephaly
    B. Schizencephaly
    C. Dandy-Walker syndrome
    D. Arnold-Chiari type I
       malformation
    E. Arnold-Chiari type II
       malformation

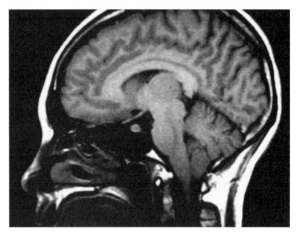

57. A schizophrenic man on an inpatient psychiatric unit develops a fever of 102.3°F, a high WBC count, unstable pulse and blood pressure, and rigidity in the arms and legs. The most likely diagnosis is:

    A. Meningitis
    B. Serotonin-specific reuptake inhibitor withdrawal
    C. Lithium toxicity
    D. Neuroleptic malignant syndrome
    E. PCP use

58. Internal carotid artery stenosis should be treated surgically by endarterectomy if the stenosis is symptomatic and above:

    A. 50%
    B. 60%
    C. 70%
    D. 80%
    E. 90%

59. A patient comes into the clinic because his family (whom he only sees one or two times per year) keeps telling him to "go see a shrink". He has no close relationships. He participates mainly in solitary activities. He has no desire for sexual activity with others. He is indifferent to the praise or criticism of others. On examination his affect is flat. His most likely diagnosis is:

    A. Schizoid personality disorder
    B. Schizotypal personality disorder
    C. Narcissistic personality disorder
    D. Major depressive disorder
    E. Dysthymic disorder

60. Poor outcome in Guillain-Barré syndrome is often associated with a preceding infection by which one of the following pathogens?

    A. *H. influenzae*
    B. *S. pneumoniae*
    C. *E. coli*
    D. *C. jejuni*
    E. *C. difficile*

61. All of the following are true regarding the Pearson correlation coefficient, EXCEPT:

    A. It spans from −1 to +1
    B. A positive value means that one variable moves the other variable in the same direction
    C. It can give information about cause and effect
    D. It indicates the degree of relationship
    E. A negative value means that one variable moves the other variable in the opposite direction

62. Which one of the following solid tumors metastasizes most frequently to the brain?

    A. Breast
    B. Colon
    C. Prostate
    D. Lung
    E. Thyroid

63. A pervasive pattern of social inhibition, feelings of inadequacy, and hypersensitivity to negative evaluation is most characteristic of:

    A. Obsessive-compulsive personality disorder
    B. Avoidant personality disorder
    C. Schizoid personality disorder
    D. Dependent personality disorder
    E. Passive-aggressive personality disorder

64. The most useful treatment for intractable post-lumbar puncture headache is:
    A. Repeat lumbar puncture with blood patch
    B. Bed-rest for two weeks
    C. Acetaminophen
    D. Hydrocodone
    E. Sumatriptan

65. Which one of the following baseline lab values would be the least important to obtain on a patient starting lithium therapy:
    A. Thyroid function tests
    B. Electrocardiogram
    C. White blood cell count
    D. Renal function tests
    E. VDRL

66. Compression of which one of the following peripheral nerves results in meralgia paresthetica?
    A. Sciatic
    B. Lateral femoral cutaneous
    C. Obturator
    D. Superior gluteal
    E. Common peroneal

67. Following a long day in the hospital, you visit your best friend from college who has recently had a baby. The child has been spending more of her time asleep than awake and is not particularly aware of the environment. If your friend were to ask you which of Mahler's stages of separation-individuation the child fits into, you would confidently answer:
    A. Normal autism
    B. Symbiosis
    C. Object constancy
    D. Practicing
    E. Differentiation

68. The classic finding on needle electromyography (EMG) that denotes the presence of a radiculopathy is:
    A. High-frequency, short-duration potentials
    B. Positive sharp waves and fibrillations
    C. Fasciculations
    D. Small, short motor unit potentials
    E. Myotonia

69. Which one of the following brain structure's dopaminergic neurons have been linked with Tourette's syndrome and the development of tics?

    A. Caudate
    B. Substantia nigra
    C. Amygdaloid body
    D. Frontal cortex
    E. Hippocampus

70. A 35 year-old woman delivers her baby at 40 weeks gestation without complication. Seven days later she experiences an acute onset of pancephalic headache, behavioral and personality changes, irritability, intermittent seizures and diplopia. The most likely diagnosis of her problem is:

    A. Aseptic meningitis
    B. Cerebral venous thrombosis
    C. Complicated migraine
    D. Bacterial meningoencephalitis
    E. Pseudotumor cerebri

71. When should advanced directives be discussed with a patient?

    A. At a time when the patient is competent
    B. When admitted to the hospital
    C. When a question of capacity arises
    D. When the patient is in pre-op
    E. When in the outpatient office

72. The most common congenital viral infection in newborns is caused by which one of the followed pathogens?

    A. Cytomegalovirus (CMV)
    B. Herpes simplex (HSV)
    C. Human immunodeficiency virus (HIV)
    D. Rubella
    E. Measles

73. A pervasive and excessive need to be taken care of that leads to submissive and clinging behavior as well as fears of separation, is characteristic of which one of the following?

    A. Obsessive-compulsive personality disorder
    B. Avoidant personality disorder
    C. Schizoid personality disorder
    D. Dependent personality disorder
    E. Passive aggressive personality disorder

74. The most frequent myopathy in patients over 50 years of age is:
   A. Dermatomyositis
   B. Polymyositis
   C. Fascioscapulohumeral dystrophy
   D. Inclusion body myositis
   E. Oculopharyngeal muscular dystrophy

75. Which one of the following is a behavioral effect of opioids?
   A. Miosis
   B. Increased arousal
   C. Euphoria
   D. Diarrhea
   E. Tachycardia

76. Duchenne's and Becker's muscular dystrophies are both disorders linked to an absence or deficiency of which one of the following muscle membrane proteins?
   A. Dystrophin
   B. Laminin
   C. Dystroglycan
   D. Spectrin
   E. Merosin

77. A 60 year-old woman is 63 pounds overweight. She comes to her psychiatrist's office with a complaint of increased irritability, noting a fight with her husband over how much sugar he put in her coffee one morning. She is fatigued and naps several times each day. She has no history of psychiatric problems, but adds that her husband now sleeps in the living room because of her snoring. Which one of the following is the most likely cause of the patient's symptoms?
   A. Night terrors
   B. Major depressive disorder
   C. Bipolar disorder
   D. Narcolepsy
   E. Sleep apnea

78. The rate-limiting enzyme in the dopamine synthetic pathway is:
   A. Dopa decarboxylase
   B. Tyrosine hydroxylase
   C. Dopamine β-hydroxylase
   D. Phenylethanolamine N-methyltransferase (PNMT)
   E. Catechol-O-methyltransferase

157

79. Which one of the following is the therapeutic range for lithium?
    A. 6–12 mEq/L
    B. 0.5–1.9 mEq/L
    C. 0.6–1.2 mEq/L
    D. 2–4 mEq/L
    E. >4 mEq/L

80. Alcohol, benzodiazepine sedative-hypnotic agents, and barbiturates all predominantly exert their clinical effects on the brain at which one of the following receptor sites?
    A. Cholinergic nicotinic
    B. *N*-methyl-D-aspartate (NMDA)
    C. Glycine
    D. GABA-A
    E. GABA-B

81. An elderly man comes into his doctor's office with symptoms of dementia and notable loss of executive functioning. Dysfunction of which one of the following brain regions would be most closely associated with the patient's loss of executive functioning?
    A. Caudate nucleus
    B. Putamen
    C. Globus palladus
    D. Frontal lobes
    E. Temporal lobes

82. A patient who is not malingering, but is believed to be producing the symptoms and signs of confusion or dementia involuntarily or unconsciously and believes that the symptoms are real is thought to have which one of the following conditions?
    A. Conversion disorder
    B. Ganser's syndrome
    C. Capgras syndrome
    D. Hypochondriasis
    E. Folie-à-deux

83. A child in school fails test after test. No matter how hard he studies, he fails. Over time he views himself as destined to fail and stops trying. Which one of the following theories best applies to this child's situation?
    A. The epigenetic principle
    B. Industry theory
    C. Cognition theory
    D. Learned helplessness
    E. Sensory deprivation

84. Entacopone and tolcapone exert their antiparkinsonian effects on which one of the following enzymes?
    A. Catechol-O-methyltransferase
    B. Monamine oxidase type A
    C. Monoamine oxidase type B
    D. Dopa decarboxylase
    E. Dopamine β-hydroxylase

85. Which one of the following could drastically increase lithium levels?
    A. Citalopram
    B. Carbamazepine
    C. Sertraline
    D. Ibuprofen
    E. Acetominophen

86. The neurologic examination finding of Argyll Robertson pupils occurs in a majority of patients with which one of the following conditions:
    A. Lyme disease
    B. Multiple sclerosis
    C. Tabes dorsalis
    D. Bubonic plague
    E. Intracerebral aneurysm

87. A patient on paroxetine complains of nausea, insomnia, muscle aches, anxiety, and dizziness. Which one of the following is the most likely explanation?
    A. He has the flu
    B. He has irritable bowel syndrome
    C. He stopped taking his antidepressant abruptly
    D. He is faking the symptoms
    E. He has multiple sclerosis

88. A 33 year-old man with known epilepsy has a 45-second generalized tonic-clonic seizure at a bus stop outdoors. He is brought to the nearest ER and once he is arousable and awake is found to have a marked right-sided hemiparesis. What is the best explanation of this occurrence?
    A. Postictal stroke
    B. Todd's paralysis
    C. Complicated postictal migraine
    D. Conversion disorder
    E. Transient ischemic attack (TIA)

159

89. All of the following have active metabolites, EXCEPT:
    A. Oxazepam
    B. Chlordiazepoxide
    C. Triazolam
    D. Clonazepam
    E. Quazepam

90. The disease known as tropical spastic paraparesis is considered to be a _____ caused by the _____ virus.
    A. Myelopathy; HTLV-1
    B. Neuropathy; HTLV-1
    C. Myelopathy; herpes simplex
    D. Neuropathy; herpes simplex
    E. Neuropathy; HIV type 1

91. To control aggression in a mentally retarded child, which one of the following would be most effective?
    A. Clonazepam
    B. Mirtazepine
    C. Doxepin
    D. Lithium
    E. Naltrexone

92. All of the following diseases are associated with expansion of trinucleotide repeat sequences, EXCEPT:
    A. Friedrich's ataxia
    B. Myotonic dystrophy
    C. Multiple system atrophy
    D. Fragile X syndrome
    E. Huntington's disease

93. Which one of the following dopaminergic pathways or areas is associated with the antipsychotic effects of the antipsychotic medications?
    A. Nigrostriatal pathway
    B. Mesolimbic-mesocortical pathway
    C. Tuberoinfundibular pathway
    D. Caudate nucleus
    E. Amygdaloid body

94. The characteristic bedside neurologic diagnostic sign known as the "battle sign" is indicative of which one of the following pathologies:
    A. Basilar skull fracture
    B. Frontal lobe damage
    C. Increased intracranial pressure
    D. Hypocalcemia
    E. Impending transtentorial cerebral herniation

95. Of the following combinations of medications, which one would the knowledgeable psychiatrist most want to avoid?
    A. Fluoxetine-lithium
    B. Fluoxetine-phenelzine
    C. Citalopram-valproic acid
    D. Citalopram-aripiprazole
    E. Mirtazapine-lamotrigine

96. Which one of the following agents is the best choice for treating attention-deficit hyperactivity disorder in a patient with Tourette's syndrome?
    A. Bupropion
    B. Methylphenidate
    C. Dextroamphetamine
    D. Atomoxatine
    E. Clonidine

97. A method of obtaining a prediction for the value of one variable in relation to another variable is called:
    A. Correlation coefficient
    B. Control group
    C. Analysis of variance (ANOVA)
    D. Regression analysis
    E. Null hypothesis

98. Which one of the following oral agents would be most beneficial in the treatment of limb spasticity related to multiple sclerosis?
    A. Clonazepam
    B. Phenytoin
    C. Lioresal
    D. Phenobarbital
    E. Cyproheptadine

99. A measurement of the direction and strength of the relationship between two variables is called:

    A. Correlation coefficient
    B. Control group
    C. Analysis of variance (ANOVA)
    D. Regression analysis
    E. Null hypothesis

100. A patient in the intensive care unit is delirious and agitated. The electro-encephalogram demonstrates a characteristic pattern of triphasic waves and some generalized background slowing. What other clinical bedside sign would you be most likely to see in this patient on physical examination?

    A. Herpetic skin vesicles
    B. Penile chancre
    C. Asterixis
    D. Dupuytren's contractures
    E. Pulmonary rales

101. A researcher at a university hospital takes rats and randomly crowds them, shocks them, feeds them at different times, and uses bright lights and loud noise to interrupt their sleep. The rats eventually decrease their movement and exploratory behavior. What can be learned from this?

    A. This researcher has serious psychological problems and really needs a girl-friend
    B. This is evidence for Freud's theory of coercive electrocution
    C. Unpredictability and lack of environmental control play a large role in the generation of stress
    D. Rats enjoy loud noise and bright lights, especially when accompanied by electric shocks
    E. Aggression among members of the same species is common

102. All of the following are possible side effects of valproic acid, EXCEPT:

    A. Weight gain
    B. Alopecia
    C. Hemorrhagic pancreatitis
    D. Thrombocytosis
    E. Liver failure

103. A patient is admitted to the hospital for suicidal behavior. The insurance company refuses to pay for the stay after the third day, and the patient is still suicidal. Which one of the following answer choices is the most ethical way to proceed?

    A. Send the patient home because the insurance company refuses to pay
    B. Secretly tell the patient to sign out against medical advice
    C. Make the patient pay out of pocket, and if they can't afford it, discharge them
    D. Sue the insurance company
    E. Continue to treat the patient as long as necessary, and file an appeal with the insurance company after discharge

104. The mechanism by which clonidine can help alleviate the symptoms of opioid withdrawal is through mediation of:

    A. Norepinephrine reuptake inhibition
    B. Alpha-2 adrenergic agonism
    C. Alpha-1 adrenergic antagonism
    D. Dopamine antagonism
    E. Serotonin antagonism

105. On a urine toxicology screen, how long can heroin be detected?

    A. 12 hours
    B. 48 hours
    C. 4 weeks
    D. 72 hours
    E. 8 days

163

106. An elderly hospitalized patient with vascular risk factors has a stroke. The patient's behavior following the stroke is noted to be unusually calm and markedly hypersexual. This presentation likely resulted from a stroke to the:

    A. Hippocampi
    B. Nucleus accumbens
    C. Hypothalamus
    D. Occipital lobes
    E. Amygdaloid bodies

107. A psychiatrist is working on an inpatient unit and one of her patients has a very resistant case of depression. She considers the option of giving the patient electro-convulsive therapy (ECT). Which one of the following should make her most concerned about giving this patient ECT?

    A. Pregnancy
    B. Past seizures
    C. Family history of severe depression
    D. Psychotic symptoms
    E. Recent myocardial infarction

108. A 20 year-old man comes to your office with his mother because of behavioral problems. On examination you note that he is verbally inappropriate, mildly mentally retarded, very tall and somewhat obese and has a small penis and scrotum. His condition is most likely due to which one of the following?

    A. Absence of an X chromosome (XO)
    B. Presence of an extra X chromosome (XXY)
    C. Trisomy 21
    D. Deletion on the paternal chromosome 15
    E. Trisomy 18

109. A psychiatrist is consulted on a medical unit because there is a patient with a substance abuse history who is in need of pain control. Which one of the following answer choices would be the best way to treat this patient's pain?

    A. Large doses of opiates
    B. A mixture of opiates and benzodiazepines
    C. Patient-controlled analgesia
    D. No opiates of any kind
    E. PRN (as needed) buprenorphine

110. A 35 year-old woman presents to your office with her husband. He tells you that she has experienced discrete episodes of physical and verbal aggression directed toward other people and property for the past year. Her husband states that the aggressiveness is not precipitated by any particular trigger and is completely unpredictable and intermittent. In between these bouts of aggression, the patient is otherwise fine and leads a normal life as a wife and mother. The most plausible diagnosis is:

    A. Borderline personality disorder
    B. Intermittent explosive disorder
    C. Antisocial personality disorder
    D. Psychotic disorder due to temporal lobe seizures
    E. Bipolar I disorder, with manic and psychotic episodes

111. While working on the ward of a state hospital, a psychiatrist comes across a patient with catatonic schizophrenia. The patient sits in one spot for extended periods of time, without changing position. This phenomenon is best described as:

    A. Psychomotor retardation
    B. Catalepsy
    C. Cataplexy
    D. Catatonia
    E. Stereotypy

112. Which one of the following agents has the unique mechanism of action of being a dopamine and norepinephrine reuptake inhibitor?
    A. Tiagabine
    B. Venlafaxine
    C. Duloxetine
    D. Bupropion
    E. Atomoxetine

113. Harry Harlow conducted a series of experiments with Rhesus monkeys. Some of his monkeys would stare vacantly into space, engage in self mutilation, and follow stereotyped behavior patterns. To which one of the following groups did these monkeys belong?
    A. Total isolation (no caretaker or peer bond)
    B. Mother-only reared
    C. Peer-only reared
    D. Partial isolation (can see, hear and smell other monkeys)
    E. Separation (taken from caretaker after developing bond)

114. Sildenafil, vardenafil and tadalafil all improve erectile dysfunction by which one of the following mechanisms?
    A. Phosphodiesterase 5 inhibition
    B. Calcium channel antagonism
    C. Nitric oxide antagonism
    D. Alpha 1 adrenergic antagonism
    E. Carbonic anhydrase inhibition

115. Which one of the following medications is the most likely to cause parkinsonian symptoms?
    A. Maprotiline
    B. Amoxapine
    C. Venlafaxine
    D. Doxepin
    E. Clomipramine

116. If you divide the incidence of a disease in those with risk factors by the incidence of the same disease in those without risk factors, the result is called the:
    A. Relative incidence
    B. Attributable risk
    C. Relative risk
    D. Period incidence
    E. Incidence risk

117. Cingulotomy is a treatment used for which one of the following choices?
    A. Psychosis
    B. Depression
    C. Obsessive-compulsive disorder
    D. Generalized anxiety disorder
    E. Pedophilia

118. All of the following causative etiologic factors are believed to contribute to the genesis of dissociative identity disorder, EXCEPT:
    A. A traumatic life event
    B. A vulnerability for the disorder
    C. Environmental factors
    D. Absence of external support
    E. Prior viral infection or exposure

119. Which one of the following is considered first-line of treatment for a mute catatonic patient who is brought into the emergency room?
    A. Haloperidol
    B. Methylphenidate
    C. Risperidone
    D. Lorazepam
    E. Paroxetine

120. All of the following are features of malingering, EXCEPT:
    A. Findings are compatible with self-inflicted injuries
    B. Medical records may have been tampered with or altered
    C. Family members are able to verify the consistency of symptoms
    D. Symptoms are vague or ill defined
    E. History and examination do not yield complaints or problems

121. Which one of the following answer choices is most true concerning mutism?
    A. It is a psychiatric disorder only
    B. It is a neurological disorder only
    C. It is a function of a high-energy environment
    D. It is associated with both psychiatric and neurological conditions
    E. It is most frequently the result of head trauma

122. Therapy that is focused on the measurement of autonomic processes and teaching patients to gain voluntary control over these physiological parameters through operant conditioning is called:

    A. Stimulus-response therapy
    B. Biofeedback
    C. Relaxation training
    D. Behavior therapy
    E. Desensitization

123. A patient has overdosed on lithium following a fight with her boyfriend. Her lithium level is 2.8 mEq/L. She is exhibiting severe signs of lithium toxicity. Which one of the following answer choices is the best treatment at this time?

    A. IV fluids
    B. Celecoxib
    C. Wait and watch
    D. Hemodialysis
    E. Gastric lavage

124. The most useful long-term treatment parameter for a noncompliant patient with schizophrenia and history of violence would be:

    A. Long-term state psychiatric hospitalization
    B. Partial hospitalization
    C. Day treatment program
    D. Outpatient commitment program
    E. Social skills training

125. Which one of the following is a dangerous combination?

    A. MAOI-lorazepam
    B. MAOI-acetominophen
    C. MAOI-meperidine
    D. MAOI-ziprasidone
    E. MAOI-loxapine

126. The psychiatrist's right to maintain a patient's secrecy in the face of a subpoena is known as:

    A. Privilege
    B. Confidentiality
    C. Communication rights
    D. Private rights
    E. Clinical responsibility

127. Which one of the following is NOT a requirement for treatment with clozapine?
    A. Baseline white blood cell (WBC) count before starting treatment
    B. Two WBC counts during the first seven days of treatment
    C. Weekly WBC count during the first six months of treatment
    D. WBC counts every two weeks after the first six months of treatment
    E. WBC count every week for four weeks following discontinuation of clozapine

128. All of the following are changes in sleep architecture noted in patients over age 65 years, EXCEPT:
    A. Lower percentage of stages 3 and 4 sleep
    B. Less total REM sleep
    C. Fewer REM episodes
    D. Increased awakening after sleep onset
    E. Shorter REM episodes

129. Which one of the following will increase clozapine levels?
    A. Red wine
    B. Cimetidine
    C. Cheese
    D. Acetaminophen
    E. Aripiprazole

130. The most widely abused recreational substance among US high school students is:
    A. Alcohol
    B. Cocaine
    C. Lysergic acid diethylamide (LSD)
    D. Inhalants
    E. Cannabis

131. Beck, in the theory supporting his cognitive triad, felt that "distorted negative thoughts" lead to:
    A. Failure of good enough mothering
    B. Transitional object development
    C. Mania
    D. Depression
    E. Aggression toward the primary caregiver

132. The mechanism of action of the sleeping aid ramelteon involves which one of the following receptor systems?

    A. Acetylcholine
    B. GABA-A
    C. Histamine
    D. Melatonin
    E. Norepinephrine

133. What is alogia?

    A. Poverty of movement
    B. Poverty of emotion
    C. Poverty of speech only
    D. Poverty of thought content only
    E. Poverty of speech and thought content

134. The rapid-cycling specifier in bipolar I disorder applies to patients who have had _____ mood disturbance episodes over the previous _____ .

    A. 4; 6 months
    B. 4; 12 months
    C. 6; 24 months
    D. 6; 12 months
    E. 3; 12 months

135. Which one of the following best explains pathological gambling?

    A. Primary reinforcement
    B. Random reinforcement
    C. Poor response to dexamethasone suppression testing
    D. Continuous reinforcement
    E. Cerebellar dysfunction

136. Late-onset schizophrenia is characterized by a more favorable prognosis and the onset of symptoms after age:

    A. 40 years
    B. 45 years
    C. 50 years
    D. 55 years
    E. 60 years

137. A group that does not receive treatment and is the standard for comparison is called the:
    A. Correlation coefficient
    B. Control group
    C. Analysis of variance (ANOVA)
    D. Regression analysis
    E. Null hypothesis

138. Bowlby's stages of childhood attachment disorder, after a lengthy departure of the child's mother, include all of the following, EXCEPT:
    A. Protest
    B. Despair
    C. Detachment
    D. Denial of affection
    E. Acceptance

139. You have a patient whom you think has both depression and attention-deficit/hyperactivity disorder. Which one of the following medications would be the best choice for this patient?
    A. Fluoxetine
    B. Paroxetine
    C. Buproprion
    D. Venlafaxine
    E. Imipramine

140. Which one of the following agents is FDA approved for use in the pediatric population under 18 years of age?
    A. Paroxetine
    B. Citalopram
    C. Sertraline
    D. Mirtazapine
    E. Velafaxine

141. During a session a therapist tells the patient "I know you feel terrible right now, but things are going to get better with the passage of time". This type of statement is characteristic of which type of therapy?
    A. Supportive psychotherapy
    B. Psychodynamic psychotherapy
    C. Psychoanalysis
    D. Play therapy
    E. Cognitive behavioral therapy

142. All of the following statements regarding risperidone intramuscular injection (Risperdal Consta) are true, EXCEPT:

    A. The formulation comes in three doses: 25, 37.5 and 50 mg
    B. The drug must be refrigerated before reconstitution
    C. The drug must be reconstituted with sterile water
    D. The drug must be administered only to the deltoid or the gluteus muscles
    E. The drug is dosed to be administered every two weeks

143. A patient is brought into the emergency room unconscious with signs of respiratory depression. The patient was found unconscious on the bathroom floor and has written a suicide note saying that he wanted to die. An empty pill bottle which had contained his mother's prescription for morphine was found on the bathroom floor. Which one of the following would the knowledgeable physician use to treat this patient?

    A. Buprenorphine
    B. Benztropine
    C. Naloxone
    D. Naltrexone
    E. Bromocriptine

144. Which one of Kübler-Ross' stages of reaction to impending death corresponds to a period when a patient goes through self-blame for his illness and asks "Why me?"

    A. Shock and denial
    B. Anger
    C. Bargaining
    D. Depression
    E. Acceptance

145. Asking patients if they are suicidal will:

    A. Increase the chance that they will kill themselves
    B. Help them plan out their suicide
    C. Scare the patients
    D. Have no influence on whether patients will attempt suicide
    E. Make patients refuse to speak to their therapist any further

146. The usual and accepted length of a period of grief following the death of a loved one can last up to:

    A. 3 months
    B. 6 months
    C. 9 months
    D. 12 months
    E. 24 months

147. In which one of the following groups has suicide increased dramatically over the past 40+ years?
    A. Geriatrics
    B. Married men
    C. Married women
    D. Adolescents
    E. Chronic alcoholics

148. Which one of the following sleep-promoting agents has the longest half-life?
    A. Ramelteon
    B. Zolpidem
    C. Zaleplon
    D. Eszopiclone
    E. Triazolam

149. What is the therapeutic range for valproic acid?
    A. 50–150 ng/mL
    B. 25–50 ng/mL
    C. 200–250 ng/mL
    D. 1000–1500 ng/mL
    E. 0.5–0.15 ng/mL

150. A psychiatrist interviews a Japanese immigrant who was brought to the hospital by her family for depression. In the meeting with her she does not endorse any significant symptoms. When speaking to the family, they state that she has been having many of the symptoms that she previously denied. Which one of the following is the most likely explanation for this situation?
    A. She is lying
    B. She is psychotic and paranoid
    C. Culture
    D. Mental retardation
    E. The family is lying

Answers

Test Number **THREE**
ANSWER KEY   ③

1	C	51	E	101	C
2	A	52	E	102	D
3	B	53	C	103	E
4	B	54	A	104	B
5	E	55	C	105	D
6	D	56	D	106	E
7	E	57	D	107	E
8	E	58	C	108	B
9	D	59	A	109	C
10	C	60	D	110	B
11	D	61	C	111	B
12	A	62	D	112	D
13	E	63	B	113	D
14	E	64	A	114	A
15	E	65	E	115	B
16	A	66	B	116	C
17	D	67	A	117	C
18	B	68	B	118	E
19	E	69	A	119	D
20	D	70	B	120	C
21	C	71	A	121	D
22	B	72	A	122	B
23	E	73	D	123	D
24	B	74	D	124	D
25	B	75	C	125	C
26	E	76	A	126	A
27	C	77	E	127	B
28	B	78	B	128	C
29	B	79	C	129	B
30	C	80	D	130	E
31	D	81	D	131	D
32	D	82	B	132	D
33	D	83	D	133	E
34	B	84	A	134	B
35	D	85	D	135	B
36	D	86	C	136	B
37	B	87	C	137	B
38	B	88	B	138	E
39	B	89	A	139	C
40	B	90	A	140	C
41	D	91	D	141	A
42	D	92	C	142	D
43	E	93	B	143	C
44	A	94	A	144	B
45	E	95	B	145	D
46	B	96	D	146	D
47	D	97	D	147	D
48	B	98	C	148	D
49	C	99	A	149	A
50	A	100	C	150	C

35   34   33

ANSWER EXPLANATIONS

Question 1. C. This question focuses on Piaget's stages of cognitive development. (Just in case you don't have it mastered after Test Two.) In the concrete operations stage, egocentric thought changes to operational thought where another's point of view can be taken into consideration. In concrete operations children can put things in order and group objects according to common characteristics. They develop the understanding of conservation (a tall cup and a wide cup can both hold equal volumes of water) and reversibility (ice can change to water and back to ice again).
K&S Ch. 2

Question 2. A. Transient global amnesia (TGA) presents with a reversible anterograde and retrograde memory loss. It is accompanied by inability to learn newly acquired information and total amnesia of events occurring during the attacks. Patients remain awake and alert during attacks, without motor or sensory deficits. Patients retain their personal information and identity and can carry on personal activities as usual. The patient may ask the same question repeatedly. Affected patients are usually in their fifties or older. Men are more often affected than women. Attacks are acute in onset and can last for several hours, but rarely greater than 12 hours. The true mechanism of TGA is unknown. One potential theory is a relationship between TGA and bilateral hippocampal ischemia, possibly migrainous in nature. Other theories postulate a relationship of TGA to epilepsy, migraine, brain tumor, and cerebrovascular events or risk factors. Onset often occurs after physical exertion, sexual exertion or exposure to extremes of temperature. The prognosis of patients with TGA is generally benign. There is no noted increased risk for future ischemic attacks or stroke. Recurrence is uncommon and there is no need for extensive workup. No particular treatment is indicated.
B&D Ch. 57

Question 3. B. GABA is the major inhibitory neurotransmitter of the CNS. It is thought to decrease seizure activity, decrease mania, and lessen anxiety. It has three receptors, GABA-A, GABA-B, and GABA-C. Topiramate works on the GABA-A receptor, potentiating its activity. Gabapentin decreases seizure activity, but does not work directly on the GABA receptors or transporter. Tiagabine is an anticonvulsant which works by blocking the GABA transporter.
K&S Ch. 3

Question 4. B. The case described in this question is a classic presentation of Lyme disease. The offending organism in Lyme infection is the spirochete *Borrelia burgdorferi*, whose vector is the deer tick: *Ixodes dammini*

175

in the eastern USA, *Ixodes pacificus* in the western USA and *Ixodes ricinus* in Europe. Lyme is the great mimicker of other neurologic conditions and it can manifest in many different ways. Early infection can appear as a meningitis, a unilateral or bilateral Bell's palsy (as in this question), a painful radiculoneuritis, optic neuritis, mononeuritis multiplex, or Guillain-Barré syndrome. After initial infection, in about two-thirds of patients a classic Lyme rash can be noted (erythema chronicum migrans), a painless expanding macular patch. Diagnosis begins with initial ELISA serologic screening, which, if positive, can be confirmed by Western blot testing. Cerebrospinal fluid lyme antibody can also be titred by polymerase chain reaction (PCR). Treatments of first choice are parenteral antibiotics: ceftriaxone or penicillin intravenously for two to four weeks. Tetracycline and chloramphenicol are treatment alternatives in penicillin or cephalosporin allergic patients. Cerebrospinal fluid persistence of antibody production may continue for years after successful treatment and remission and in isolation does not indicate active disease.

Rocky Mountain spotted fever is caused by the tick-borne spirochete *R. rickettsii*. Different tick species can carry this organism and the disease can be seen all over the world. The condition starts with fever, headache, muscle aches and gastrointestinal symptoms about 2–14 days after the tick bite. There is a rash that appears initially around the wrists and hands and spreads over days to the feet and forearms. Systemic symptoms can also appear and include meningoencephalitis, renal failure and pulmonary edema. Retinal vasculitis may be seen on fundoscopic examination. Diagnosis is confirmed by direct immunofluorescence or immunoperoxidase skin biopsy staining. Treatment is undertaken with oral or parenteral tetracycline or chloramphenicol and a switch to oral doxycycline for a total of about 10–14 days of therapy.

Yersinia pestis is an organism causing the plague, a zoonotic infection of wild rodents, transmitted by the bites of infected fleas to human victims. Human infection can result in infectious lymphadenitis (bubonic plague), pneumonic, septicemic, or meningeal plague. Primary or secondary meningitis can occur from *Y. pestis* infection. Diagnosis is confirmed by cerebrospinal fluid Gram stain and culture. Treatment of primary infection is undertaken with intramuscular streptomycin twice daily for ten days. Meningitis is treated with intravenous chloramphenicol for at least ten days.

Leptospirosis is caused by zoonotic infection from *Leptospira interrogans*. This spirochete is transmitted to humans by contact with urine from infected rodents or farm animals or soil or water that contains the infected urine. About 15% of patients develop a meningitic picture. Severe systemic symptoms include jaundice, hemorrhage and renal failure. Diagnosis can be confirmed by organism isolation from blood or cerebrospinal fluid. Severe disease is treated with at least a week-long course of parenteral penicillin G. Less severe illness can be treated with a week-long course of oral doxycycline.

Treponema pallidum is the spirochete associated with syphilis, which is explained in depth elsewhere in this volume.

B&D Ch. 59

Question 5. E. This is a clear case of body dysmorphic disorder. It is characterized by an imagined belief that there is a defect in part or all of the body. The belief does not approach delusional proportions. The patient complains of the defect and his perception is out of proportion to any minor physical abnormality that exists. The person's concern is grossly excessive, but when pressed he can admit that it may be excessive (this is why it is not delusional). Treatment with serotonergic drugs and therapy is usually helpful; plastic surgery is not.

K&S Ch. 17

Question 6. D. Tourette's syndrome (TS) is a tic disorder that occurs in about 10 to 700 in 100 000 individuals. Boys are affected more often than girls. The manifestations begin between 2 and 10 years of age. Early signs include cranial motor tics, including eye blinks, stretching of the lower face and head-shaking. Vocal tics can include throat clearing, grunting, coughing, sniffing and involuntary swearing (coprolalia). Both motor and vocal tics must be present to meet criteria for the disorder. Symptoms tend to peak in severity during adolescence and often wane during adulthood. Behavioral manifestations are common in TS and can include attention-deficit/hyperactivity disorder (ADHD), obsessive-compulsive disorder, and conduct disorder. Obsessions and rituals often revolve around counting and symmetry. The diagnosis is clinical and is based on the appropriate history and physical examination.

Evidence suggests that TS is hereditary and likely follows an autosomal dominant pattern of inheritance. Concordance in monozygotic twins is greater than 85%. Exact mendelian inheritance pattern for the disorder is not yet elucidated. Positron emission tomography studies suggest increased dopaminergic activity in the ventral striatum and abnormal release and reuptake of dopamine as being probable pathophysiologic mechanisms.

Treatment of TS is symptomatic. Tics can be treated with conventional or atypical neuroleptic agents, such as haloperidol, pimozide, fluphenazine, risperidone, quetiapine, and olanzapine. Guanfacine and clonidine are useful for both tics and ADHD symptoms. Obsessive-compulsive disorder can be treated with the selective serotonin reuptake inhibitors. The stimulants methylphenidate, pemoline, and dextroamphetamine, must be used carefully as they can either alleviate or exacerbate tics. Atomoxetine, a non-stimulant ADHD medication that is a norepinephrine reuptake inhibitor, is an excellent choice for ADHD in TS because it does not exacerbate tics.

B&D Ch. 77

Question 7. E. In order to diagnose schizoaffective disorder (as opposed to bipolar), one needs a two-week period where the patient has had psychotic symptoms in the absence of mood symptoms. The patient must also have had periods of mania or depression during which psychotic symptoms are present. A bipolar patient may have psychotic symptoms during periods of mania or depression, but these psychotic symptoms cease when the mood disturbance resolves.

K&S Ch. 14

Question 8. E. The safest choice of all the answers is of course electroconvulsive shock therapy (ECT). There is no real contraindication to ECT in the normal pregnancy. If the pregnancy is high-risk or complicated, fetal monitoring can be carried out during the procedure. Haloperidol would be the next best choice and is of course a butyrophenone antipsychotic agent. Haloperidol can pass into breast milk and so mothers should not breast feed if they are taking this drug. Haloperidol is a category C agent in pregnancy and it has been shown to cause teratogenicity in animals. Human studies are inadequate in this regard and the benefit needs to outweigh the risk before the drug is given to a pregnant patient. The first trimester is the most vulnerable period of pregnancy for teratogenic fetal effects. Lithium is of course contraindicated in pregnancy because of the risk of Ebstein's anomaly of the tricuspid valves. The risk of Ebstein's anomaly is 1 in 1000. Lithium is also excreted into breast milk. Lithium is a category D agent in pregnancy. Divalproex sodium is also dangerous in pregnancy because of the first trimester risk of fetal spina bifida and neural tube defects in about 1–2% of those taking the drug in their first trimester. Folic acid supplementation (1–4 mg daily) taken during the first trimester of pregnancy reduces the risk of neural tube defects

with divalproex sodium. Divalproex is a category D agent in pregnancy. Aripiprazole has not been well studied in pregnancy, but is a category C agent in pregnancy. There are animal studies that have revealed fetal abnormalities as a direct result of maternal exposure to aripiprazole.
K&S Ch. 36

Question 9. D. This is a case of delirium. Delirium presents as confusion, impaired consciousness (often fluctuating), emotional lability, hallucinations or illusions, and irrational behavior. Its onset is rapid and its course fluctuates. Thinking is often disordered, and attention and awareness are often impaired. Causes are usually medical or organic in nature (metabolic imbalance, infection, intracranial bleed, etc.). The patient's increased age makes him more susceptible to a delirium. Dementia and depression are incorrect because the time of onset of symptoms for these disorders is over weeks to months, not days.
K&S Ch. 10

Question 10. C. Metoclopramide (Reglan) is a potent antiemetic agent that is a benzamide derivative, has phenothiazine-like properties, and can cause extrapyramidal side effects. It is a potent antagonist of dopamine type 2 (D2) receptors and blocks these receptors on the chemoreceptor trigger zone of the area postrema which prevents nausea and emesis. Because of it's affinity for the D2 receptor it has been known to cause extrapyramidal side effects (EPS), especially at higher doses, and can also cause tardive dyskinesia after long-term use and discontinuation.
Ondansetron (Zofran) is a potent antiemetic like metoclopramide, but its mechanism does not involve D2 so it does not have the potential to cause EPS or tardive dyskinesia. It is a potent 5-HT3 antagonist and also works in the area postrema and likely on peripheral vagal nerve receptors.
Hydroxyzine (Atarax, Vistaril), like diphenhydramine (Benadryl) is an antihistamine that also has analgesic and antiemetic properties. Is has no effect on dopamine receptors and therefore does not cause EPS or tardive dyskinesia.
Tizanidine (Zanaflex) is a potent sedating muscle relaxant that works via α-2 adrenergic agonism. It can lower blood pressure, much like clonidine which has this same mechanism of action. It does not affect dopamine receptors and does not cause EPS or tardive dyskinesia.
K&S Ch. 36

Question 11. D. Sleep attacks are the most common symptom of narcolepsy. Narcolepsy is also characterized by cataplexy (a sudden loss of muscle tone) and hallucinations while falling asleep and waking up. Patients with narcolepsy can have sleep paralysis where they wake up and are often unable to move. Their sleep also characteristically goes into REM cycles when sleep begins. Treatments involve taking regular naps during the day, stimulants, and antidepressants.
K&S Ch. 24

Question 12. A. The primary auditory cortex localizes to the superior temporal gyrus (Heschl's gyrus) in both temporal lobes. Cortical deafness can result from bilateral strokes to the temporal lobes destroying Heschl's gyri. The thalamus is of course the relay station for much of the sensory input to the brain. The frontal lobes are responsible for attention, concentration, set-shifting, organization and executive functioning and planning. The occipital lobes are the location of the calcarine cortex that is responsible for interpreting and processing visual input and stimuli.
B&D Chs. 11&12

Question 13. E. Glycine is a neurotransmitter synthesized from serine. It is a necessary adjunctive neurotransmitter at the NMDA receptor that binds with glutamate. It is also an independent inhibitory neurotransmitter with its own receptors that open chloride ion channels. The activity of glycine on the NMDA receptor is an area of research for schizophrenia, with some studies showing improvement in negative symptoms with the use of glycine or glycine analogues. The highest concentrations of glycine receptors have been found in the spinal cord. Mutations of this receptor lead to a rare condition called hyperekplexia where the main symptom is an exaggerated startle response.

K&S Ch. 3

Question 14. E. Gabapentin and pregabalin are both FDA-approved for the systemic oral treatment of postherpetic neuralgia. The lidocaine transdermal patch (Lidoderm) is FDA-approved for the topical and local treatment of postherpetic neuralgic pain. Carbamazepine and oxcarbazepine are not FDA-approved, but both have been shown to be acceptable alternatives for the treatment of trigeminal and postherpetic neuralgia. Phenytoin, an anticonvulsant agent, has no place in the treatment of postherpetic neuralgia.

B&D Ch. 59

Question 15. E. This is a clear case of acute stress disorder. Acute stress disorder occurs after a person is exposed to a traumatic event. The patient then feels anxiety, detachment, derealization, feelings of being "in a daze", dissociative amnesia, and numbing. Flashbacks and avoidance of stimuli can occur. The symptoms do not last longer than 4 weeks, and occur within 4 weeks of the traumatic event (as opposed to PTSD where symptoms must last more than 1 month).

K&S Ch. 16

Question 16. A. Epidural hematomas result most often from head trauma and skull fracture that cause a tear to the middle meningeal artery or one of its branches. They occur between the dura and the skull table and appear as a biconvex or lens-shaped hyperdensity on CT scan of the brain. Most epidural hematomas are localized to the temporal or parietal areas, but they can occur elsewhere in the brain as well.
Subdural hematoma is the most common intracranial hematoma, found in 20–25% of all traumatic brain injury patients who are comatose. The subdural hematoma is believed to result from tearing of the bridging veins over the cortical surface, or from trauma to the venous sinuses or their tributaries. Subdural hematoma is more common in patients over 60, particularly alcoholics, presumably because the dura is tightly adhered to the skull table in this population. The other answer choices are distracters.

B&D Ch. 56

Question 17. D. Though one could argue for bits and pieces of other diagnoses, when taking the whole picture into consideration, this patient is a case of borderline personality disorder. Borderline personality disorder is characterized by frantic efforts to avoid abandonment, unstable interpersonal relationships, disturbed self image, impulsive behavior, recurrent suicidality or self mutilation, affective instability, chronic feelings of emptiness, intense anger, and stress related paranoia or severe dissociative symptoms. The woman in the question clearly presents with many of these symptoms.

K&S Ch. 27

Question 18. B. Electroencephalograms (EEG) of patients with Creutzfeld-Jakob disease (CJD) classically demonstrate theta and delta waves with periodic burst-suppression pattern and periodic, rhythmic paroxysmal sharp-wave complexes. These high-amplitude sharp wave-forms are present in up to 80% of patients with CJD. This pattern can also be noted in subacute sclerosing panencephalitis, but with longer interburst intervals.

179

The 3-per-second spike and wave pattern is indicative of absence seizures (petit mal epilepsy). Temporal spikes would be indicative of a seizure focus in the temporal lobe, most often of the partial-complex variety. Generalized background slowing can be noted in postictal states, coma, delirium, or following anoxic brain injury. It usually indicates a decrease in the level of consciousness. Periodic lateralizing epileptiform discharges (PLEDS) are characteristic of herpes simplex encephalitis, but can also be seen in acute hemispheric stroke, tumors, abscesses and meningitis.

B&D Chs. 36&59

Question 19. E. The criteria for polysubstance dependence state that during a 12 month period the patient repeatedly used at least three groups of substances (excluding caffeine and nicotine), but no single substance predominated. During this period, the dependence criteria need to be met for groups of substances, but not for any one particular substance.

K&S Ch. 12

Question 20. D. Aseptic or viral meningitis tends to produce a cerebrospinal fluid (CSF) assay with mild to moderate lymphocytic pleocytosis, normal glucose and normal to mildly elevated protein. Gram stain and cultures would be negative. A bacterial meningitis would produce a CSF as in answer choice C, with marked lymphocytosis, particularly polymorphonuclear neutrophils, markedly increased protein and decreased glucose. A fungal meningitis would produce a CSF as in answer choice B, with moderate lymphocytic pleocytosis, mildly decreased glucose and mildly increased protein. Tuberculous meningitis would produce a CSF with mild lymphocytic pleocytosis, mildly decreased glucose and markedly increased protein, as in answer choice A. Herpetic meningitis would produce a similar CSF picture to that in aseptic meningitis, but may also reveal a predominance of red blood cells in the CSF. Answer choice E is a CSF assay indicative of Guillain-Barré syndrome (acute inflammatory demyelinating polyneuropathy) which is characterized by a cytoalbuminergic dissociation with high protein (> 55 mg/dL) and an absence of significant pleocytosis.

B&D Ch. 59

Question 21. C. This question focuses on Mahler's stages of separation-individuation. The first stage is normal autism, lasting from birth to 2 months. In this stage the baby spends more time asleep than awake. The next stage is symbiosis, from 2 months to 5 months. In this stage the baby is developing the ability to distinguish the inner from the outer world. The child perceives himself as being part of a single entity with his mother. The following stage is differentiation, from 5 to 10 months. Here the child is drawn further into the outside world and begins to distinguish himself from his mother. Next is practicing. Practicing is from 10 to 18 months and is characterized by the baby's ability to move independently and explore the outside world. Practicing is followed by rapprochement between 18 and 24 months. In rapprochement the child's independence vacillates with his need for his mother. The child moves away from the mother, then quickly returns for reassurance. Mahler's last stage is object constancy, from 2 to 5 years. In this stage the child understands the permanence of other people, even when they are not present. It would be wise to know all of Mahler's stages well. You never know where you might see them again!

K&S Ch. 2

Question 22. B. Arsenic poisoning has both central and peripheral nervous system manifestations. Systemic manifestations include nausea, vomiting, diarrhea, hypotension, tachycardia, and vasomotor collapse that can lead to death. Stupor or encephalopathy may develop. Peripherally, arsenic causes a distal axonal neuropathy. Symptoms of the neuropathy may develop after two to three weeks following initial exposure. Skin manifestations may develop with more chronic exposure, particularly keratosis, melanosis, malignancies and characteristic Mees' lines of the fingernails. Mees' lines are white transverse striations of the fingernails that occur about 3 to 6 weeks after initial arsenic exposure. Mees' lines can also be noted in thallium poisoning and from chemotherapy exposure.

Lead poisoning occurs in those who work with metal, soldering, battery manufacturing, and in smelting factories. Children tend to develop an acute encephalopathy and adults a polyneuropathy with lead poisoning. Children can get exposed to lead by ingestion of old paint that contains lead. They develop an acute gastrointestinal illness and ultimately behavioral manifestations with confusion, drowsiness, generalized seizures and intracranial hypertension. In adults, the lead neuropathy manifests predominantly as a motor neuropathy which presents as bilateral wrist drop and/or foot drop. A rare sign of lead poisoning is the appearance of a blue line at the gingival margin in patients with poor oral hygiene. Adults sometimes develop a gastrointestinal illness and a hypochromic, microcytic anemia. Lead encephalopathy is managed supportively. Systemic corticosteroids can be given to reduce brain edema and chelating agents like dimercaprol (British anti-Lewisite) are also prescribed.

Mercury poisoning can occur from mercury vapor inhalation in the making of batteries, electronics manufacturing and in the past in the hat-making industry. Clinical manifestations include personality changes ("mad as a hatter"), irritability, insomnia, drowsiness, confusion and stupor. Other systemic symptoms and signs include intention tremors ("hatter's shakes"), proteinuria, glycosuria, hyperhidrosis, and muscle weakness. Chronic exposure can lead to visual field deficits, sensory disturbances, progressive ataxia, tremor, and cognitive impairment. Treatment using chelating agents does not always increase rate or extent of recovery.

Organophosphate poisoning can occur from exposure to pesticides, herbicides, and flame retardants. Organophosphates inhibit acetylcholinesterase by phosphorylation and result in cholinergic toxicity. Clinical manifestations include salivation, lacrimation, nausea, bronchospasm, headache, weakness and in severe cases, bradycardia, tremor, diarrhea, pulmonary edema, cyanosis, and convulsions. Coma can ensue and death can result from respiratory or cardiac failure. The treatment of choice is pralidoxime and atropine. Pralidoxime helps restore acetylcholinesterase and atropine helps to counteract muscarinic adverse effects.

Ionizing radiation is a risk factor for central nervous system tumor formation, particularly meningiomas and nerve sheath tumors. Electromagnetic radiation is a likely risk factor for both leukemia and brain tumor.

B&D Chs. 58&64

Question 23. E. This question covers some of the statistical terms that could be fair game for an exam. Learn them well. A control group is a group that does not receive treatment and is a standard of comparison. Analysis of variance is a set of statistical procedures which compares two groups and determines if the differences are due to experimental influence or chance. Regression analysis is a method of using data to predict the value of one variable in relation to another. The null hypothesis is the assumption that there are no differences between two samples of a population. When the null hypothesis is rejected, differences between the groups are not attributable to chance alone. Correlation coefficient will be covered in detail in future questions.

K&S Ch. 4

Question 24. B. Organophosphates inhibit acetylcholinesterase and cause cholinergic toxicity. Organophosphates are found predominantly in pesticides and herbicides and poisoning generally occurs in agriculture workers who are exposed following spraying in fields. Pralidoxime and atropine are the agents of choice to treat organophosphate toxicity. The other answer choices are simply distracters. For a more detailed explanation of the organophosphates, see Question 22.

B&D Ch. 64

Question 25. B. Emil Kraepelin used the term dementia praecox to describe schizophrenia. It referred to the early onset of memory loss or decreased cognitive function often seen in patients with schizophrenia. Patients with dementia praecox were found to have a long deteriorating course with hallucinations and delusions. It was Eugen Bleuler who coined the term schizophrenia. The term schizophrenia is often misconstrued to mean split personality, which in modern times is referred to as dissociative identity disorder. Other answer choices given are unrelated distracters.

K&S Ch. 13

Question 26. E. Lead poisoning can cause a rare appearance of a blue line at the gingival margin in patients with poor oral hygiene. Lead can also cause a microcytic, hypochromic anemia. A more detailed explanation of lead poisoning appears in Question 22 above.

Manganese classically causes neurotoxicity after months or years of exposure. Manganese miners are particularly at risk due to their prolonged inhalation of the toxin. Parkinsonism and motor symptoms can develop from manganese poisoning and usually follow initial manifestations of behavioral changes, headache and cognitive disturbances ("manganese madness"). A characteristic gait, walking on the toes with spine erect and elbows flexed, called the "cock-walk," can emerge. The condition is generally poorly-responsive to L-dopa therapy.

Thallium poisoning results in a severe neuropathy and central nervous system degeneration. A chronic, progressive sensory polyneuropathy can develop. Thallium causes potassium depletion which can result in cardiac abnormalities, such as sinus tachycardia, T-wave changes and U waves. Alopecia can develop two to four weeks after initial exposure. Treatment with intravenous potassium chloride and oral potassium ferric ferrocyanide, and hemodialysis and forced diuresis can help in recovery from acute thallium intoxication. Arsenic and mercury poisonings are discussed in more detail in Question 22.

B&D Ch. 64

Question 27. C. This is a case of shared psychotic disorder (folie-à-deux). In shared psychotic disorder, a delusion develops in an individual who is in a close relationship with someone who already has an established delusion. This delusion is similar to that of the person who already has the established delusion.

K&S Ch. 14

Question 28. B. Ataxia results from cerebellar lesions. Midline cerebellar vermian lesions cause truncal ataxia. Head tremor and truncal instability leading to oscillation of the head and trunk in a seated or standing posture (titubation) may result from lesions of the cerebellar vermis. In lateralized lesions to the cerebellar hemisphere, signs and symptoms occur ipsilateral to the lesion. Cerebellar hemispheric lesions would be expected to cause ipsilateral limb ataxia and/or dysmetria, either of the arm or leg, or both, depending on the location of the lesion. Dysdiadochokinesis can result from a cerebellar hemispheric lesion. This refers to a deficit in the ability to perform smooth rapid alternating movements of the hands or feet. A disturbance in both rhythm and amplitude of these alternating movements can be noted with cerebellar lesions.

Lesions arising in the cerebellopontine angle area can result in cranial neuropathy particularly to nerves V, VII and VIII. Manifestations include ipsilateral peripheral facial palsy (Bell's palsy, VII nerve palsy), ipsilateral facial numbness and weakness of masseter muscles (V nerve palsy) and ipsilateral hearing loss, tinnitus and vertigo (VIII nerve palsy).

Thalamic lesions can cause any number of deficits. Lacunar thalamic infarcts can lead to a pure sensory stroke (contralateral to the lesion), or to a sensorimotor stroke if the lesion also invades the internal capsule. Thalamic lesions can cause a rare disorder of central thalamic pain (again contralateral to the lesion and usually in the extremities and/or the face) known as the thalamic syndrome of Déjerine-Roussy.

Strokes or lesions to the midbrain can cause a variety of symptoms and syndromes. One such classic presentation is the Parinaud's syndrome which can result from a midbrain lesion arising from ischemia to the posterior cerebral artery (PCA) penetrating branches. This manifests with supranuclear paresis of eye elevation, eyelid retraction, skew deviation of the eyes, defective convergence and convergence-retraction nystagmus and light-near dissociation. Another midbrain stroke syndrome is Weber's syndrome, also arising from ischemia in the PCA territory. There is a contralateral hemiplegia of the face, arm and leg and ipsilateral oculomotor (III nerve) paresis with a dilated fixed pupil.

B&D Chs. 18,23&57

Question 29. B. Here is another chance to understand glycine if you did not master it after Question 13. Glycine is a neurotransmitter synthesized from serine. It is a necessary adjunctive neurotransmitter at the NMDA receptor that binds with glutamate. It is also an independent inhibitory neurotransmitter with its own receptors that open chloride ion channels. The activity of glycine on the NMDA receptor is an area of research for schizophrenia, with some studies showing improvement in negative symptoms with the use of glycine or glycine analogues. The highest concentrations of glycine receptors have been found in the spinal cord. Mutations of this receptor lead to a rare condition called hyperekplexia where the main symptom is an exaggerated startle response.

K&S Ch. 3

Question 30. C. Suspected meningitis with obtundation is not a contraindication to performing a lumbar puncture (LP). All of the other answer choices are indeed absolute or relative contraindications to LP. A localized infection at the level of the puncture would be a contraindication to performing the procedure, due to a risk of the LP needle seeding the infection into a meningitis. Thrombocytopenia may lead to excessive and uncontrollable bleeding if LP is performed. Fresh frozen plasma or platelet transfusion may need to be given prior to the procedure, if the LP is deemed to be essential to further diagnosis and management of the patient. Cerebral mass lesion is generally an absolute contraindication to LP because of the risk of cerebral or cerebellar herniation following the procedure. Transtentorial herniation can arise if a LP suddenly releases elevated cerebrospinal fluid pressure forcing the medial temporal lobe downwards causing the midbrain or the cerebellum to compress the cervicomedullary junction through the foramen magnum. Papilledema is a sign of increased intracranial pressure and a possible mass lesion. Fundoscopic examination must be conducted before LP is performed. Head trauma is also a contraindication to LP, because it too may lead to a herniation syndrome because of increased intracranial pressure.

B&D Ch. 35

183

Question 31. D. In case Question 15 didn't solidify acute stress disorder and posttraumatic stress disorder in your mind, take advantage of this question to clarify your understanding. Acute stress disorder occurs when a person is exposed

to a traumatic event. The patient then feels anxiety, detachment, derealization, feelings of being "in a daze", dissociative amnesia, and numbing. Flashbacks and avoidance of stimuli can occur. The symptoms do not last longer than 4 weeks, and occur within four weeks of the traumatic event (as opposed to PTSD where symptoms must last more than one month).
K&S Ch. 16

Question 32. D. Fragile X syndrome is believed to be the most frequent cause of mental retardation (MR) in the general population. The syndrome is characterized by moderate to severe MR, macroorchidism, prominent jaw, large ears, and jocular high-pitched speech. Hyperactivity and inattention are characteristic in affected males with Fragile X syndrome. The chromosomal anomaly lies at Xq28.

Down's syndrome results generally from chromosomal nondisjunction that leads to a trisomy 21. This is most often due to advanced maternal age. Manifestations include infantile hypotonia, hyperlaxity of the joints, brachycephaly, flattened occiput, mental retardation, upslanting palpebral fissures, flattened nasal bridge, epicanthal folds, small ears, hypoplastic teeth, short neck, lenticular cataracts, speckling of the iris (Brushfield's spots), brachydactyly, simian creases and congenital cardiac anomalies (in 30–40% of cases). Down's syndrome patients acquire Alzheimer-like dementia much earlier than in the general population at large.

Trisomy 18 occurs in about 1 in 6000 live births. Fifty per cent of infants do not survive past the first week of life. Manifestations include low-set ears, small jaw, hypoplastic fingernails, mental retardation, cryptorchidism, congenital heart disease (patent ductus arteriosus, atrial septal defect, ventricular septal defect), microcephaly, and renal anomalies such as polycystic kidneys.

Cri-du-chat syndrome is a hereditary congenital mental retardation syndrome caused by a deletion at the short arm of chromosome 5p15.2. It occurs in 1 in 20 000 to 50 000 live births. Manifestations include severe mental retardation, microcephaly, round face, hypertelorism, micrognathia, epicanthal folds, hypotonia, and low-set ears. Newborns present with a cat-like high-pitched cry that is considered to be diagnostic of the disorder. A majority of these patients do not live past early childhood.

Prader-Willi syndrome is considered to be an autosomal dominant disorder resulting in a deletion to chromosome 15q11-13. Clinical stigmata include decreased fetal activity, obesity, mental retardation, hypotonia, short stature, hypogonadism, and small hands and feet. High caloric intake leads to diabetes and cardiac failure in many patients and many Prader-Willi syndrome patients do not survive past 25 to 30 years of age.
B&D Ch. 67

Question 33. D. Dissociation is a disturbance in which a person fails to recall important information. There are a number of dissociative disorders including dissociative amnesia, dissociative fugue, and dissociative identity disorder. In all of these situations the patient's lack of recall is in excess of what could be explained by ordinary forgetfulness. Used as a defense mechanism, the term dissociation represents an unconscious process involving the segregation of mental or behavioral processes from the rest of the person's psychological activity. It can involve the separation of an idea from its emotional tone, as one sees in conversion disorder.
K&S Ch. 20

Question 34. B. Shaken-baby syndrome from child abuse can lead to death from intracranial, subarachnoid, and subdural hemorrhages. These result from vascular shearing and tearing due to the violent back-and-forth movement that results in cerebral trauma. Retinal hemorrhages are often noted as well in these cases. Hemorrhages can lead to seizures and ischemic cerebral infarction due to vasospasm of intracranial vessels. Ninety five per cent of severe intracranial injuries in children 1 year of age or younger are due to child abuse. The other answer choices are of less pathological importance in cases of child abuse.

B&D Ch. 57

Question 35. D. This is a case of normal bereavement. Crying, weight loss, decreased libido, withdrawal, insomnia, irritability, and poor concentration and attention can all be part of normal bereavement. Keys to normal bereavement are that suicidality is rare, it improves with social contacts, and it lacks global feelings of worthlessness. In depression, one finds anger and ambivalence towards the deceased, suicidality is common, and social contacts do not help, thus the person isolates. In addition others find the depressed person irritating or annoying, whereas the bereavement patient evokes sympathy from others. In depression the patient may feel that he or she is worthless, which is not the case in bereavement. With respect to the other answer choices, these symptoms aren't going on long enough for dysthymic disorder. There are no anxiety symptoms described to argue for acute stress disorder. There is no mania described, and the patient does not meet criteria for major depression.

K&S Ch. 2

Question 36. D. Lower motor neuron signs include hypotonia, muscle atrophy, fasciculations, hyporeflexia, flaccidity, muscle cramps, and marked motor weakness. These are considered to arise from lesions that are distal (i.e., peripheral) to the anterior horn cells where the upper and lower motor neurons synapse. Upper motor neuron signs include hyperreflexia, spasticity, Babinski's sign, clonus, pseudobulbar palsy, loss of dexterity, and mild motor weakness. Both upper and lower motor neuron signs can be demonstrated in amyotrophic lateral sclerosis (Lou Gehrig's disease), a disease which carries both sets of characteristics. Poliomyelitis is a classic disease of the lower motor neurons and carries the manifestations of lower motor neuron disease as noted above.

B&D Ch. 80

Question 37. B. Mahler's stages of separation-individuation are back again! This question describes symbiosis, which lasts from 2 months to 5 months. In this stage the baby is developing the ability to distinguish the inner from the outer world. The child perceives himself as being part of a single entity with his mother. For more details on Mahler, see Question 21.

K&S Ch. 2

Question 38. B. Brandt-Daroff exercises can be extremely helpful in the treatment of benign paroxysmal positional vertigo (BPPV). The exercises involve rapidly lying down on one side from a seated position and remaining there for about thirty seconds before sitting up for thirty seconds and repeating the maneuver in the opposite direction. Patients are supposed to complete 20 full repetitions twice daily. Most patients see relief within a week, but it may take three months or more to achieve complete symptom remission. Once in remission, most patients are cured of the disorder. Benign paroxysmal positional vertigo is a vestibulopathy that is believed to be a result of sludge deposition or otoliths in the utricle of the posterior semicircular canal of the inner ear. When the patient moves his head, the movement of the material in the semicircular canal irritates the hair cells in the inner ear and triggers a severe acute onset of rotational vertigo, with nausea, possible vomiting, and characteristic rotatory nystagmus. Diagnosis is clinical and is suggested by the history. Symptoms can usually be evoked acutely by the Dix-Hallpike maneuver in which the patient's head is rapidly lowered to the bed by the examiner. The head is then turned with one ear down to the bed. The examiner notes the reproduction of vertigo and nystagmus, which are generally pathognomonic

for BPPV. The fast phase of the nystagmus is noted in the direction of the lower ear (the ear with the vestibular problem) when the patient looks toward the affected side. In primary gaze, the fast rotational phase is vertical and upward, rotating toward the affected (lower) ear. Other treatments include meclizine, an antiemetic agent, that helps with nausea and vomiting, but not generally with the vertigo. Metoclopramide (Reglan) is also an antiemetic agent that can help in a similar way to meclizine. Diazepam can lessen anxiety that can be associated with severe symptoms. Gabapentin is not indicated, nor is it particularly useful, in BPPV.
B&D Chs. 18&41

Question 39. B. All of this question's answer choices are criteria for diagnosis of kleptomania, except that, before the theft, the patient has an increased sense of tension. Kleptomania is found within the larger heading of impulse control disorders. In kleptomania the patient engages in repeated stealing of objects that they do not need. An important part of the disorder is the sense of tension before the act and the sense of pleasure or relief afterward.
K&S Ch. 25

Question 40. B. The persistent vegetative state usually follows from a period of coma and is believed to signal the onset of severe cerebral cortical damage, often due to brain anoxia, trauma, or both. A period of one month of coma needs to elapse before the patient can be said to be in a persistent vegetative state. The condition is characterized by absence of cognitive function and absent awareness of the surrounding environment, despite a preserved sleep-wake cycle. Spontaneous movements can be noted and eye opening can be preserved, but the patient does not speak and cannot obey commands. Eye tracking and swallowing can also be preserved. There is no response to noxious stimulation in the persistent vegetative state. Permanent irreversible brain damage is believed to set in after about 12 months of a persistent vegetative state that follows brain trauma and usually after about 3 or more months following anoxic brain injury.
B&D Ch. 5

Question 41. D. Attaque de nervios is a culture bound anxiety syndrome associated with those from Latin-American cultures. Its symptoms include headache, insomnia, anorexia, fear, anger, despair, and diarrhea.
The question says nothing about psychosis, so schizophrenia and schizoaffective disorder are incorrect. This case does not meet criteria for panic disorder. Myoclonic sleep disorder is not even remotely related to the symptoms given. Add in the fact that the patient is Hispanic, and the answer choice is clear, attaque de nervios.
K&S Ch. 14

Question 42. D. Depression classically disrupts rapid eye movement (REM) sleep patterns. The most typical effect of depression on sleep however, is early morning awakening. Depression can also shorten REM latency (one hour or less). Depression can increase the total percentage of REM sleep and flip the predominance of REM from the early morning near awakening, to the beginning of the night.
K&S Ch. 24

Question 43. E. In pyromania the patient sets fires repeatedly because of the tension before the act and the relief after. There is also a fascination with fire and its various uses. If the patient is setting fires for gain such as money or to make a political statement, then it is not a case of pyromania. One can not make the diagnosis in the presence of conduct disorder, mania, or antisocial personality disorder. Pyromania is included in the impulse control disorders.
K&S Ch. 25

Question 44. A. Apoptosis is the phenomenon of programmed cell death. Apoptosis can be triggered by exposure to antigens, exposure to corticosteroids, withdrawal of growth factors and cytokines. NMDA receptor channels, when opened, lead to calcium influx into neuronal cells and this triggers the apoptotic cascade known as hyperexcitability and excitotoxicity that leads to neuronal compromise and demise. This mechanism of cellular death is not well-understood, but is believed to be implicit in the mediation of such neurologic conditions as epilepsy, stroke and neurodegenerative diseases like Alzheimer's dementia and amyotrophic lateral sclerosis.
B&D Ch. 49

Question 45. E. This is a case of intermittent explosive disorder. The patient has a history of violent outbursts that are out of proportion to the severity of the situation in which they occur. He has no other signs or symptoms that would suggest another axis I or II diagnosis. He has no medical history that would suggest that he could have a seizure disorder or that would otherwise explain his behavior.
K&S Ch. 25

Question 46. B. The treatment of choice for acute benzodiazepine overdose is flumazenil (Romazicon). Flumazenil is administered intravenously and has a short half-life of 7–15 minutes. The initial dosage in suspected benzodiazepine overdose is 0.2 mg IV over 30 seconds. An additional 0.3 mg can be given for more efficacy. Further doses of 0.5 mg can be given to a maximum total of 3 mg. The most common serious side effect of flumazenil administration is the onset of seizures, particularly in those patients who are dependent on benzodiazepines, or in those who have ingested large quantities of benzodiazepines.
Naloxone (Narcan) is administered in cases of acute opioid intoxication or overdose. Dimercaprol (British Anti-Lewisite) is a chelating agent that is administered in cases of acute lead poisoning and lead encephalopathy. Atropine is a potent anticholinergic agent that is administered in cases of organophosphate or herbicide poisoning. Epinephrine injection is administered in cases of allergic anaphylactic shock.
K&S Ch. 36

Question 47. D. All of the answer choices in this question are potential considerations for the differential diagnosis of intermittent explosive disorder except obsessive-compulsive disorder (OCD). OCD patients do not have a particular likelihood to become intermittently violent and destructive. Other things to include in the differential would be personality change from a medical condition, oppositional defiant disorder, antisocial personality disorder, mania, malingering, and schizophrenia.
K&S Ch. 25

Question 48. B. The clinical triad of infantile spasms, hypsarrhythmia and psychomotor developmental arrest is known as West's syndrome. The incidence is about 1 in 5000 live births. The onset of symptoms is generally before 1 year of age. Spasms occur intermittently and involve rapid flexor/extensor movements of the body. Developmental arrest occurs prior to or at the onset of spasms. Electroencephalography reveals a characteristic interictal hypsarrhythmia pattern, which is a pattern with predominant posterior diffuse slow and sharp waves and spikes. Treatment of choice is adrenocorticotropic hormone, prednisone, or prednisolone. Prognosis is extremely poor. Only 5% of affected children achieve normal development.
The 3-per-second spike and wave pattern is characteristic of absence seizures. PLEDS are characteristic of herpes simplex virus encephalitis. Triphasic sharp waves are characteristic of Creutzfeld-Jakob disease.

Burst-suppression pattern is indicative of severe diffuse brain damage, such as in anoxic brain injury, severe drug overdose and head injury.
B&D Ch. 73

Question 49. C. Heat intolerance is a symptom of hyperthyroidism, not AIDS. The other symptoms in this question, such as progressive dementia, personality changes, depression, and loss of libido are all worth considering in a patient with AIDS. More than 60% of AIDS patients have neuropsychiatric symptoms. They also show impaired memory, decreased concentration, and may have seizures.
K&S Ch. 11

Question 50. A. Papez' circuit connects the hippocampus with the thalamus, hypothalamus and cortex. The pathway includes all of the answer choices noted, plus the mammillothalamic tract and anterior nucleus of the thalamus. The amygdala is not considered part of Papez' circuit.
B&D Ch. 6

Question 51. E. Oh joy! Mahler's stages of separation-individuation are back again! This question focuses on Mahler's last stage of object constancy, which lasts from 2 to 5 years. In this stage the child understands the permanence of other people, even when they are not present. For more information on Mahler's stages, see Question 21.
K&S Ch. 2

Question 52. E. Benign familial neonatal convulsions is a rare, autosomal dominant hereditary disorder resulting from a defect in voltage-gated potassium channels. Generalized tonic-clonic seizures occur after about the third day of life and disappear spontaneously in most cases in a few weeks to months. Lambert-Eaton myasthenic syndrome is a paraneoplastic autoimmune disorder affecting P/Q-type voltage gated calcium channels at the motor neuron terminal. Malignant hyperthermia, hypokalemic periodic paralysis and familial hemiplegic migraine are all genetic disorders involving gene mutations that result in abnormal voltage-gated calcium channels.
B&D Ch. 70

188

Question 53. C. The patient in this question has paranoid personality disorder. Symptoms not listed in this question include reluctance to confide in others for fear that the information will be used maliciously against one, perceiving attacks on one's character that others do not see, and having recurrent suspicions regarding fidelity of sexual partners. The patient in the question does not present with the usual grouping of positive and negative symptoms used to diagnose schizophrenia. Although there is a great deal of suspiciousness present she does not present with frank psychosis. There is an absence of bizarre beliefs on a number of subjects, magical thinking, and excessive social anxiety as would be expected in schizotypal personality disorder. She does not exhibit ego-syntonic social isolation, as would be expected in schizoid personality disorder. There is no suggestion of memory loss as would be noted in dementia.
K&S Ch. 27

Question 54. A. Phenylketonuria (PKU) is an autosomal recessive heritable inborn error of metabolism resulting from a deficiency in phenylalanine hydroxylase that can cause mental retardation. The prevalence of the disorder is about 1 in 10 000 to 20 000 live births. Phenylalanine levels increase dramatically because it cannot be converted to tyrosine due to the missing enzyme. The defect localizes to chromosome 12. Classic clinical features include microcephaly, a characteristic 'mousy' odor, infantile spasms, and light hair and skin pigmentation. Sensorineural deafness is not a feature of PKU. Diagnosis can be established by measurement of blood levels of phenylalanine which are elevated. The treatment of choice is a phenyl-alanine free diet, which must begin during gestation in order to prevent mental retardation.

B&D Ch. 68

Question 55. C. The nigrostriatal tract projects from the substantia nigra to the corpus striatum. When the D2 receptors in this tract are blocked, parkinsonian side effects emerge. This tract degenerates in Parkinson's disease. Choices A, B, and C are all tracts involved in some way with antipsychotic medications. The antipsychotic medications effect both positive and negative symptoms of schizophrenia through the mesolimbic–mesocortical tract. They also lead to increased prolactin, amenorrhea, and galactorrhea through the tuberoinfundibular tract. The caudate neurons have many D2 receptors as well, and regulate motor activity. With blockade of the caudate D2 receptors bradykinesia develops. With their over stimulation tics and extraneous motor movements develop.

K&S Ch. 3

Question 56. D. The photo depicts a classic Arnold-Chiari type I malformation. The Chiari I malformation presents as a descent of the cerebellar tonsils below the level of the foramen magnum with or without forward displacement of the medulla. This manifestation is believed to be caused by a low intracranial pressure state. The defect is often accompanied by syringomyelia, syringobulbia, and hydrocephalus. Common clinical features include headache, cranial neuropathies, and visual disturbances. Some cases present with motor and sensory complaints, particularly myelopathy with a "shawl" distribution pattern of sensory deficit over the shoulders due to the syrinx. Surgical decompression of the brainstem may be needed if the patient is highly symptomatic. Chiari type II malformation has similar features as type I, with caudal displacement of the medulla and fourth ventricle and the addition of a lumbar myelomeningocele. Lissencephaly, also known as agyria, is a disorder of early neuroblast migration. It results from the developmental failure of the gyri of the cerebral cortex. The cortex remains smooth and lacks the convolutions that are typical of normal neuronal migration and development. Schizencephaly is a disorder associated with defective genetic expression of the EMX2 gene. It results in clefts in the cerebral hemispheres. There are two types of schizencephaly: closed lip (the edges of the cleft are closed) and open lip (the edges of the cleft are open). Schizencephaly can be symmetrical or asymmetrical. Dandy-Walker syndrome presents as a cystic enlargement or pouching of the fourth ventricle. In addition, the posterior portion of the cerebellar vermis is hypoplastic or aplastic. Noncommunicating hydrocephalus invariably results from this anomaly. Mental retardation and spastic diplegia are frequent clinical manifestations.

B&D Ch. 66

189

Question 57. D. Neuroleptic malignant syndrome is a life threatening condition resulting from the use of antipsychotic medications. Its symptoms are muscular rigidity, dystonia, akinesia, obtundation, or agitation. It also involves autonomic instability such as fever, sweating, unstable blood pressure, or unstable heart rate. Patients are given supportive medical treatment and medications such as dantrolene and bromocriptine may be used. Mortality is around 10–20%. The syndrome is a result of dopamine blockade, and some postulate it may be the result of a precipitous withdrawal of dopamine receptor stimulation. The other answer choices would not present with the grouping of symptoms listed, and the fact that the patient has schizophrenia and is on a psychiatric inpatient unit should point the test-taker in the direction of a side effect to antipsychotics.

K&S Ch. 36

Question 58. C. About 15% of ischemic strokes are caused by extracranial internal carotid artery (ICA) stenosis. Endarterectomy, surgical removal of the atherosclerotic plaque, has been deemed to be indicated and useful in symptomatic ICA stenosis of 70–99%. Symptomatic stenosis implies the prior occurrence of ipsilateral ischemic events such as transient ischemic attacks, amaurosis fugax, or completed nondisabling carotid territory stroke within the past 6 months. Asymptomatic ICA stenosis is a more difficult and controversial issue with respect to its optimal surgical management. European stroke trials and many stroke experts feel that asymptomatic ICA stenosis of 80% or greater presents a high enough risk to warrant endarterectomy only if carried out by a surgeon with morbidity statistics indicating less than a 3% complication rate.
B&D Ch. 57

Question 59. A. The patient in this question has schizoid personality disorder. He has a pervasive pattern of detachment from social relationships and a restricted range of emotional expression. Other symptoms include taking little to no pleasure in activities, lacking close friends or confidants, and showing emotional coldness or detachment. Schizotypal patients have odd behaviors and beliefs such as magical thinking. Narcissistic patients are grandiose, need admiration, and lack empathy. This patient is socially isolated but has none of the other criteria that one would expect to find with a major depressive disorder or dysthymic disorder, and as such they are not the correct answers.
K&S Ch. 27.

Question 60. D. *Campylobacter jejuni* is the most common bacterial infection that precedes the onset of Guillain-Barré syndrome (acute inflammatory demyelinating polyneuropathy; AIDP). It accounts for about 20–40% of all cases of AIDP. *C. jejuni* causes an acute enteric and systemic illness and the onset of AIDP occurs about two to three weeks after this initial diarrheal condition. AIDP tends to follow about 1 in 1000 to 2000 cases of known *C. jejuni* infections. *C. jejuni* infection can be diagnosed by stool or blood cultures and is treated with a week-long course of oral erythromycin 250 mg four times daily.
AIDP is preceded by an upper respiratory or gastrointestinal infection, a surgical intervention, or an immunization about 1 to 4 weeks prior to the illness onset in about two-thirds of cases. *C. jejuni* infection has been linked to a worse prognosis because it tends to be associated with the more severe axonal form of AIDP.
B&D Chs 59&82

Question 61. C. The correlation coefficient is a measurement of the direction and strength of the relationship between two variables. The Pearson correlation coefficient is on a scale from –1 to +1. A positive correlation means that one variable moves the other in the same direction. A negative value means that one moves the other in the opposite direction. A correlation close to –1 or +1 shows a strong relationship. A correlation close to 0 shows a weak relationship. Correlation coefficients indicate the degree of relationship only; they say nothing about cause and effect.
K&S Ch. 4

Question 62. D. Brain metastases are the most common form of neurologic complication from systemic cancer and they account for about 20–40% of all central nervous system tumors. Lung cancer is the most common cause of metastases to the brain and accounts for about two-thirds of all such metastases. In particular, non-small cell lung carcinoma accounts for about two-thirds of all metastases to the brain originating from the lung. Breast cancer leads to about 15–20% of patients with brain metastases.

Melanoma, gastrointestinal carcinoma and renal cell carcinoma each account for about 5–10% of metastatic brain tumors.
B&D Ch. 58

Question 63. B. This question gives a description of avoidant personality disorder. These patients avoid interpersonal contact for fear of criticism. They are unwilling to get involved with others without assurance of being liked. They show restraint in interpersonal relationships for fear of being shamed or ridiculed. They are inhibited interpersonally because of fears of inadequacy. They see themselves as inferior to others. Of the other choices, the only one that comes close is schizoid personality disorder, but in schizoid personality disorder the person doesn't care that he is isolated, and he has a blunted affect. Passive-aggressive personality disorder is only in the DSM-IV-TR as a subject for further research. Obsessive-compulsive personality disorder (OCPD) presents as a pervasive pattern of preoccupation with orderliness, perfectionism, and control. This preoccupation comes at the expense of openness, efficiency, and flexibility. The OCPD patient's perfectionism interferes with task completion. These patients are inflexible regarding moral and ethical issues. They devote time to work at the expense of leisure activities. They are reluctant to delegate tasks to others. They are characteristically rigid and stubborn. OCPD patients often can not discard old or worn-out objects even when they have no value.
K&S Ch. 27

Question 64. A. A post-lumbar puncture (LP) headache is a frequent adverse event resulting from diagnostic or therapeutic LP. The headache is considered to be due to low cerebrospinal fluid (CSF) pressure because the needle bevel (usually a Quincke needle) leaves an open dural tear from shearing as it is pulled out of the patient. This dural tear results in a chronic CSF leak from the puncture site and an intractable headache that is noted particularly when the patient is upright. The headache is generally relieved when the patient lies recumbent. Loss of CSF results in a traction of the brain on sensory nerves and bridging veins, which causes pain.
The pain often resolves in several days if the patient lies recumbent and receives adequate hydration. A blood patch is often immediately curative of the post-LP headache and involves the gentle injection of 10 to 20 mL of the patient's own blood into the epidural space at the same site of the LP. Bed-rest for two weeks is far too long a period to wait before undertaking a blood patch. Acetaminophen and hydrocodone may be helpful, but are not curative therapy for post-LP headache. Sumatriptan is indicated for migraine only and not for post-LP headache.
B&D Ch. 75

Question 65. E. Patients starting lithium should obtain baseline thyroid function tests, electrolytes, white blood cell count, renal function tests, and a baseline electrocardiogram. Why? Because lithium can cause renal damage, hypothyroidism, increased WBC count, and ECG changes (T wave flattening or inversion). Low sodium can lead to toxic lithium levels. VDRL is a distracter which is unrelated to starting a patient on lithium.
K&S Ch. 7

Question 66. B. Compression of the lateral femoral cutaneous nerve as it passes beneath the inguinal ligament results in a painful sensory syndrome known as meralgia paresthetica. Predisposing factors include obesity, pregnancy and the wearing of pants that are tight at the waist or a heavy belt, such as those worn by workmen carrying heavy tools. Clinically there is pain and sensory loss (numbness) to the lateral thigh. Motor deficits are absent. Treatment is conservative and involves weight loss (if that is the cause), wearing looser clothing, or the use of tricyclic antidepressants or anticonvulsants to treat the neuropathic pain. Surgery is not generally

needed in these cases. The other peripheral nerves listed as answer choices are simply distracters.
B&D Ch. 34

Question 67. A. Your new friend Mahler is back again! If you didn't get this right it's time to memorize her stages! Mahler's first stage is normal autism, lasting from birth to 2 months. In this stage the baby spends more time asleep than awake. For more information on Mahler's stages, see Question 21.
K&S Ch. 2

Question 68. B. Fibrillation potentials are the electromyographic (EMG) hallmarks of muscle denervation. Positive sharp waves are spontaneous activity emanating from groups of denervated muscle fibers. Fibrillation potentials, combined with the finding of positive sharp waves, and decreased recruitment in a segmental myotomal distribution are characteristic of a radiculopathy. Fasciculations are commonly characteristic of anterior horn cell diseases such as poliomyelitis and amyotrophic lateral sclerosis. They can also be benign and can be seen in normal healthy individuals. They represent spontaneous discharges of a single motor unit. High-frequency, short-duration potentials are seen when the EMG needle is very close to or embedded in the motor endplate. This is not a pathologic finding. Myotonia is the phenomenon of delayed muscle relaxation after needle insertion or contraction. It is the pattern noted in myotonic dystrophy and is characterized by a "dive-bomber" pattern heard on the speaker. Small, short motor unit potentials are noted in myopathies (polymyositis, muscular dystrophies). This pattern occurs from reduction in size of the muscle fibers.
B&D Ch. 36

Question 69. A. The caudate nucleus neurons have many D2 receptors. They regulate motor activity by determining which motor acts get carried out. With blockade of the caudate D2 receptors, bradykinesia develops from excessive dampening of motor activity. With caudate D2 receptor over-stimulation, tics and extraneous motor movements develop.
K&S Ch. 3

Question 70. B. Cerebral venous thrombosis (CVT) generally occurs one day to four weeks postpartum, with a peak in incidence about 7–14 days after delivery. Clinical features include puerperal headache that worsens over days, seizures, neurologic deficits, and behavior or personality changes. The condition is believed to be due to the hypercoagulable state induced by pregnancy with likely decreased protein S activity and to a possible presence of circulating antiphospholipid antibodies during the puerperal period. Brain MRI with MRI venography is the imaging modality of choice to clinch the diagnosis. Heparin anticoagulation may be helpful. Thrombolysis by either intravenous infusion or invasive venographic approach has also proved to be useful treatment, especially in severe cases where prognosis is deemed to be poor.
Meningitis and meningoencephalitis are certainly in the differential diagnosis when considering CVT, but both would be expected to be accompanied by high fever and possibly obtundation. A migraine, even when complicated, is rarely accompanied by seizures. Pseudotumor cerebri does not cause seizures and usually presents with intermittent visual obscurations and papilledema rather than diplopia.
B&D Ch. 87

Question 71. A. Patients must make decisions regarding advanced directives at a time when they are competent to do so. At the time of admission to the hospital they may or may not be competent. If the question of capacity arises they may or may not have capacity and therefore lack competence. When immediately prior to an operation, or in the office, they may or may not be competent. Competence is a legal decision, made by the courts, that a patient has sufficient ability to manage their own affairs. Capacity is a medical decision made by a psychiatrist that says whether at a given point in time the patient is thinking clearly enough to make certain medical decisions for himself. In order to make an advanced directive one would want the patient to have both capacity and be competent at the time of the decision.

K&S Ch. 57

Question 72. A. Cytomegalovirus (CMV) is the most common congenital viral infection in newborns and is the result of either primary maternal infection or from viral reactivation in the mother. Most affected newborns are asymptomatic and most develop normally. Less than 10% of patients with CMV have complications such as jaundice, hepatosplenomegaly, microcephaly, chorioretinitis, ataxia, and seizures. The mortality rate is about 20–30% in symptomatic newborns. The other neonatal infections noted in this question occur less frequently than CMV.

B&D Ch. 86

Question 73. D. Patients with dependent personality disorder have trouble making decisions without excessive amounts of advice from others. They need others to assume responsibility for most areas of their life. They do not express disagreement with others for fear of disapproval. They feel helpless and uncomfortable when alone. They urgently seek new relationships when a prior one ends, and can be unrealistically preoccupied with fears of being left alone to care for themselves. None of the other answer choices fit these parameters. Passive-aggressive personality disorder is in the DSM as a subject for further research.

K&S Ch. 27

Question 74. D. Inclusion body myositis is the most common myopathy in those over 50 years of age and it rarely occurs in those younger than 50 years of age. Men are more frequently affected than women. The disorder affects strength in the distal muscles of the arms and legs. Wrist and finger flexors and quadriceps muscles are preferentially weak. There are no muscle pains noted in the disorder. The disorder is generally chronic, progressive and poorly responsive to corticosteroid or immunosuppressive therapies. Muscle biopsy helps confirm the diagnosis in about 80% or more cases if done properly. It classically reveals endomysial inflammation, macrophage invasion of muscle, rimmed vacuoles, and characteristic inclusion bodies in the nuclei.

Fascioscapulohumeral dystrophy (FSHD) is an autosomal dominant inherited disease of muscle with a prevalence of about 1 to 2 per 100 000. The genetic anomaly localizes to 4q35 in most cases. The phenomenon of *anticipation* is noted in FSHD, which implies that as successive generations acquire the disease, the onset of the condition occurs earlier and the disease becomes more severe. Clinical features include weakness of orofacial muscles, with inability to pucker or whistle. Shoulder muscles are weak and winging of the scapula can be noted when the arms are outstretched. Biceps and triceps are often weak, as are the hip flexors and quadriceps. DNA studies establish the diagnosis. Treatment is supportive as the condition is irreversible.

Oculopharyngeal muscular dystrophy (OPMD) is an autosomal dominant inherited disease of muscle. The disorder localizes to chromosome 14q11.2-13. The disease begins in the fifth or sixth decade most often and presents initially with eye muscle weakness and ptosis. Difficulty swallowing soon follows and swallowing may become impossible. Death can occur from starvation if nutritional support is not given. DNA testing proves the diagnosis. Treatment is supportive.

Dermatomyositis and polymyositis are discussed at length in other questions in this volume.
B&D Ch. 85

Question 75. C. Euphoria is a behavioral effect of opioids, as are drowsiness, decreased sex drive, hypoactivity, and personality changes. Miosis is a physical effect of opioid use. Increased arousal is not an effect of opioid intoxication, drowsiness is. Diarrhea can come from withdrawal, but opioids themselves cause constipation. Bradycardia is also a physical effect of opioids, and as such tachycardia is incorrect.
K&S Ch. 12

Question 76. A. Duchenne's and Becker's muscular dystrophies are X-linked inherited disorders of muscle. The gene locus is Xp21 on the short arm of the X chromosome. This abnormality results in a deficiency in dystrophin, a structural muscle membrane protein located in the subsarcolemmal region of muscle fibers. These two disorders are explained in greater detail as part of other questions in this volume. The other answer choices are all muscle proteins that work together with dystrophin to stabilize the muscle membrane, but they are not implicated in the pathophysiology of the two muscular dystrophies mentioned in this question.
B&D Ch. 85

Question 77. E. Sleep apnea is a disorder in which there is a cessation of airflow in and out of the lungs during sleep. These stoppages of airflow must last for ten seconds or more. In central sleep apnea, both respiratory effort and airflow stop. In obstructive sleep apnea, air stops flowing but respiratory effort increases. It is considered pathological if patients have five or more apneic episodes per hour or 30 or more episodes per night. Sleep apnea can lead to cardiovascular changes including arrhythmia and blood pressure changes. Long-standing sleep apnea can lead to pulmonary hypertension. The characteristic pattern of sleep apnea involves an older person who reports tiredness or inability to stay awake during the daytime. It can be associated with depression, irritability, and daytime sleepiness. Bed partners often report loud snoring. Patients may also awaken during the night as a result of the cessation of breathing. Patients suspected of sleep apnea should undergo sleep studies, and should be treated with a CPAP machine (continuous positive airway pressure). Losing weight helps many people, and for some surgery is the appropriate option to remove the obstruction in the airway. Now looking at the test question, the patient is not dropping into "sleep attacks" while in the middle of activities, as such narcolepsy is incorrect. There is no substantial evidence of mania given. The patient does not meet criteria for major depression. Behaviors associated with sleep terrors are not described. The snoring that drove her husband out of the bedroom should immediately point you in the direction of sleep apnea. The fact that she is overweight clinches the diagnosis.
K&S Ch. 24

Question 78. B. Tyrosine hydroxylase is the rate-limiting enzyme in the dopamine synthetic pathway. Dopamine synthesis occurs as follows: L-tyrosine is converted to L-dopa by tyrosine hydroxylase. Dopa decarboxylase converts L-dopa to dopamine. Once dopamine is extruded into the synaptic cleft, its termination of action is carried out by monoamine oxidase, catechol-O-methyltransferase, as well as reuptake into the presynaptic bouton where it is initially synthesized. Norepinephrine synthesis occurs when dopamine β-hydroxylase converts dopamine to norepinephrine. Norepinephrine in turn is converted to epinephrine by phenylethanolamine N-methyltransferase (PNMT).
B&D Ch. 49

Question 79. C. The therapeutic range for lithium is 0.6–1.2 mEq/L. Toxic levels are 2 mEq/L or higher. Lethal levels are 4.0 mEq/L or higher.
K&S Ch. 7

Question 80. D. GABA-A is a complex receptor with multiple binding sites. GABA is found throughout the central and peripheral nervous systems and is the predominant inhibitory neurotransmitter in the brain. When the GABA receptor is agonized, there is a rapid influx of negatively charged chloride ions through the postsynaptic cellular membrane. This results in fast inhibitory postsynaptic potentials. The GABA-A receptor is believed to be responsible for the clinical effects of benzodiazepines, barbiturates and alcohol. Only sodium oxybate (gamma hydroxybutyrate; GHB; Xyrem), which is a "date-rape" drug that is FDA-approved for narcolepsy and cataplexy, and lioresal, a potent anti-spasticity agent, act in the central nervous system by agonism of the GABA-B receptor. The other receptor types mentioned in this question are simply distracters.
B&D Ch. 49

Question 81. D. It is the frontal lobes that determine how the brain acts on information. The relatively large size of the human frontal lobes is what distinguishes our brains from those of primates. It is in the frontal lobes that executive functioning takes place, and injury of the frontal lobes leads to impairment in motivation, attention, and sequencing of actions. A "frontal lobe syndrome" exists, and consists of slowed thinking, poor judgment, decreased curiosity, social withdrawal, and irritability. Patients with frontal lobe dysfunction may have normal IQ, as IQ has been found to be mostly a parietal lobe function.
K&S Ch. 3

Question 82. B. Ganser's syndrome, considered to be a dissociative disorder, is the voluntary production of symptoms that involve giving approximate answers or talking past the point. This syndrome is often associated with other psychopathy such as conversion, perceptual disturbances, and dissociative symptoms like amnesia and fugue. Males and prisoners are most commonly affected. The major contributory factor is the presence of a severe personality disorder. Recovery is most often sudden and patients claim amnesia of the symptoms. It is believed to be a variant of malingering, with possible secondary gain.
Conversion disorder is a somatoform disorder characterized by the presence of one or more neurologic symptoms that are not explained by any known neurologic or medical disorder. Capgras' syndrome is a specific type of systematized delusion in which the patient feels that a familiar person is mistakenly thought to be an unfamiliar imposter. Hypochondriasis is a somatoform disorder in which the patient misinterprets bodily symptoms and functions and becomes preoccupied with the fear of contracting or having a serious disease even after reassurance to the contrary is given by a physician. Folie-à-deux is a delusional disorder, now termed a shared psychotic disorder in DSM-IV-TR. It involves the transfer of delusions from a patient to another person who has a close relationship with the patient. The associated person's delusion is similar in content to that of the patient.
K&S Ch. 20

Question 83. D. Learned helplessness is a behavioral model for depression developed by Martin Seligman. He took dogs and gave them electric shocks from which they could not escape. Eventually they gave up and stopped trying to escape. In time this spread to other areas of functioning until they were always helpless and apathetic. This behavioral pattern has also been seen in humans with repeated setbacks or failures in their lives, as the question stem demonstrates. Industry is part of Erikson's stages and is irrelevant to the question. Cognition is the process of obtaining, learning, and using intellectual knowledge. This has some relation to the test taking but is not the explanation for the child's behavior. Sensory deprivation is removing a person or animal from external stimuli of any kind. Again, it is unrelated to the question. The epigenetic principle states that development occurs in sequential, clearly defined stages. This is clearly unrelated to the question.

K&S Ch. 4

Question 84. A. Entacapone (Comtan) and tolcapone (Tasmar) are catechol-O-methyl-tranferase (COMT) inhibitors. COMT inhibitors block peripheral degradation of peripheral levodopa and central degradation of L-dopa and dopamine, thereby increasing L-dopa and dopamine levels centrally. The COMT inhibitor is generally given concomitantly with each dose of carbidopa-levodopa (Sinemet) throughout the day to improve parkinsonian symptoms.

Selegiline (Eldepryl) is the classic monoamine oxidase type-B (MAO-B) inhibitor. It has some potentiating effects on dopamine and prevents MAO-B dependent dopamine degradation. Phenelzine (Nardil) and tranylcypromine (Parnate) are nonspecific MAO inhibitors that affect both MAO-A and MAO-B. There are reversible MAO-A inhibitors (moclobemide and befloxatone) that are only available outside the USA. These agents do not require the strict dietary restrictions on tyramine that the nonselective MAO inhibitors require in order to avoid a hypertensive crisis. There are no specific pharmacologic agents that act upon dopa decarboxylase or dopamine β-hydroxylase. These two answer choices are simply distracters.

B&D Ch. 77

Question 85. D. The commonly used drug ibuprofen can drastically increase lithium levels. Many diuretics can increase lithium levels, as can ACE inhibitors and other non-steroidal anti-inflammatory drugs such as naproxen. Aspirin will not affect lithium levels. Lithium combined with anticonvulsants can increase lithium levels and worsen neurotoxic effects.

K&S Ch. 36

Question 86. C. Argyll Robertson pupils are a characteristic of late syphilis, particularly in either general paresis or tabes dorsalis. Argyll Robertson pupils are small, irregular pupils that constrict to accommodation, but not to light. Tabes dorsalis is the spinal form of syphilis and develops about 15 to 20 years after the initial infection. The clinical triad is that of sensory ataxia, lightning pains and urinary incontinence. Lower extremity deep tendon reflexes are absent. There is impaired proprioception with a positive Romberg's sign. Ninety per cent of patients have pupillary abnormalities and about one-half have Argyll Robertson pupils. Another classic characteristic is the presence of Charcot's (neuropathic) joints.

The pupillary abnormality seen in optic neuritis or multiple sclerosis is called the Marcus Gunn pupil and is revealed when a swinging light is moved away from the affected eye. Both eyes should constrict because of consensual innervation, but the affected pupil enlarges when the flashlight is moved away to the unaffected eye. Lyme disease and bubonic plague do not present with characteristic pupillary abnormalities. Intracerebral aneurysm, particularly of the posterior communicating artery, presents with a complete third nerve palsy that involves the pupil which is fixed and slightly dilated.

B&D Ch. 59

Question 87. C. The symptoms given in this question are most likely the result of a serotonin withdrawal syndrome, which is possible with most serotonin-selective reuptake inhibitors (SSRIs), but which occurs particularly with paroxetine due to its shorter half-life. Symptoms include nausea, insomnia, muscle aches, anxiety and dizziness. The way to prevent this uncomfortable situation is to taper the drug off slowly. Patients on paroxetine should be warned against abruptly stopping the drug.

K&S Ch. 36

Question 88. B. Todd's paralysis is a brief period of transient hemiparesis or hemiplegia following a seizure. The symptoms usually dissipate within 48 hours and treatment is expectant and supportive. The weakness is generally contralateral to the side of the brain with the epileptic focus. The condition may also affect speech and vision, but again the deficits are temporary. Certain studies have pointed to Todd's paralysis being the result of arteriovenous shunting that leads to transient cerebral ischemia following an ictal event. The other answer choices are distracters.

B&D Ch. 73

Question 89. A. The 3-hydroxy benzodiazepines are directly metabolized by glucuronidation and have no active metabolites. The 3-hydroxy benzodiazepines include oxazepam, lorazepam, and temazepam. Know these three well, as they are often the subject of questions on standardized exams. Some of the longest half lives are found with the 2-keto benzodiazepines (chlordiazepoxide, diazepam, prazepam) because they have multiple active metabolites that can keep working in the body from 30 hours to over 200 hours in patients who are slow metabolizers.

K&S Ch. 36

Question 90. A. Tropical spastic paraparesis is a chronic progressive myelopathy associated with infection by human T-lymphotropic virus type-1 (HTLV-1). The condition affects men more often than women and the onset is usually after 30 years of age. Diagnosis is confirmed by cerebrospinal fluid polymerase chain reaction and detection of HTLV-1 antibodies. Clinical features include upper motor neuron weakness, bladder disturbance and variable sensory loss. By ten years out, 60–70% of patients cannot walk. Treatment can be undertaken with corticosteroids, interferon-α, or plasmapheresis, but has proven only minimally beneficial.

B&D Ch. 80

Question 91. D. Lithium is often used to treat aggression in patients with schizophrenia, prisoners, those with conduct disorder, and the mentally retarded. It is less useful in aggression associated with head trauma and epilepsy. Other drugs used for aggression include anticonvulsants and antipsychotics.

K&S Ch. 36

Question 92. C. The neurodegenerative disorders that are associated with expansion of genetic trinucleotide repeat sequences are: fragile X syndrome, myotonic dystrophy, Huntington's disease, X-linked spinobulbar muscular atrophy, dentatorubral-pallido-luysian atrophy, spinocerebellar atrophies types 1, 2, 3, 6 and 7, and Friedrich's ataxia. Multiple system atrophy is a Parkinson's plus syndrome that is not associated with an expansion of trinucleotide repeat sequences.

B&D Ch. 44

Question 93. B. The mesolimbic-mesocortical pathway projects from the ventral tegmental area (VTA) to many areas of the cortex and limbic system. This is the tract that is thought to mediate the antipsychotic effects of the antipsychotic medications. The nigrostriatal pathway is associated with parkinsonian effects of the antipsychotics. The caudate is associated with Tourette's disorder and tics (see Question 69). The tuberoinfundibular pathway is associated with prolactin increase and lactation from antipsychotics.

K&S Ch. 3

Question 94. A. The "battle sign" is a hematoma overlying the mastoid that results from a basilar skull fracture extending into the mastoid portion of the temporal bone. The lesion is not usually visible until 2 to 3 days after the trauma. Frontal lobe damage would be expected to yield classic frontal lobe signs on examination, such as a Meyerson's sign, rooting reflex, snout reflex, palmomental reflex, and grasp reflex. These signal extensive damage to the frontal lobe (or lobes if the sign is bilateral). Increased intracranial pressure presents with obtundation of level of consciousness, papilledema, and signs of brainstem compromise. Hypocalcemia that is chronic may result in the clinical observation of a Chvostek's sign. The sign is positive when the cheek is tapped with the examiner's finger and the corner of the mouth involuntarily contracts. Impending cerebral herniation usually presents with all of the signs of increased intracranial pressure as noted above. Systemic hypertension and respiratory compromise are also often noted.

B&D Chs 5&62

Question 95. B. Fluoxetine and phenelzine should not be combined because one is a serotonin-selective reuptake inhibitor (SSRI) and the other is a monoamine oxidase inhibitor (MAOI). SSRIs should not be combined with MAOIs because of the possibility of causing a fatal serotonin syndrome. Using an SSRI with selegeline, which only inhibits MAO-B, is tolerated by some patients. But the general rule to remember is: do not mix SSRIs and MAOIs. If you give one followed by the other there must be a washout period in between. It would be a good idea for the well-prepared test taker to know the symptoms of a serotonin syndrome and how to distinguish it from neuroleptic malignant syndrome. Both conditions are covered elsewhere in this volume.

K&S Ch. 36

Question 96. D. Atomoxatine (Strattera) is FDA-approved for symptoms of attention deficit-hyperactivity disorder (ADHD) in both adults and children. Its mechanism of action is by norepinephrine reuptake inhibition. It is the most useful choice when trying to treat both tics and ADHD, as it does not worsen the tic condition and may in fact help the tic symptoms. Bupropion (Wellbutrin) is not specifically FDA-approved for ADHD and its use in the disorder has not been shown to be consistently beneficial. The amphetamine-like stimulant medications methylphenidate (Ritalin, Metadate, Concerta) and dextroamphetamine (Dexedrine), although approved, well-studied and efficacious in ADHD, have been known to worsen underlying tics in concomitant Tourette's syndrome. Clonidine (Catapres) is an alpha-2 adrenergic agonist that has little place in ADHD, although it may certainly help alleviate tics in Tourette's syndrome.

B&D Ch. 67

Question 97. D. More statistics! Regression analysis is a method of using data to predict the value of one variable in relation to another. The other distracters are explained elsewhere in this volume.

K&S Ch. 4

Question 98. C. Lioresal (Baclofen) is one of the most potent of the oral muscle relaxing agents and treats spasticity highly effectively. Its full mechanism of action is not well-understood, but it is believed to have predominant effect as a GABA-B agonist. It can cause muscular weakness and difficulty with weight-bearing because of its potency. Other first-line agents to treat symptomatic spasticity include gabapentin, diazepam, clonidine, tizanidine, and dantrolene. Second-line agents include intrathecal lioresal, marinol, chlorpromazine, cyproheptadine, phenytoin, and phenobarbital.

B&D Ch. 54

Question 99. A. Just in case Question 61 wasn't enough, here it is again. Correlation coefficient is a measurement of the direction and strength of the relationship between two variables. The Pearson correlation coefficient is on a scale from −1 to +1. A positive correlation means that one variable moves the other in the same direction. A negative value means that one moves the other in the opposite direction.
K&S Ch. 4

Question 100. C. Triphasic waves on electroencephalogram are characteristic of hepatic or metabolic encephalopathy. Of course, hepatic encephalopathy is often accompanied by asterixis, particularly when the condition is severe. Asterixis is a sudden loss of postural tone and manifests as a flapping tremor of the hands. It is exhibited when the arms are fully extended. Herpetic skin vesicles would of course be expected with herpes simplex virus infections. Penile chancre can be demonstrated in cases of syphilis. Dupuytren's contractures are a form of benign progressive fibroproliferative disease of the palmar fasciae of unknown etiology. The condition is seen more often in men than women and is associated with alcoholism, hand trauma and diabetes. Pulmonary rales would be an expected sign in congestive heart failure.
B&D Ch. 62

Question 101. C. Experiments such as the one in this question have been used to give behavioral models for depression and stress. In this situation it is the unpredictability of the insults and the animal's inability to control them that leads to a state of chronic stress. Animals put under chronic stress become restless, tense, irritable, or very inhibited. The concept of unpredictable stress is important to understand in conjunction with the theory of learned helplessness proposed by Martin Seligman. In learned helplessness experiments, animals are exposed to electric shocks from which they can not escape. They eventually become apathetic and make no attempts to escape. This can be generalized to human behavior as seen in a child who consistently fails in school and then gives up trying and becomes depressed. Learned helplessness is a proposed animal model for human depression. The other answer choices are unrelated, or are simply ridiculous.
K&S Ch. 4

Question 102. D. Common side effects of valproic acid include weight gain, tremor, thinning of the hair, and ankle swelling. Other noted adverse effects are gastrointestinal distress, sedation, pancreatitis, bone marrow suppression (pancytopenia), and hepatotoxicity. The agent is teratogenic and the most worrisome fetotoxic effect is the neural tube defect (spina bifida) which is dangerous during neurogenesis in the first trimester of gestation.
B&D Ch. 73

Question 103. E. It is the doctor's ethical obligation to treat the patient in question regardless of ability to pay. It is unethical to allow a suicidal patient to leave the hospital due to a dispute with the insurance company. Should the patient go and kill himself, the doctor, not the insurance company, is liable. After the patient is treated and released, the issue can be taken up more aggressively with the insurance company. As a physician, your first and most important obligation is to the patient, not to the insurance company or to your wallet.
K&S Ch. 58

Question 104. B. Clonidine (Catapres) is a presynaptic $\alpha2$-receptor agonist. It is FDA-approved as an antihypertensive agent. It acts by reducing the amount of norepinephrine that is released from the synaptic bouton. This effect decreases sympathetic tone and bodily arousal and activation. The agent diminishes the autonomic symptoms associated with opioid withdrawal, such as tachycardia, hypertension, sweating, and lacrimation. Atomoxetine (Strattera) FDA-approved for ADHD in children and adults is a norepinephrine reuptake inhibitor. The neuroleptic medications, both conventional and atypical, can cause α-1 adrenergic antagonism and thereby cause orthostatic hypotension. Dopamine type 2 antagonism is the putative antipsychotic mechanism of all of the neuroleptic agents, both conventional and atypical. Serotonin antagonism is what makes an atypical antipsychotic atypical. It is in fact the ratio of D2 to 5-HT2 blockade that reduces the extrapyramidal side effects of the atypical neuroleptics.

K&S Ch. 36

Question 105. D. Heroin can be detected on a urine toxicology screen for 36–72 hours. Alcohol can be detected for up to 12 hours. Amphetamines can be detected for up to 48 hours. Cannabis can be detected for up to 4 weeks. PCP can be detected for up to 8 days.

K&S Ch. 7

Question 106. E. The Klüver-Bucy syndrome results from bilateral destruction of the amygdaloid bodies and the inferior temporal cortex. Clinical features include hypersexuality, placidity and hyperorality. One of the causes of the syndrome is Pick's disease (frontotemporal dementia). Other causes include stroke and Alzheimer's dementia. Other associated features include visual agnosia (psychic blindness), hyperphagia and prosopagnosia (the inability to recognize faces). The rest of the answer choices are simply distracters.

K&S Ch. 10

Question 107. E. Patients at high risk during electro-convulsive therapy (ECT) include the following: those with space occupying lesions in the CNS, those with increased intracranial pressure, those at risk for cerebral bleed, those who have had a recent myocardial infarction, and those with uncontrolled hypertension. There are no absolute contraindications for ECT, but patients who fall into any of the above mentioned categories should be screened carefully and decisions made on a case by case basis depending on risks, benefits, and ability to control risk factors.

K&S Ch. 36

Question 108. B. Klinefelter's syndrome results from the presence of an extra X chromosome (XXY triploidy). It is noted in about 1 in 700 men. Clinical features include small dysfunctional testes, mental retardation and pear-shaped stature. Testosterone replenishment may offset some of the stigmata of the condition. Turner's syndrome is the absence of an X chromosome in a genetic female (X0). Characteristics include short stature and lack of pubertal sexual development. Other clinical features include a webbed neck, and heart and kidney anomalies. Trisomy 21 is of course classic Down's syndrome which is explained in detail in another question in this volume. Deletion on the paternal chromosome 15 results in the Prader-Willi syndrome. The prevalence is about 1 in 12 000 to 15 000. Clinical features include profound mental retardation, hypogonadism, hypotonia, behavioral disinhibition, rapid and excessive weight gain, and facial dysmorphism. Trisomy 18 is described elsewhere in this volume.

B&D Ch. 44

Question 109. C. Patient controlled analgesia has proven to be an extremely good way of treating pain. Patients who control their own dosing end up using less pain medication than those who have to ask for the medication and wait for the doctor to write an order. They also have far better pain control. Some patients, particularly cancer patients may need large and escalating doses of medication to control their pain. Under these circumstances, this

should not be viewed as addiction, but as a necessary part of the treatment of their illness. Cancer patients have been shown to wean themselves off of the pain medication once the pain decreases. The use of pain control in a drug addict with a painful medical illness is as important as it is in a non-addict with the same illness. They may need higher doses to control their pain, but the doctor has as much of an obligation to manage their pain as they do to manage the pain of the non-addict. The other answer choices do not address the issue of using as little medication as necessary while obtaining the best pain control. This is why patient-controlled analgesia is the best choice.
K&S Ch. 28

Question 110. B. This vignette points to a diagnosis of intermittent explosive disorder. Intermittent explosive disorder manifests as discrete episodes of failure to resist aggressive impulses that lead to extreme physical aggression directed towards people and/or property. The degree of aggression is completely out of proportion to any particular psychosocial stressor that may trigger such an episode.
Episodes are unpredictable and often arise without cause or particular trigger and remit as spontaneously as they begin. There are no signs or symptoms of aggressivity noted in between these discrete episodes. The disorder is more common in men than in women. Predisposing psychosocial factors include an underprivileged or tempestuous childhood, childhood abuse, and early frustration and deprivation. Biological predisposing factors are believed to be decreased cerebral serotonergic transmission, low cerebrospinal fluid (CSF) levels of 5-hydroxyindoleacetic acid (5-HIAA) and high CSF levels of testosterone in men. There is strong comorbidity with fire setting, substance use and the eating disorders.
The personality disorders such as borderline and antisocial, are distinguished from intermittent explosive disorder by a pervasive pattern of maladaptive behavior that would be expected to occur in between episodes and affect the patient's life adversely in more areas of functioning. Aggressive patients with bipolar mania would be expected to present with evidence of manic symptoms, including elevated/irritable mood, increased energy, rapid pressured speech, sleeplessness, racing thoughts, distractability, increased goal-directed behavior, and perhaps even psychosis. Temporal-lobe seizures are a remote possibility and can certainly result in aggression, most often interictally, but there is no evidence of this presented in this question.
Treatment of intermittent explosive disorder can be undertaken with mood stabilizers such as lithium, carbamazepine, divalproex sodium, and gabapentin. Selective serotonin reuptake inhibitors and tricyclic antidepressants can also be effective in reducing aggression.
K&S Ch. 25

Question 111. B. Catalepsy is an immobile position that is constantly maintained. Cataplexy is temporary loss of muscle tone precipitated by an emotional state. Psychomotor retardation is decreased motor and cognitive activity often seen with depression. Catatonia is markedly slowed motor activity to the point of immobility and unawareness of surroundings. Stereotypy is a repetitive fixed pattern of movement or speech.
K&S Ch. 8

Question 112. D. Bupropion (Wellbutrin) is the only antidepressant agent that is believed to be a dopamine and norepinephrine reuptake inhibitor. It is FDA-approved for both depression and smoking cessation. It has a unique side effect profile and is unlikely to cause the sexual dysfunction or weight gain noted with the serotonergic antidepressants. Bupropion is a noncompetitive inhibitor of nicotinic cholinergic receptors and in this way can reduce tobacco cravings in smokers. Bupropion is less likely to precipitate a bipolar manic episode than the tricyclic antidepressants. It is also less likely to induce rapid cycling in bipolar patients than other antidepressants.

Tiagabine (Gabitril) is a selective GABA reuptake inhibitor. It is FDA-approved for adjunctive therapy in partial complex seizures in adolescents and adults. Duloxetine (Cymbalta) is a serotonin and norepinephrine reuptake inhibitor. It is approved in both major depressive disorder and diabetic neuropathic pain. It works on pain modulation via the brainstem and spinal cord efferent noradrenergic tracts originating in the locus ceruleus. Venlafaxine XR is also a serotonin and norepinephrine reuptake inhibitor and is FDA-approved in major depressive disorder, generalized anxiety disorder, social anxiety disorder, and most recently obtained an indication in panic disorder. Atomoxetine (Strattera) is a norepinephrine reuptake inhibitor that is FDA-approved for the treatment of attention deficit-hyperactivity disorder in both children and adults.

K&S Ch. 36

Question 113. D. The description in this question is of partial isolation monkeys. Those totally isolated from other monkeys were very fearful, unable to copulate, and unable to raise young. Mother-only raised monkeys failed to copulate, didn't leave the mother to explore, and were scared of their peers. The peer-only raised monkeys were easily frightened, timid, had little playfulness, and grasped other monkeys in a clinging manner. In monkeys separated from their mothers, there was an initial protest stage followed by despair. Many of these behavior patterns can be correlated with human behaviors that are seen in our patients.

K&S Ch. 4

Question 114. A. Sildenafil, vardenafil and tadalafil are nonselective phosphodiesterase 5 (PDE5) inhibitors. They also have some agonistic effects on nitric oxide (NO). PDE5 blockade causes arterial smooth muscle dilatation and facilitates cavernosal blood filling which potentiates penile erection. These agents cannot be used with nitrates because the combined effect of NO agonism with nitrates can cause significant vasodilatation and precipitous lowering of the blood pressure than can result in diminished cardiac perfusion and myocardial infarction. The other answer choices are simply distracters.

K&S Ch. 36

Question 115. B. Amoxapine is one of the tricyclic antidepressants. What sets it apart from the others is that one of its metabolites has dopamine blocking activity. Because of this amoxapine has the potential to cause parkinsonian symptoms, akathesia, and even neuroleptic malignant syndrome. None of the other drugs listed has dopamine blocking activity.

K&S Ch. 36

Question 116. C. The relative risk of an illness is the ratio of the incidence of the condition in those with risk factors to the incidence of the condition in those without risk factors. Attributable risk refers to the absolute incidence of the illness in patients exposed to the condition that can be attributed to the exposure. The other answer choices are nonsense distracters and are not true biostatistical terms.

K&S Ch. 4

Question 117. C. Cingulotomy is a surgical treatment for obsessive-compulsive disorder. It is successful in treating about 30% of otherwise treatment resistant patients. Some patients who fail medication, and then subsequently fail surgery, will respond to medication after surgery. Complications of cingulotomy include seizures, which are then managed with anticonvulsants. The other disorders listed in this question do not have surgical treatments.

K&S Ch. 16

Question 118. E.   Dissociative identity disorder (DID) also known as multiple personality disorder, is a chronic dissociative disorder. The origins of the disorder are believed to stem from early childhood trauma, most often sexual or physical. The hallmark of the disorder is the presence of two or more distinct identities or personality states that recurrently take over the person's behavior. There is also a presence of dissociative amnesia, with a noted inability to recall important personal information that is too extensive to be explained solely by forgetfulness.

The true cause of DID is unknown. Some research points to a possible connection between DID and epilepsy, with some patients having abnormal electroencephalograms. The absence of external supports, particularly from parents, siblings, relatives and significant others, seems to play a pivotal role in the genesis of the disorder. The patient's lack of stress coping mechanisms is also a likely contributory factor. The differential diagnosis includes borderline personality disorder, rapidly-cycling bipolar disorder, and schizophrenia. The disorder can start at almost any age and an early age of onset is predictive of a worse prognosis.

Treatment is focused on insight-oriented psychotherapy. Hypnotherapy may also be helpful. Antipsychotic medications are often unhelpful. Antidepressant and anxiolytic medications can be useful in addition to psychotherapy. Anticonvulsant mood stabilizers have shown some efficacy in certain studies. Viral exposure or infection has nothing to do with the etiology of DID.

K&S Ch. 20

Question 119. D.   The first-line therapy for the catatonic patient is intramuscular lorazepam. Many patients will respond to this treatment and will come out of their catatonic state. They can then be given subsequent treatment with antipsychotic drugs for the underlying psychotic disorder that is the most likely cause of the catatonia. Antidepressants and stimulants are not indicated for catatonia.

K&S Ch. 36

Question 120. C.   Malingering is diagnosed in the presence of intentional production of symptoms that are exaggerated and either physical or psychological in nature. These symptoms are motivated by secondary gain and incentives to avoid responsibility or danger, or to obtain compensation or some other benefit that is material or monetary. Symptoms are vague, ill-defined, overdramatized and do not conform to known clinical conditions. Patients seek secondary gain most often in the form of drugs, money, or the avoidance of work or jail. History and examination typically do not reveal complaints from the patient. The patient is often uncooperative and refuses to accept a good prognosis or clean bill of health. Findings can be compatible with self-inflicted injuries. Medical records may have been tampered with or altered. Family members are usually unable to verify the consistency of symptoms.

K&S Ch. 33

Question 121. D.   Mutism refers to a patient who is voiceless without abnormalities in the structures which produce speech. Mutism is common in catatonic schizophrenia. It can be seen in conversion disorder. There is also a diagnosis known as selective mutism for children who consistently fail to speak in social situations despite speaking in other situations. Other causes of mutism include mental retardation, pervasive developmental disorder, and expressive language disorders. It can also be a component of bucco-facial apraxia, locked-in syndrome, and a persistent vegetative state.

K&S Ch. 48

Question 122. B. Biofeedback is a therapy in which instruments are used to measure autonomic parameters in patients who are provided with "real-time" feedback from the instrumentation about their bodily physiologic processes. This feedback enables patients to control their own physiologic functions and alter them in positive ways to alleviate symptoms using operant conditioning techniques. Feedback is provided to the patient by measuring physiologic parameters such as heart rate, blood pressure, galvanic skin response and skin temperature. The measurement is translated into a visual or auditory output signal that patients can rely on to gauge their responses. Patients can alter the tone by using guided imagery, breathing techniques, cognitive techniques and other relaxation techniques. The modality is useful for anxiety disorders, migraine, and tension-type headache in particular.

Stimulus-response therapy is a nonsense distracter, as there is no such thing. Relaxation training is a form of behavior therapy that basically encompasses techniques such as meditation and yoga to help patients to dispel anxiety by tapping into their own physiologic parameters such as heart rate and breathing rate. Guided mental imagery also helps patients to enter a relaxed state of mind. Behavior therapy is the global term used to describe different therapeutic modalities that employ either operant or classical conditioning techniques to help patients overcome their fears, phobias and anxieties. Flooding, systematic desensitization, and aversion therapy are all examples of behavior therapy. Desensitization refers to the technique that helps patients gradually overcome their fears, phobias and anxieties, by graded exposure to the very stimulus that is the source of their fears. The patient is exposed to more and more anxiety-provoking stimuli, but relaxation training helps patients to cope with their maladaptive responses and eventually ideally respond to the stimulus without it evoking anxiety.

K&S Ch. 35

Question 123. D. Lithium toxicity is a medical emergency and can result in permanent neuronal damage and death. Toxicity occurs at lithium levels above 2.5 mEq/L. Treatment includes discontinuation of lithium as well as vigorous hydration. If the level is above 4 mEq/L, or the patient shows serious signs of lithium toxicity (nephrotoxicity, convulsions, coma) the patient must have hemodialysis. Hemodialysis can be repeated every 6–10 hours until the level is no longer toxic and the patient's symptoms remit. If the patient in question was not showing serious signs of toxicity, labs to assess the situation could be sent, neurological examination done, EKG obtained, gastric lavage performed, activated charcoal given, and vigorous hydration used. The patient could then be monitored and given time to clear the lithium.

K&S Ch. 36

Question 124. D. The most useful long-term treatment parameter for the noncompliant patient with schizophrenia who has a history of violence would be the use of an outpatient commitment program. Certain states have such laws in place, but others do not. Treating clinicians can petition the court to place refractory, potentially dangerous patients on this status. A judge mandates the patient's cooperativeness and the patient is compelled to report for outpatient follow-up. If the patient is noncompliant, a psychiatrist can order that the patient be picked up against his wishes and brought in for psychiatric evaluation to an emergency room where the patient can be held for a period of time. Certain states use an alternative to outpatient commitment called conservatorship. This modality involves the court appointing a conservator, often a family member, to look after the patient and make decisions on the patient's behalf, including placing the patient in involuntary hospitalization if it is deemed necessary.

Partial hospitalization is quite similar to inpatient hospitalization, except the patient sleeps at home. This modality is often a good transition between inpatient and outpatient services and patients can stay in such a program over extended periods of time if necessary. Patients have a case manager assigned to them in partial programs. The case manager helps coordinate and facilitate the patient's care and helps make the patient's transition easier to the less restrictive setting. Day treatment programs are somewhat less intense and less structured than partial hospital programs. Patients again sleep at home, but they participate in facility-based care five or more days a week. Case management and social work also play pivotal roles in the day treatment program setting.

Social skills training refers to a program that is dedicated to helping low-functioning patients, such as those with schizophrenia, to gain key skills that will enable them to function more independently in the community. The focus is on improving patients' interactions with other people in their environment.

K&S Ch. 35&59

Question 125. C. Monoamine oxidase inhibitors (MAOIs) have several serious drug–drug interactions than must be kept in mind. Meperidine (Demerol) can *never* be given with an MAOI, as this combination has led to death in several patients (common exam question!). MAOIs should never be used with anesthetics (no spinal anesthetics, no anesthetics containing epinephrine, lidocaine is OK). MAOIs should not be combined with asthma medication or over the counter drugs that contain dextromethorphan (cold and flu medications). They can not be given with sympathomimetics (epinephrine, amphetamines, cocaine). They can not be given with SSRIs or clomipramine as this will precipitate a serotonin syndrome. There are also many food restrictions with MAOIs which will, no doubt, be the subject of another question.

K&S Ch. 36

Question 126. A. Privilege refers to the psychiatrist's right to maintain a patient's secrecy or confidentiality even in the face of a subpoena. This implies that the right of privilege belongs to the patient, not the psychiatrist and therefore the patient can wave the right. There are many exceptions to medical privilege, and many physicians are not aware that they do not legally enjoy the same privilege that exists between husband and wife, priest and parishioner, and a client and an attorney.

Confidentiality is the professional obligation of the physician to maintain secrecy regarding all information given to him by the patient.

A psychiatrist may be asked to appear in court and testify by subpoena and thereby be forced to break a patient's confidentiality. A patient may release the clinician from the obligation of confidentiality by signing a consent to release information. Each release pertains to a specific matter or piece of information and may need to be reobtained for subsequent disclosures.

Communication rights refers to the patient's right to free and open communication with the outside world by either telephone or mail, while hospitalized. Private rights refers to the patient's right to privacy. In a hospital setting, this applies to patients having private toileting and bathing space, secure storage space for personal effects, and adequate personal floor space per person. Patients also have the right to wear their own clothing and carry their own money if they desire to do so. Certain restrictions to this right may apply based on dangerousness to self or others. Clinical responsibility is not a forensic term per se, but it refers to the responsibility of the physician to the patient to provide the patient with the best care possible in any clinical setting, irrespective of the patient's financial, racial, or personal status.

K&S Ch. 57

Question 127. B. Patients being started on clozapine should have a baseline white blood cell (WBC) count with differential before treatment. A WBC count with differential is taken every week during treatment for the first six months, then every two weeks thereafter. When treatment is stopped WBC counts should be taken every week for four weeks. It is not a part of standard monitoring to take 2 WBC counts in one week. The US Food and Drug Administration recently approved monthly monitoring of WBC count after 12 months of therapy on clozapine.
K&S Ch. 7

Question 128. C. Patients over 65 years of age undergo sleep problems that affect both rapid eye movement (REM) sleep and non-rapid eye movement (NREM) sleep. There are more REM episodes noted. REM episodes are shorter in duration. There is less total REM sleep. In NREM sleep there is a decreased amplitude of delta waves. There is a lower percentage of stages three and four sleep. There is a higher percentage of stage one and two sleep. The elderly experience increased awakening after sleep onset.
K&S Ch. 55

Question 129. B. Clozapine has several drug–drug interactions that are noteworthy. Cimetidine, SSRIs, tricyclics, valproic acid, and erythromycin will all increase clozaril levels. Phenytoin and carbamazepine will decrease clozapine levels. Clozapine should not be combined with any medication that can cause agranulocytosis (carbamazepine, propylthiouracil, sulfonamides, and captopril). CNS depressants (alcohol, benzodiazepines, and tricyclics) cause even more depression when combined with clozapine. The combination of lithium and clozaril can increase neuroleptic malignant syndrome, seizures, confusion, and movement disorders. Other answer choices are distracters. The foods given should be avoided when taking MAOIs. Acetaminophen and aripiprazole have no interaction.
K&S Ch. 36

Question 130. E. Cannabis is the most widely abused recreational drug among US high school students. Cannabis use has been demonstrated to lead to future cocaine abuse in adolescents. About 35% of high school seniors reported using cannabis. Alcohol is also a pervasive problem among high school teens, but only in about 10–20% of students surveyed. Over 85% of high school seniors have reported that they have tried alcohol at some time. About 15% of adolescents have reported using inhalants. Fewer than 2% of high school students report having used cocaine. About 9% of high school seniors have reported trying LSD at some time.
K&S Ch. 51

Question 131. D. Aaron Beck is the originator of cognitive therapy. It is based on the theory that affect and behavior are determined by the way in which patients structure the world. Patients have assumptions, on which they base cognitions, which lead to affect and behavior. In depression specifically, Beck feels that there is a triad consisting of the following:

1. Depressed people see themselves as defective, inadequate, and worthless.
2. Depressed people experience the world as negative and self-defeating.
3. Depressed people have an expectation of continued hardship and failure.

It is this triad of distorted negative thoughts that Beck feels leads to depression. The goal of cognitive therapy is to help test the cognitions and develop more productive alternatives. Other answer choices given are distracters. Good enough mothering and transitional object are terms associated with the child development theory of Winnicott. Mania is not associated with Beck's cognitive triad. Aggression toward the primary caregiver has nothing to do with Beck.
K&S Ch. 35

Question 132. D. Ramelteon (Rozerem) is a novel sleeping agent that was FDA-approved in 2005 for insomnia with sleep onset difficulties. It has a unique mechanism of action: it is a melatonin agonist. It works by stimulating melatonin type 1 and type 2 receptors in the suprachiasmatic nucleus of the hypothalamus. It has no addictive or abuse potential, because it is not a GABA-A agonist and has no activity at the benzodiazepine receptor whatsoever. It has no effects at histamine, acetylcholine, dopamine, serotonin, or norepinephrine receptors. The dosage is the same for all patients: one 8 mg tablet at bedtime. Recall that zolpidem, zaleplon and eszopiclone are all benzodiazepine receptor agonists and as such have sedative-hypnotic effects and potential for tolerance, withdrawal and abuse.
K&S Ch. 36; also see www.rozerem.com

Question 133. E. Alogia is a lack of speech that results from a mental deficiency or dementia. Poverty of movement is called akinesia. Poverty of emotion is described using the term "flat affect."
K&S Ch. 8

Question 134. B. To meet criteria for the rapid cycling specifier in bipolar disorder, the patient must present with at least 4 mood episodes over the past 12 months. The mood episodes must meet criteria for a major depressive, manic, mixed, or hypomanic episode. Female patients are more likely than men to have rapid cycling bipolar disorder. There is no evidence to suggest that rapid cycling is a heritable phenomenon in bipolar disorder. It is therefore likely to be a result of external factors such as stress or medication.
K&S Ch. 15

Question 135. B. Random reinforcement is seen with the gambler. In random reinforcement the reward is only given a fraction of the time at random intervals. The money from a slot machine is won at random times. This keeps the gambler guessing and trying to anticipate when they will win. This is a very good way to maintain a behavior. Continuous reinforcement is when every action is rewarded, and is the best way to teach a new behavior. Primary reinforcers are independent of previous learning, for example, the need to eat is biological and not based on previous learning. Secondary reinforcers are based on previous learning, such as rewarding a child with a present when they do something well. The dexamethasone suppression test is an experimental measure associated with depression, and is unrelated to pathological gambling. Cerebellar dysfunction would lead to ataxia and gait disturbance, again, unrelated to pathological gambling.
K&S Ch. 4

Question 136. B. Late-onset schizophrenia is noted more often in women than in men. The prognosis seems to be more favorable when the onset is late. There is a tendency to see more paranoia in these late-onset schizophrenic patients. Schizophrenia is considered late-onset when symptoms begin after 45 years of age. It is clinically identical to schizophrenia that has normal onset.
K&S Ch. 13

Question 137. B. One might think that this one was too easy, but it's just the kind of question that could show up on an exam. A control group is a group in a study that does not receive treatment and is used as a standard of comparison.
K&S Ch. 4

Question 138. E. Bowlby and Robertson identified three essential stages of separation response among children. The first stage is that of protest. The child protests the mother's departure by crying, calling out and searching for

her. The second stage is despair and pain. The child loses faith that the mother will return. The third stage is detachment and denial of affection to the mother figure upon her return. These phases are noted universally in children who go through separation by loss of parents to death, divorce, or going off to boarding school. Acceptance is not one of Bowlby's stages of the separation response. It is the fifth and final stage of Kübler-Ross' stages of reaction to impending death.
K&S Ch. 4

Question 139. C. Buproprion has been shown in studies to be efficacious for the treatment of attention-deficit/hyperactivity disorder (ADHD) in children and adults. It is also a very good antidepressant, which is its most common use. It has also been found very useful in patients who do not respond to a serotonin-selective reuptake inhibitor. When buproprion is added to SSRIs up to 70% of these cases improve, as both drugs together hit more neurotransmitter systems than either drug alone. The other drugs listed have no proven usefulness in ADHD.
K&S Ch. 36

Question 140. C. Of the agents listed in this question, only sertraline (Zoloft) is FDA-approved in the pediatric population. It is only approved for obsessive-compulsive disorder (OCD) in patients ages 6 to 17 years. It is not indicated for depression or any of the other anxiety disorders in children. Fluoxetine (Prozac) is the only SSRI that is FDA-approved for the treatment of major depressive disorder in patients age 8 years and older. Fluvoxamine (Luvox) is also FDA-approved for OCD in patients 8 years of age and older. Paroxetine and venlafaxine are FDA-approved for depression and anxiety only in the adult population 18 years of age and older. Citalopram is FDA-approved for major depressive disorder only in adults over 18 years of age. Mirtazapine is only indicated for major depressive disorder and only in the adult population over 18 years of age.
K&S Ch. 36

Question 141. A. This question contains a supportive statement which acknowledges how difficult things are for the patient currently, but gives her hope for the future. It is characteristic of supportive psychotherapy. In psychodynamic therapy and psychoanalysis, the therapist would wish to remain more neutral and not make statements that expressed opinion or boosted the patient's mood. The question does not involve playing with children, so play therapy is incorrect. Cognitive behavioral therapy would involve looking at the patient's assumptions and cognitions and seeing how they affect the patient's mood. That is not happening in this question stem. Supportive psychotherapy seeks to stabilize the self and the patient's ability to cope. Defenses are strengthened. Symptom relief is sought. Neutrality is suspended. Direction by the therapist is encouraged. Free association is not part of this technique. Supportive psychotherapy can be used with those who have severe character pathology, psychosis, or are in the midst of an acute crisis or a physical illness.
K&S Ch. 35

Question 142. D. Risperidone decanoate injection (Risperdal Consta) is the only atypical antipsychotic currently available in long-acting injectable form. The drug is FDA-approved for schizophrenia, particularly in noncompliant and refractory cases. The formulation comes in three dosing strengths: 25 mg, 37.5 mg, and 50 mg. The recommended dosing interval is two weeks. The product comes prepared in a dose-pack with sterile water in a vial and a syringe for reconstituting the drug. The powdered, unreconstituted drug must be refrigerated prior to adding water. Sterile water is necessary for reconstitution. Once reconstituted, the drug must be administered within 6 hours. The drug must only be injected to the gluteus muscle.

The deltoid is not a recommended injection site because it is too small a muscle to accommodate proper timed dissipation of the agent. It is advisable to keep patients on their oral medication for at least three to four weeks while initiating risperidone Consta. This prevents possible decompensation from too rapid cross titration of antipsychotic agents.
K&S Ch. 13; also see www.risperdalconsta.com

Question 143. C. Naloxone is an opioid antagonist. An opioid overdose is a medical emergency. Respiratory depression ensues leading to coma and shock. Naloxone is given IV and can be repeated 4–5 times in the first 30 minutes. Care must be used as the half-life is short and the patient can relapse back into coma, plus severe withdrawal can ensue from the use of an opioid antagonist.
Naltrexone is a longer acting antagonist with a half-life of 72 hours. It is a preventative measure for those with opioid addiction. It is used for blocking the euphoric effects of opioid use and thus decreases craving. Because of its long half life it is not the best choice for an emergency.
Buprenorphine is a mixed opioid agonist-antagonist. It is used in place of morphine to keep people off of heroin, and is not used in emergencies.
Benztropine is also known as Cogentin, an anticholinergic medication used to mitigate the side effects of antipsychotic drugs. It has nothing to do with opium overdose.
Bromocriptine is a mixed dopamine agonist-antagonist which is approved in the US for treatment of Parkinson's disease.
K&S Ch. 12

Question 144. B. Elisabeth Kübler-Ross developed a comprehensive paradigm to classify the stages of a person's reactions to impending death. Stage one is that of shock and denial. Upon learning the news that they are dying, people are initially in a state of shock and may deny that the diagnosis is correct. Stage two is that of anger. During this stage patients get frustrated, angry and irritable about their condition. They often ask: "Why me?" They typically undergo a lot of self-blame about their illness. Stage three is that of bargaining. Patients may try to negotiate or bargain with doctors, friends, family and even God to alleviate their illness in exchange for good deeds or fulfillment of certain pledges. Stage four is that of depression. During this stage patients demonstrate frank signs and symptoms of depression, including hopelessness, suicidal ideation, social withdrawal, and sleep problems. If the symptoms are severe enough to qualify as a major depressive disorder, the patient should be treated with an antidepressant. Stage five is that of acceptance. Patients acknowledge and come to terms with the inevitability of their death during this stage. Patients can begin to talk about facing the unknown without fear and with resolution.
K&S Ch. 2

209

Question 145. D. Asking patients about suicide will have no effect on whether they are actually suicidal. Talking about suicide will not make patients suicidal. Most patients, when asked, are relieved to have permission to speak about something they have already thought about but were uncomfortable talking about with friends or family. The question is not frightening to them, nor will the mention of the word suicide help them plan their death.
K&S Ch. 34

Question 146. D. Patients can display their grief over the death of loved ones in different ways and with different intensity. It is generally believed that a period of grief or mourning typically lasts about six months to one year. Some symptoms and signs of mourning may persist for a longer period, even up to two years or more. In most cases, the acute symptoms of grief improve over a period of about one to two months, after which time the individual returns to a more normal level of functioning.

K&S Ch. 2

Question 147. D. The suicide rate for adolescents has quadrupled since 1950. Suicide accounts for 12% of deaths in the adolescent age group. The suicide rate has gone up more in this group than in any other group over the same time period.

K&S Ch. 49

Question 148. D. Ramelteon (Rozerem) is a melatonin agonist and has a short half-life ranging from one to 2.5 hours. Ramelteon has an active metabolite, M-II, that has a half-life of about 5 hours. Zolpidem (Ambien) has a half-life of about 2.5 hours, but the duration of action can range from one to 4.5 hours. Zolpidem has no active metabolite. Zaleplon (Sonata) is a benzodiazepine receptor agonist that has the shortest half-life of all these agents at about one hour. It is therefore very useful for the treatment of middle insomnia. Eszopiclone (Lunesta) has the longest half-life of all these sleeping agents at about 6 hours. It is therefore, at least theoretically, the one most likely to cause next-day drowsiness. Triazolam (Halcion) is a benzodiazepine sedative-hypnotic agent with high potency and a short half-life ranging in duration from 2–4 hours.

K&S Ch. 36

Question 149. A. The therapeutic range for valproic acid is 50–150 ng/mL. At doses as high as 125 ng/mL, side effects including thrombocytopenia may occur. Liver function tests should be obtained at the start of treatment and every 6–12 months thereafter, and valproic acid levels should be checked periodically.

K&S Ch. 7

Question 150. C. This is a question based on an understanding of the importance of culture. Different cultures view health and sickness differently. They view the medical system differently, and these differences must be taken into account when dealing with a multi-cultural population. In Japanese culture it is customary to minimize distress in front of an authority figure. This is the explanation for the patient's behavior in this question. If the doctor involved was unaware of cultural issues, the patient's behavior could be misinterpreted as psychosis or malingering, or the family could be seen as manipulative.

K&S Ch. 4

Test Number **FOUR**

1. All of the following are true regarding Freud's theories of human development, EXCEPT:

   A. During development, sexual energy shifts to different areas of the body that are usually associated with eroticism

   B. The anal phase is from age 1 year to 3 years

   C. Latency is marked by a sharp increase in sexual interest

   D. Freud thought that resolution of his stages was essential to normal adult functioning

   E. The phallic stage is from age 3 to 5 years

2. Ischemia to which one of the following arterial territories is responsible for the phenomenon known as amaurosis fugax?

   A. Carotid

   B. Vertebrobasilar

   C. Lenticulostriate

   D. Anterior cerebral

   E. Middle cerebral

3. Which one of the following is true regarding norepinephrine (NE) and/or the locus caeruleus?

   A. NE is synthesized in the locus caeruleus

   B. Dopamine is synthesized in the locus caeruleus, NE in the dorsal raphe nuclei

   C. Acetylcholine is synthesized with NE in the substantia nigra

   D. GABA is synthesized in the locus caeruleus

   E. The locus caeruleus is the site of formation of serotonin

4. A 75 year-old man with a recent history of influenza vaccination presents to the emergency room with an acute onset of paraparesis and urinary incontinence. He reported that his symptoms began a week earlier with dull, progressive low back pain that soon resulted in bilateral leg weakness. The most likely diagnosis in this case is:

   A. Spinal cord metastases

   B. Acute spinal cord compression

   C. Vacuolar myelopathy

   D. Transverse myelitis

   E. Acute disseminated encephalomyelitis

5. A doctor in a certain hospital makes a diagnosis for a particular patient. That diagnosis is considered reliable if:

   A. It is accurate

   B. Many different doctors in different locations would agree upon the same diagnosis

   C. The disorder has features characteristic enough to distinguish it from other disorders

   D. The disorder allows doctors to predict the clinical course and treatment response

   E. The diagnosis is based on an understanding of the underlying pathophysiology and has biological markers

6. Which one of the following set of symptoms and signs correctly identifies the Horner's syndrome?

   A. Ptosis, miosis, sweating

   B. Ptosis, mydriasis, sweating

   C. Ptosis, miosis, anhydrosis

   D. Ptosis, mydriasis, anhydrosis

   E. Lid-lag, miosis, anhydrosis

7. A patient presents with the following symptoms: tremor, halitosis, dry mouth, tachycardia, hypertension, fever, euphoria, alertness, agitation, paranoia, hallucinations, and irritability. Which one of the following substances is the most likely cause?

   A. Amphetamines

   B. Opioids

   C. Alcohol

   D. Barbiturates

   E. Benzodiazepines

8. The inability to recognize familiar faces is known as:
    A. Anosognosia
    B. Simultanagnosia
    C. Aprosodia
    D. Prosopagnosia
    E. Astereognosis

9. Effects resulting from PCP use include all of the following, EXCEPT:
    A. Paranoia
    B. Nystagmus
    C. Catatonia
    D. Convulsions
    E. Hypotension

10. A characteristic of a facial nerve (Bell's) palsy that clearly distinguishes it from a stroke-related facial paresis is:
    A. The presence of miosis
    B. The involvement of the whole face
    C. Anhydrosis
    D. Rapid recovery of motor functioning
    E. A post-infectious onset

11. Object permanence develops during which one of Piaget's developmental stages?
    A. Sensorimotor
    B. Preoperational thought
    C. Concrete operations
    D. Formal thought
    E. Rapprochement

12. Classic features of syringomyelia include all of the following, EXCEPT:
    A. Spasticity
    B. Muscular atrophy
    C. Fasciculations
    D. Loss of temperature and pain sensation
    E. Preservation of proprioception

13. A patient comes into the emergency room and admits to sniffing glue daily for the past eight months. Which one of the following is NOT your concern as this patient's physician?
    A. Liver damage
    B. Permanent brain damage
    C. Kidney damage
    D. Myocardial damage
    E. Urinary retention

14. One of the most common causes of the movement disorder of opsoclonus-myoclonus in the infant is:

     A. Neonatal seizures
     B. Craniopharyngioma
     C. Prematurity
     D. Neuroblastoma
     E. Meningioma

15. A physician examines a patient in the emergency room who has recently been diagnosed with a social phobia. Which one of the following answer choices would most likely be the greatest fear for this patient?

     A. Having to take responsibility for planning a dinner with her husband
     B. Being in a relationship with a new boyfriend
     C. Going to a state fair and being around thousands of people
     D. Being scrutinized by others
     E. Competing for a new position that just opened up in her company

16. The Ramsay-Hunt syndrome classically affects which one of the following pairs of cranial nerves?

     A. III and VI
     B. IV and VI
     C. V and VII
     D. V and VIII
     E. VII and VIII

17. All of the following statements are true regarding body dysmorphic disorder, EXCEPT:

     A. It is a preoccupation with an imagined defect in appearance
     B. It is most commonly associated with a comorbid mood disorder
     C. The most common concerns involve facial flaws
     D. Treatment with surgical, medical, dental or dermatological care is usually successful
     E. If a slight physical anomaly is present the concern is markedly excessive

18. Which one of the following primary brain tumors is the most common in patients over 60 years of age?

     A. Anaplastic astrocytoma
     B. Glioblastoma multiforme
     C. Meningioma
     D. Ependymoma
     E. Acoustic neuroma

19. Patients with obsessive-compulsive disorder are noted to have anomalies of which one of the following brain regions?

    A. Corpus callosum
    B. Striatum
    C. Hippocampus
    D. Caudate nucleus
    E. Cerebellum

20. Anton's syndrome results from a stroke that localizes to the:

    A. Frontal lobes
    B. Temporal lobes
    C. Parietal lobes
    D. Occipital lobes
    E. Cerebellar hemispheres

21. All of the following should be considered to be predictive factors for violence, EXCEPT:

    A. Alcohol intoxication
    B. Recent acts of violence
    C. Command auditory hallucinations
    D. High socioeconomic status
    E. Menacing other people

22. Riluzole, the only agent FDA-approved in the treatment of amyotrophic lateral sclerosis, affects which one of the following neurotransmitters?

    A. Glutamate
    B. GABA
    C. Acetylcholine
    D. Dopamine
    E. Norepinephrine

23. A 29 year-old patient is admitted to the neurology unit for evaluation of seizures. Workup is negative and there has not been any seizure activity captured on electroencephalogram during his seizure episodes. Neurological examination is negative. The patient is noted to be very sad, and a psychiatric consult is called. Nurses have noted conflict between the patient and his wife during her visits. As the consultant, which one of the following would be the highest on your list of differential diagnoses?

    A. Obsessive-compulsive disorder
    B. Conversion disorder
    C. Somatization disorder
    D. Social phobia
    E. Panic disorder

24. What is the most common CNS cancer noted in patients with advanced AIDS?
    A. Glioblastoma multiforme
    B. Lymphoma
    C. Meningioma
    D. High-grade brainstem glioma
    E. Epidermoid tumor

25. The highest rate of synapse formation in the brain takes place during which one of the following time periods?
    A. Adolescence
    B. Weeks 32 to 35 of gestation
    C. Weeks 13 to 26 of gestation
    D. Within the first six weeks of gestation
    E. As a toddler

26. Presenting features of AIDS dementia complex include all of the following, EXCEPT:
    A. Poor attention and concentration
    B. Slowness of thinking
    C. Personality changes
    D. Apathy
    E. Hemiparesis

27. All of the following are medical complications of weight loss in eating disorders, EXCEPT:
    A. Cachexia
    B. Loss of cardiac muscle
    C. Delayed gastric emptying
    D. Lanugo
    E. Increased bone density

28. The most frequent opportunistic CNS infection in the AIDS patient is:
    A. CNS toxoplasmosis
    B. Cryptococcal meningitis
    C. Herpes meningitis
    D. Cytomegalovirus encephalitis
    E. Neurosyphilis

29. All of the following are medical complications of purging seen in eating disorders, EXCEPT:

    A. Electrolyte abnormalities

    B. Salivary gland inflammation

    C. Erosion of dental enamel

    D. Hyperkalemia

    E. Seizures

30. A 45 year-old man with end-stage AIDS and CD4 count of 50/μL presents to the ER with a complaint of rapidly progressive onset of gait difficulty, spasticity, leg weakness, sphincter dysfunction and loss of proprioception to both feet and legs. The most likely diagnosis in this case is:

    A. Progressive multifocal leukoencephalopathy

    B. Distal sensory polyneuropathy

    C. Vacuolar myelopathy

    D. Neurosyphilis

    E. HTLV-1 myelopathy

31. All of the following medical conditions should be considered when evaluating patients with anxiety disorders, EXCEPT:

    A. Carcinoid syndrome

    B. Hyperventilation syndrome

    C. Hypoglycemia

    D. Hyperthyroidism

    E. Central serous chorioretinopathy

32. A 45 year-old man with end-stage AIDS and CD4 count of 0/μL presents to the ER with a complaint of progressive onset over the past few weeks of ataxia, visual field deficits, altered mental status, aphasia and fluctuating sensory deficits. T2-weighted brain MRI reveals the image noted below. The most likely diagnosis in this case is:

    A. CNS toxoplasmosis

    B. Lymphoma

    C. Neurosyphilis

    D. AIDS dementia complex

    E. Progressive multifocal leukoencephalopathy

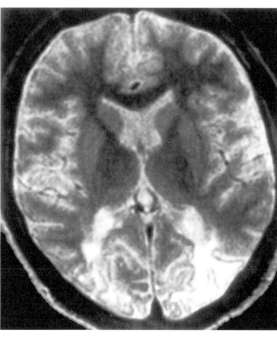

33. When diagnosing a patient with social phobia, which axis II diagnosis is it most important for the treating psychiatrist to keep in mind?
    A. Paranoid personality disorder
    B. Schizoid personality disorder
    C. Obsessive compulsive personality disorder
    D. Avoidant personality disorder
    E. Borderline personality disorder

34. All of the following are prion diseases, EXCEPT:
    A. Kuru
    B. Gerstmann-Sträussler-Scheinker syndrome
    C. Fatal familial insomnia
    D. Devic's syndrome
    E. Creutzfeldt-Jakob disease

35. A psychiatrist is covering the emergency room and a patient comes in who has a previous diagnosis of bipolar II disorder. Based on this diagnosis which one of the following symptoms would the knowledgeable psychiatrist expect to see in this patient over time?
    A. Psychotic features
    B. Manic episodes that do not respond to treatment with mood stabilizers
    C. Rapid cycling between severe depression and mania
    D. Recurrent manic episodes in the absence of depression
    E. Recurrence of both depressive and hypomanic episodes

36. The classic triad of headache, ipsilateral Horner's syndrome and contralateral hemiparesis is generally due to:
    A. Carotid artery occlusion
    B. Giant cell arteritis
    C. Wallenberg's syndrome
    D. Pontine hemorrhage
    E. Cerebral aneurysmal rupture

37. A set of statistical procedures designed to compare two or more groups of observations and determine whether the differences are due to chance or experimental difference is called:
    A. Correlation coefficient
    B. Control group
    C. Analysis of variance (ANOVA)
    D. Regression analysis
    E. Null hypothesis

38. A 55 year-old woman presents to the emergency room with a sudden and acute onset of right-sided painless complete facial paralysis, involving both the upper and lower parts of the face. The symptoms began earlier that day and were initially accompanied by a mild ache behind the ear which resolved. The organism most likely responsible for this condition is:

   A. B. burgdorferi
   B. Herpes simplex virus
   C. Epstein-Barr virus
   D. West Nile virus
   E. Varicella zoster virus

39. A psychiatrist is asked to evaluate a child who does not make appropriate eye contact, fails to respond to the social cues of others, lacks the ability for spontaneous make-believe play, and on close examination has a delay in language development. What is this child's most likely diagnosis?

   A. Schizophrenia
   B. Avoidant personality disorder
   C. Asperger's disorder
   D. Conduct disorder
   E. Autism

40. A veterinary radiologist presents to the emergency room with a four-week history of headache, vague fever, and paresthesias in the fingers and toes. His temperature is 103.5°F. He complains of difficulty swallowing with pharyngeal spasms for the past three days. The most likely diagnosis is:

   A. West Nile virus infection
   B. Tetanus infection
   C. Acute botulism
   D. Rabies
   E. Epstein-Barr virus infection

41. Which one of the following receptor subtypes is associated with the neurotransmitter glutamate?

   A. Nicotinic
   B. Muscarinic
   C. Alpha 1
   D. AMPA
   E. GABA

42. A 60 year-old woman presents to the emergency room with a progressive downward course over the past six months characterized by behavioral disinhibition, emotional lability, severe naming and word-finding difficulties, hyperorality, stubbornness, inability to plan, and poor judgment. Autopsy of this patient's brain would most likely reveal:

    A. Hirano bodies
    B. Pick's inclusion bodies and gliosis
    C. Lewy bodies
    D. Neurofibrillary plaques and tangles
    E. Severe white-matter demyelination

43. Your friend just had a baby that is 8 months old. You and she talk about the child and note its temperament. At this point in the child's development you tell your friend that the child's temperament is most likely a function of:

    A. Biological factors
    B. The parent's culture
    C. The grandmother's influence on weekends
    D. The baby's birth month
    E. The influence of the child's siblings

44. The neuropathological hallmark of idiopathic Parkinson's disease is:

    A. Brainstem Lewy bodies
    B. Hirano bodies
    C. Amyloid plaques
    D. Mesial temporal sclerosis
    E. Caudate nucleus atrophy

45. A young woman comes to a psychiatrist's office seeking help because of problems on her job. She describes nervousness talking in front of other coworkers at conferences, and difficulty at social events. She thinks that her boss knows her inner feelings and that there was wording put in everyone's contracts with her specifically in mind. Her dress is eccentric and out of date. She complains that she does not have any friends at the office. Given this picture, she most likely has which one of the following diagnoses?

    A. Borderline personality disorder
    B. Dependent personality disorder
    C. Schizotypal personality disorder
    D. Histrionic personality disorder
    E. Schizoid personality disorder

46. All of the following are possible symptoms of fibromyalgia, EXCEPT:

    A. Headache
    B. Psychosis
    C. Depression
    D. Sleep disturbance
    E. Paresthesias

47. Pancreatic cancer is most often associated with which one of the following psychiatric disorders?

    A. Psychosis
    B. Anxiety
    C. Depression
    D. Impulse control disorders
    E. Bulimia

48. A 75 year-old man with known history of prostate cancer presents to the emergency room with an acute onset of bilateral leg weakness, leg spasticity, sensory loss to pain and temperature below the waist, and acute bladder and bowel incontinence. The first test of choice to perform in the emergency room setting is:

    A. Noncontrast head CT
    B. Brain MRI
    C. Screening spine MRI
    D. Spinal X-rays
    E. HTLV-1 antibody titer

49. Which one of the following symptoms would a psychiatrist look for in a child to make the diagnosis of conduct disorder rather than depression, ADHD, or bipolar disorder?

    A. Irritable mood
    B. Difficulty organizing tasks
    C. Excessive activity
    D. Starting fights with other children
    E. Sleep disturbance

50. Subacute combined degeneration of the spinal cord is a result of deficiency in which one of the following:

    A. Vitamin B12
    B. Vitamin B1
    C. Vitamin B6
    D. Niacin
    E. Folic acid

51. When patients who have been victim to childhood incest become adults, which one of the following disorders are they most prone to develop?

    A. Anorexia
    B. Bipolar disorder
    C. Social phobia
    D. Major depression
    E. Conversion disorder

52. A patient presents to the emergency room with an acute onset of pure right hemiparesis that on examination is noted to affect the face, arm and leg equally. There is no sensory deficit, and no cortical signs are noted. This stroke most likely localizes to the:

    A. Left thalamus and internal capsule
    B. Left internal capsule
    C. Right basis pontis
    D. Right medulla
    E. Left midbrain

53. Which one of the following statements is true regarding the amino acid neurotransmitters?

    A. Histamine is an amino acid neurotransmitter
    B. GABA is an excitatory amino acid neurotransmitter
    C. Glutamate is an inhibitory amino acid neurotransmitter
    D. Glutamate receptors have been found to be important in the mechanism of action for cocaine
    E. Benzodiazepines, barbiturates and several anticonvulsants work through mechanisms involving GABA-B

54. All of the following are symptoms or signs of Parkinson's disease, EXCEPT:

    A. Bradykinesia
    B. Loss of postural reflexes
    C. Tremor
    D. Choreoathetosis
    E. Rigidity

55. A psychiatrist is asked to evaluate an 8 year-old girl. She does not want to go to school, and refuses to do her homework. Her teacher reports that she will not read out loud in class. She likes to go and spend the weekends at friends' houses or go on over-night trips with her grandparents. Her IQ is average. What diagnosis should the informed psychiatrist most strongly consider?

    A. ADHD
    B. Conduct disorder
    C. Separation-anxiety disorder
    D. Pervasive developmental disorder
    E. Reading disorder

56. All of the following are features of botulism toxin poisoning, EXCEPT:

    A. Myoclonus
    B. Dysphagia
    C. Diplopia
    D. Nausea
    E. Urinary retention

57. A couple brings their son in to see a psychiatrist. The child fights with his mother and father and is rude and dismissive toward them. He states that he wants to leave, and when the doctor tells him he has to stay he yells, curses, cries, and rolls around on the floor. His teacher tells the psychiatrist that his work at school is good, but that he gets very nasty with her when she tells him to do a particular task, and he often refuses to cooperate with her. The child's most likely diagnosis is:

    A. ADHD
    B. Bipolar disorder
    C. Conduct disorder
    D. Oppositional defiant disorder
    E. Separation anxiety disorder

58. Balint's syndrome is the result of a lesion to which one of the following areas?

    A. Frontal lobe
    B. Temporal lobe
    C. Parietal lobe
    D. Occipital lobe
    E. Bilateral parietal-occipital lobes

59. A psychiatrist evaluates a 7 year-old patient who is brought in by his parents because of complaints they have been receiving from school. The child has been sexually provocative with other children, sexualizes play activities, and openly displays sexual behavior. The most likely cause of this behavior is:

    A. Normal development
    B. Early onset puberty
    C. Traumatic brain injury
    D. Sexual abuse
    E. Psychosis with sexual delusions

60. Which one of the following symptoms is a feature of Anton's syndrome?

    A. Aphasia
    B. Prosopagnosia
    C. Apraxia
    D. Confabulation
    E. Hiccups

61. Which one of the following personality disorders is least associated with violent behavior?

    A. Borderline personality disorder
    B. Histrionic personality disorder
    C. Narcissistic personality disorder
    D. Dependent personality disorder
    E. Antisocial personality disorder

62. Inhalant intoxication (sniffing glue) causes which one of the following neurologic conditions?
    A. Myopathy
    B. Neuropathy
    C. Myelopathy
    D. Denervation of muscle
    E. Seizures

63. A 30 year-old man presents to the emergency room with a complaint that there is a cockroach living in his rectum. He says he knows that there is a hole in the side of his rectum which was created by the roach. He has no prior psychiatric history, but states that he has felt the roach crawling around in his rectum for the past 18 months. He is a lawyer with a busy successful practice, and says he has no problems at work. During previous trips to the doctor for this complaint, he was examined and told that there was no cockroach in his rectum. He feels that they just did not examine him properly, otherwise the roach would have been found. Examination and blood work are all normal. His most likely diagnosis is:
    A. Conversion disorder
    B. Schizophrenia
    C. Depression with psychotic features
    D. Delusional disorder with somatic features
    E. Hypochondriasis

64. Which one of the following substances of abuse is the most likely to lower the seizure threshold during intoxication?
    A. Morphine
    B. PCP
    C. Cocaine
    D. Cannabis
    E. Alcohol

65. Five patients are brought into the emergency room on a Friday evening. Of the five, which one is most likely to kill themselves successfully?
    A. Bob, who has schizophrenia
    B. Carol, who has alcoholism
    C. Dave, who is mentally retarded
    D. Sally, who has borderline personality disorder
    E. Mark, who has major depressive disorder

66. Meige's syndrome comprises which one of the following sets of symptoms?
    A. Hemifacial spasm and seizures
    B. Hemifacial spasm and cervical dystonia
    C. Blepharospasm and ptosis
    D. Blepharospasm and oromandibular dystonia
    E. Lid apraxia and myokymia

67. A physician that has reason to believe a patient may kill or injure another person must notify the potential victim, authorities, or the victim's family or friends. This is the result of which one of the following answer choices?

    A. Durham rule
    B. M'Naughten rule
    C. Ford vs Wainwright
    D. Tarasoff rule
    E. Respondeat superior

68. The phenomenon of scanning speech results from a lesion to the:

    A. Cerebellum
    B. Thalamus
    C. Frontal lobes
    D. Midbrain
    E. Dominant temporal lobe

69. A friend just gave birth to a healthy baby boy five days ago. Now your friend is crying and irritable, and has been dysphoric over the past two days. Which one of the following is the most likely diagnosis based on the information given?

    A. Postpartum depression
    B. Postpartum blues
    C. Postpartum psychosis
    D. Postpartum bipolar disorder
    E. Specific phobia of being a parent

70. Which one of the following is a syndrome of near muteness with normal reading, writing and comprehension?

    A. Aphasia
    B. Apraxia
    C. Agnosia
    D. Aphemia
    E. Abulia

71. All of the following are true regarding the N-methyl-D-aspartate (NMDA) receptor, EXCEPT:

    A. The NMDA receptor has been linked with learning and memory
    B. The NMDA receptor allows for the passage of potassium only
    C. The NMDA receptor only opens when it has bound two molecules of glutamate and one molecule of glycine
    D. The NMDA receptor can be blocked by physiological concentrations of magnesium
    E. The NMDA receptor can be blocked by PCP

72. Which one of the following refers to a state of unresponsiveness from which arousal only occurs with vigorous and repeated stimulation?
    A. Alertness
    B. Lethargy
    C. Stupor
    D. Coma
    E. Persistent vegetative state

73. Of the following disorders, which one has the best prognosis?
    A. Somatization disorder
    B. Body dysmorphic disorder
    C. Pain disorder
    D. Hypochondriasis
    E. Conversion disorder

74. Which one of the following statements is true?
    A. All patients with acute Guillain-Barré syndrome should be hospitalized in an intensive care unit in case of respiratory compromise
    B. All comatose patients require a head CT scan before a lumbar puncture is performed
    C. A positive grasp reflex is always a sign of frontal lobe damage
    D. Cerebellar hemispheric lesions produce deficits that are contralateral to the lesion
    E. Bell's palsy is most often caused by *Borrelia burgdorferi* infection

75. Which one of the following choices is considered unethical by the American Psychiatric Association Ethics Committee?
    A. Closing a practice and finding follow up care for your patients
    B. Refusing to discuss a patient's case with her family unless she gives you permission
    C. Charging a colleague rent to sub-let office space from you
    D. A patient wills you their estate after death. You accept and use the money for a new car
    E. You charge a fee to supervise another psychiatrist

76. Emotional memory localizes to the:
    A. Amygdala
    B. Hippocampus
    C. Primary auditory cortex
    D. Nucleus basalis of Meynert
    E. Pons

77. Of the following medications, which one is the least anticholinergic?
    A. Amitriptyline
    B. Imipramine
    C. Desipramine
    D. Nortriptyline
    E. Maprotiline

78. By what age should a child have a six-word vocabulary, be able to self-feed, and be able to walk up steps with his hand being held?
    A. 6 months
    B. 9 months
    C. 12 months
    D. 18 months
    E. 24 months

79. A 30 year-old male is brought to the emergency room after being arrested for exposing his genitals to women on the train. He states that he has impulses to expose himself that he can't control, and that he finds the whole experience very sexually exciting. Which one of the following medications would be an appropriate treatment for this patient?
    A. Medroxyprogesterone acetate
    B. Lorazepam
    C. Ziprasidone
    D. Duloxetine
    E. Chlorpromazine

80. A 45 year-old woman presents to the emergency room with an acute left hemiparesis of the arm and leg. You ask her to lift her normal right leg while you put your hand under her paretic leg. You note that while lifting her good leg, she pushes her affected leg downwards on the bed with normal strength. You suspect a hysterical or psychogenic disorder. This phenomenon is termed:
    A. Hoffman's sign
    B. Hoover's sign
    C. Lasegue's sign
    D. Romberg sign
    E. Gegenhalten

81. Clomipramine can be used for all of the following, EXCEPT:
    A. Depression
    B. Obsessive-compulsive disorder
    C. Panic disorder
    D. Premature ejaculation
    E. Command auditory hallucinations

82. The only true emergency in neurology that requires immediate MRI imaging and evaluation in the emergency room is:
    A. Acute suspected early hemispheric stroke
    B. Acute suspected myasthenia gravis.
    C. Acute suspected spinal cord compression
    D. Acute suspected Guillain-Barré syndrome
    E. Acute suspected subarachnoid hemorrhage

83. Which one of the following terms refers to the state's right to intervene and act as a surrogate parent for those who cannot care for themselves?
    A. Actus reus
    B. Mens rea
    C. Parens patriae
    D. Durable power
    E. Respondeat superior

84. Which one of the following medications has the unique mechanism of action of being a selective GABA reuptake inhibitor?
    A. Gabapentin
    B. Tiagabine
    C. Pregabalin
    D. Vigabitrin
    E. Lioresal

85. Which one of the following answer choices is measured by the trail making test?
    A. Memory
    B. Language
    C. Social learning
    D. Psychosis
    E. Executive function

86. The principal mechanism of action of the Alzheimer's disease agent memantine involves which one of the following receptors?
    A. Acetylcholine
    B. Dopamine
    C. NMDA
    D. Glycine
    E. GABA

87. Which one of the GABA receptors is thought to be the site of action of the benzodiazepines?

  A. GABA-A
  B. GABA-B
  C. GABA-C
  D. GABA-D
  E. GABA-E

88. Vagal nerve stimulation is FDA-approved for which one of the following indications?

  A. Refractory epilepsy
  B. Bipolar mania
  C. Schizophrenia
  D. Intermittent explosive disorder
  E. Obsessive-compulsive disorder

89. Which one of the following statements is true regarding carbamazepine?

  A. Carbamazepine is approved in the US for treatment of temporal lobe epilepsy and general epilepsy, but not trigeminal neuralgia
  B. Carbamazepine is metabolized by the kidneys
  C. Carbamazepine can be associated with a transient increase in the white blood cell count
  D. Carbamazepine has been shown to be as effective as the benzodiazepines in some studies for management of alcohol withdrawal
  E. A benign pruritic rash occurs in 60–70% of patients treated with carbamazepine

90. Auscultation of the head that reveals a bruit would likely be indicative of which one of the following?

  A. Brain tumor
  B. Venous sinus thrombosis
  C. Temporal arteritis
  D. Intracranial aneurysm
  E. Arteriovenous malformation

91. Which one of the following tests is considered to be projective?

  A. Halstead-Reitan battery
  B. Stanford-Binet test
  C. Wechsler-Bellevue test
  D. Draw-a-Person test
  E. MMPI

229

92. A 47 year-old man presents to the emergency with intermittent headaches, and periodic drop attacks. His brain MRI on T1 weighted imaging reveals the scan noted below. The most likely diagnosis is:

    A. Choroid plexus papilloma
    B. Colloid cyst of the third ventricle
    C. Ependymoma
    D. Pineal region germinoma
    E. Pituitary macroadenoma

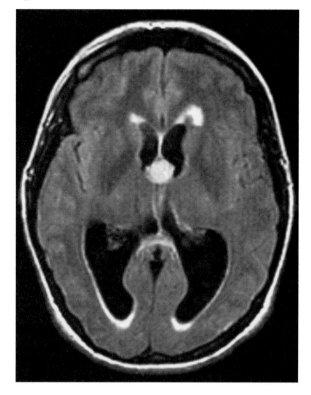

93. Which one of the following drugs is both an opioid agonist and antagonist?

    A. Aripiprazole
    B. Naltrexone
    C. Buprenorphine
    D. Methadone
    E. Gabapentin

94. Hallevorden-Spatz syndrome is a neurodegenerative disorder that results from lesions localizing to the:

    A. Frontal lobes
    B. Parietal lobes
    C. Occipital lobes
    D. Basal ganglia
    E. Hippocampus

95. A patient presents to the emergency room because of alcohol withdrawal. He and his family describe a history of alcohol-induced blackouts. Which one of the following memory problems is most consistent with alcohol induced blackouts?

    A. Making up details of how he got to work three days ago
    B. Retrograde amnesia
    C. Anterograde amnesia
    D. Loss of memories from his daughter's birthday five years ago
    E. Inability to tell you who the current president is

96. Strict vegetarians who ingest no meat products can suffer from deficits in proprioception and vibration sensation due to lesions that localize to the:

    A. Posterior spinal cord
    B. Central spinal cord
    C. Anterior spinal cord
    D. Thalamus
    E. Peripheral sensory nerves

97. A psychiatrist is treating a bipolar patient with carbamazepine. After being started on the drug he has therapeutic serum levels. Three months later the patient starts to become hypomanic and the psychiatrist decides to check a level. The level comes out below therapeutic range. Both the patient and his family reassure the psychiatrist that he has been taking the medication regularly. What should the psychiatrist do with this patient?

    A. Confront him, because he and his family are lying
    B. Stop the carbamazepine and put him on divalproex sodium
    C. Increase the dose of carbamazepine and take follow-up serum levels
    D. Add a high dose of a serotonin-selective reuptake inhibitor
    E. Hospitalize the patient

98. Patients exposed to isoniazid (INH) for tuberculosis treatment can develop a sensory polyneuropathy as a result of a deficiency in which one of the following?

    A. Vitamin B6
    B. Vitamin B12
    C. Niacin
    D. Thiamine
    E. Vitamin A

99. What is the best way to handle suicidal patients with borderline personality disorder?

    A. Take the threats seriously and take whatever steps are necessary to protect these patients
    B. Do not discuss suicide with them
    C. Isolate these patients from friends and family
    D. Make these patients promise not to hurt themselves (contract for safety)
    E. Give these patients benzodiazepine prescriptions to calm them down.

100. The West Nile virus is considered to belong to which one of the following viral families?

    A. Arenaviruses
    B. Arboviruses
    C. Filoviruses
    D. Papovaviruses
    E. Retroviruses

231

101. A patient is on lithium, risperidone, and a daily aspirin. He comes to his session confused and unsteady on his feet. He states that he has the flu, because of recent GI upset. Which one of the following should the psychiatrist do with this patient first?

    A. Refer him to an internist
    B. Get a lithium level
    C. Review the patient's recent diet
    D. Send stool for ova and parasites
    E. Obtain a complete blood count

102. Which one of the following neurotransmitters localizes predominantly to the basal forebrain and is responsible for memory, attention, and executive functioning?

    A. Serotonin
    B. Norepinephrine
    C. GABA
    D. Glycine
    E. Acetylcholine

103. All of the following drugs act by blocking the reuptake of norepinephrine into the presynaptic neuron, EXCEPT:

    A. Imipramine
    B. Venlafaxine
    C. Bupropion
    D. Nefazodone
    E. Mirtazapine

104. What is the mechanism of action of the hallucinogen PCP (phencyclidine)?

    A. Dopamine antagonism
    B. Serotonin antagonism
    C. Norepinephrine antagonism
    D. NMDA antagonism
    E. Acetylcholinesterase inhibition

105. A physician needs to give a benzodiazepine to someone with impaired liver function. Which one of the following would be the best choice of medication in this situation?

    A. Diazepam
    B. Oxazepam
    C. Clonazepam
    D. Prazepam
    E. Estazolam

106. Which one of the following fungal organisms can cause vertebrobasilar strokes by invasion of vessel walls and tends to colonize in the paranasal sinuses and cause a hypersensitivity pneumonitis?

    A. *Histoplasma*
    B. *Candida albicans*
    C. *Aspergillus*
    D. *Cryptococcus neoformans*
    E. *Pseudallescheria boydii*

107. Which one of the following side-effects is most likely to develop in a patient started on fluoxetine?

    A. Loss of consciousness
    B. Shuffling gait
    C. Headache
    D. High blood pressure
    E. Blurred vision

108. The GABA-A receptor (the most predominant GABA receptor) is which one of the following:

    A. A sodium channel
    B. A chloride channel
    C. A calcium channel
    D. A potassium channel
    E. A magnesium channel

109. A psychiatrist made a minor error in her last session with a patient. The patient comes to her for psychodynamic psychotherapy. The best approach is to:

    A. Interpret the patient's reaction
    B. Ignore the mistake
    C. Give a long but clear explanation of her reasoning
    D. Briefly acknowledge that she made a mistake
    E. Profusely apologize

110. A failure to develop a cohesive self-awareness is known as:

    A. Entrapment
    B. Climacterium
    C. Identity diffusion
    D. Activity dependent modulation
    E. All-or-none phenomenon

233

111. What is the most important step in treating separation anxiety disorder in an 11 year-old?
    A. Give methylphenidate
    B. Give risperidone
    C. Rapidly send the child back to school
    D. Thorough psychoanalysis of the mother
    E. High dose benzodiazepine treatment

112. Why do doctors use naltrexone for alcohol abuse?
    A. It is almost 100% effective
    B. It blocks the effects of alcohol at the GABA receptor
    C. It alters dopamine levels to decrease pleasure from drinking
    D. It has been shown to decrease craving and decrease alcohol consumption
    E. It is better than behavioral modification in treating alcohol abuse

113. A 30 year-old man on imipramine complains of difficulty urinating and impotence. What should his doctor do for him?
    A. Increase the dose of imipramine
    B. Tell the patient to decrease fluid intake
    C. Tell the patient to stop all sexual activity
    D. Prescribe bethanechol
    E. Prescribe melatonin

114. Which one of the following statements about mood disorders is true?
    A. Major depression is more common in men than in women
    B. Bipolar disorder has equal prevalence for men and women
    C. Higher socioeconomic status leads to increased depression
    D. There is a correlation between the hyposecretion of cortisol and depression
    E. About 90% of those with major depressive disorder receive specific treatment

115. A mother brings a 26 month-old child into the doctor's office. The child has not spoken any words yet. How should the doctor proceed?
    A. Speech therapy
    B. Audiometry
    C. Sensory evoked potentials
    D. Tell the mother to give it more time
    E. Chromosomal analysis

116. The assisted recall of information by a person in the same external environment that the information was originally acquired in is known as:

    A. Classical conditioning

    B. Social learning

    C. Partial recovery

    D. Respondent conditioning

    E. State-dependent learning

117. A 29 year-old man comes into the hospital with complaint of confusion, ataxia, disorientation and dysarthria. He has the smell of alcohol on his breath. Which one of the following is the best first step for the physician to take?

    A. Phone the patient's primary care physician

    B. Speak with the patient's family

    C. Give intravenous thiamine

    D. Sedate the patient with haloperidol

    E. Give the patient an anticonvulsant

118. Niacin deficiency (pellagra) results in which one of the following classic triads of symptoms?

    A. Gastritis, neuropathy, stroke

    B. Dementia, dermatitis, diarrhea

    C. Neuropathy, ataxia, dementia

    D. Neuropathy, retinopathy, areflexia

    E. Neuropathy, spasticity, encephalopathy

119. A psychiatrist is doing psychodynamic psychotherapy with a patient. The patient is usually on time, but missed a session last Tuesday. When he comes back, how should the psychiatrist approach this issue?

    A. Do not mention the missed appointment

    B. Refuse to treat the patient anymore

    C. "You missed your appointment Tuesday. I was wondering what happened."

    D. "I'm glad you didn't show on Tuesday. I spent the time with a patient I like better than you."

    E. "I'm going to charge you twice the normal fee because you missed your appointment last Tuesday."

120. All of the following are signs of cannabis intoxication, EXCEPT:

    A. Conjunctival injection

    B. Increased appetite

    C. Dry mouth

    D. Bradycardia

    E. Orthostatic hypotension

121. A patient comes to his psychiatrist's office with complaints consistent with akathisia. Which one of the following would be the best treatment?

    A. Bupropion
    B. Amoxapine
    C. Vitamin B6
    D. Captopril
    E. Propranolol

122. What is the mechanism by which clonidine is effective in reducing symptoms of opiate withdrawal?

    A. Indirect dopamine blockade
    B. Serotonin increase in the locus ceruleus
    C. Agonist activity at alpha-2 adrenergic receptors
    D. Generation of the metabolite trichloroethanol
    E. Decreased Free T4

123. Blockade of muscarinic cholinergic receptors may lead to all of the following, EXCEPT:

    A. Difficulty urinating
    B. Improvement in Alzheimer's symptoms
    C. Dry mouth
    D. Blurred vision
    E. Delirium

124. Which one of the following lab tests is most likely to pick up alcohol abuse?

    A. Gamma glutamyl transferase (GGT)
    B. Mean corpuscular volume (MCV)
    C. Uric acid
    D. Serum glutamic-oxaloacetic transaminase (SGOT)
    E. Serum glutamic-pyruvic transaminase (SGPT)

125. A psychiatrist is asked by a primary care physician to treat a patient with Tourette's disorder. He is suffering from several motor tics. Which one of the following would be the best medication to give him?

    A. Propranolol
    B. Pimozide
    C. Paroxetine
    D. Pindolol
    E. Piroxicam

126. On which chromosome is the gene for amyloid precursor protein found?
    A. Chromosome 19
    B. Chromosome 20
    C. Chromosome 21
    D. Chromosome 4
    E. Chromosome 13

127. Which one of the following answer choices is central to Kohut's theories of self psychology?
    A. The theory of oedipal conflict
    B. The concept of the good enough mother
    C. The paranoid-schizoid position
    D. The necessity for parental mirroring and empathic responsiveness to the child
    E. The importance of the depressive position

128. A patient with bipolar disorder is on carbamazepine. He goes to his primary care physician and is placed on erythromycin. What should be expected to happen?
    A. Carbamazepine levels will go down
    B. Erythromycin levels will go down
    C. No interaction of any kind
    D. Carbamazepine levels will go up
    E. Erythromycin levels will go up

129. A patient with bipolar disorder gives birth to a child with spina bifida and hypospadias. What is the most likely cause for the child's defects?
    A. Genetics
    B. Intrauterine infection
    C. Haloperidol use during pregnancy
    D. Valproic acid use during pregnancy
    E. Lithium use during pregnancy

130. A patient presents with decreased energy, increased appetite, weight gain, increased sleep, decreased mood, lack of interest in usual activities, and social withdrawal. Which one of the following medications would be the best choice to treat him?
    A. Citalopram
    B. Lithium
    C. Desipramine
    D. Phenelzine
    E. Venlafaxine

131. A patient states that he was given an antidepressant in the past but does not remember the name. He does remember having his blood pressure checked regularly by the psychiatrist because of the antidepressant. Which one of the following was the patient most likely taking?

    A. Mirtazepine
    B. Paroxetine
    C. Venlafaxine
    D. Citalopram
    E. Fluoxetine

132. Which one of the following is the focus of interpersonal therapy?

    A. Anxiety management
    B. Belief systems
    C. Faulty cognitions
    D. Social interactions
    E. Transference

133. All of the following are aspects of experiments carried out by Nikolaas Tinbergen, EXCEPT:

    A. Quantifying the power of certain stimuli in eliciting specific behavior
    B. Displacement activities
    C. Innate releasing mechanisms
    D. Autism
    E. Imprinting

134. Which one of the following structures is most critical to the formation of memory?

    A. Right frontal lobe
    B. Right parietal lobe
    C. Thalamus
    D. Cerebellum
    E. Hippocampus

135. All of the following are rating scales used for mood disorders, EXCEPT:

    A. Beck depression inventory
    B. Zung self-rating scale
    C. Carroll rating scale
    D. Montgomery-Asberg scale
    E. Brief psychiatric rating scale (BPRS)

136. All of the following are characteristics of sleep terror disorder, EXCEPT:
    A. Awakening from sleep and screaming
    B. Autonomic arousal
    C. Recall of a detailed dream
    D. Sweating
    E. Unresponsiveness to attempts to comfort the person during the episode

137. Thioridazine is most often associated with which one of the following side effects?
    A. Hematuria
    B. Delayed orgasm
    C. Retrograde ejaculation
    D. Priapism
    E. Hypospadias

138. What is the mechanism of action of donepizil?
    A. Dopamine blockade
    B. Serotonin reuptake inhibition
    C. Acetylcholinesterase inhibition
    D. Increasing GABA activity
    E. Prevention of beta amyloid deposition

139. Depression may present differently in different cultures. How would the knowledgeable psychiatrist predict depression would present in a 37 year-old Chinese immigrant?
    A. Concern with mood symptoms
    B. Somatic complaints
    C. Hysteria
    D. Self mutilation
    E. Paranoia

140. Which one of the following neurotransmitters is most involved in the effects of methylenedioxyamphetamine (ecstasy)?
    A. Serotonin
    B. Norepinephrine
    C. GABA
    D. Glycine
    E. Acetylcholine

141. The growth of child guidance clinics in the US in the early 1900s lead to:
    A. The development of the first medications for ADHD
    B. The development of sewage systems in major US cities
    C. The development of child psychiatry as a profession
    D. Freud's three essays on the theories of sexuality
    E. The Ryan White Care Act

239

142. The most common neurologic manifestation of neurosarcoidosis is:
    A. Cranial neuropathy
    B. Cauda equina syndrome
    C. Peripheral neuropathy
    D. Meningoencephalitis
    E. Uveitis

143. Trazodone is most often associated with which one of the following side effects?
    A. Hematuria
    B. Delayed orgasm
    C. Retrograde ejaculation
    D. Priapism
    E. Hypospadias

144. Which one of the following answer choices is true regarding aggression?
    A. High levels of cerebrospinal fluid (CSF) serotonin are associated with increased aggression
    B. Serotonin is unrelated to aggression
    C. Low levels of CSF serotonin are associated with increased aggression
    D. Low levels of CSF serotonin are associated with decreased aggression
    E. Low levels of dopamine are associated with increased aggression

145. How does mirtazapine work?
    A. Serotonin reuptake inhibition
    B. Norepinephrine reuptake inhibition
    C. Alpha-2 adrenergic receptor antagonism
    D. Partial dopamine antagonism
    E. Decreasing breakdown of serotonin in the synaptic cleft.

146. Which one of the following answer choices is most consistent with sleep changes in the elderly?
    A. Increased REM sleep only
    B. Increased slow wave sleep only
    C. Increased REM and slow wave sleep
    D. Decreased REM and slow wave sleep
    E. Decreased slow wave sleep only

147. A score of 70 on the Global Assessment of Functioning corresponds with:
    A. Persistent failure to maintain personal hygiene
    B. Major impairment in several areas
    C. Superior functioning in all areas
    D. Some difficulty functioning, but generally functioning well
    E. No friends, unable to keep a job

148. All of the following are aspects of Kleine-Levin syndrome, EXCEPT:
    A. Irritability
    B. Voracious eating
    C. Loss of libido
    D. Incoherent speech
    E. Hypersomnia

149. David works 17 hours per day. He does not have many friends because he feels that they interfere with his work schedule. He believes that he is a moral person and harshly criticizes those whom he finds to be unethical. He often starts projects but fails to complete them because he can not do them perfectly. His family describes him as stubborn and cheap, because he will never throw anything out. David's most likely diagnosis is:
    A. Generalized anxiety disorder
    B. Obsessive-compulsive disorder
    C. Obsessive-compulsive personality disorder
    D. Schizoid personality disorder
    E. Avoidant personality disorder

150. Which one of the following is an important technique of cognitive behavioral therapy?
    A. Maintaining therapeutic neutrality
    B. Offering interpretations of patients' unconscious wishes
    C. Abreaction
    D. Working through unresolved conflict
    E. Finding and testing automatic thoughts

Test Number **FOUR**
ANSWER KEY

④

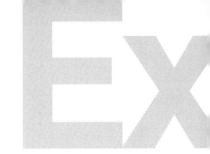

1	C	51	D	101	B
N 2	A	N 52	B	N 102	E
3	A	53	D	103	E
N 4	D	N 54	D	104	D
N 5	B	55	E	105	B
6	C	N 56	A	N 106	C
7	A	57	D	107	C
N 8	D	N 58	E	108	B
9	E	59	D	109	D
N 10	B	N 60	D	110	C
11	A	61	D	111	C
N 12	A	N 62	B	112	D
13	E	63	D	113	D
N 14	D	64	C	114	B
15	D	65	E	115	B
N 16	E	N 66	D	116	E
17	D	67	D	117	C
N 18	B	N 68	A	N 118	B
19	D	69	B	119	C
N 20	D	N 70	D	120	D
21	D	71	B	121	E
N 22	A	N 72	C	122	C
23	B	73	E	N 123	B
N 24	B	N 74	B	124	A
25	E	75	D	125	B
N 26	E	76	A	N 126	C
27	E	77	C	127	D
N 28	A	78	D	128	D
29	D	79	A	N 129	D
N 30	C	80	B	130	D
31	E	81	E	131	C
N 32	E	N 82	C	132	D
33	D	83	C	133	E
N 34	D	84	B	134	E
35	E	N 85	E	135	E
N 36	A	N 86	C	136	C
37	C	87	A	137	C
N 38	B	88	A	N 138	C
39	E	89	D	139	B
N 40	D	N 90	E	140	A
41	D	91	D	141	C
N 42	B	N 92	B	N 142	A
43	A	93	C	143	D
N 44	A	N 94	D	144	C
45	C	95	C	145	C
46	B	N 96	A	N 146	D
47	C	97	C	147	D
N 48	C	N 98	A	N 148	C
49	D	99	A	149	C
N 50	A	N 100	B	150	E
35		31		42	

ANSWER EXPLANATIONS

Question 1. C. Freud described a series of stages through which children pass as a part of normal development. These stages correspond to shifts of sexual energy from one erotic body part to the next.

The first phase is the oral phase from birth to 1 year. In the oral phase the infant's needs and expression are centered in the mouth, lips, and tongue. Tension is relieved through oral gratification. Those who do not complete the oral phase successfully can be very dependent in adulthood. Successful resolution of the oral stage allows the adult to both give and receive without excessive dependency or envy.

The next is the anal stage from ages 1 to 3 years. In the anal stage the child develops control of his anal sphincter. This phase is marked by increase in aggressive and libidinal drives. Control of feces gives the child independence, and the child struggles with the parent over separation. Successful completion of this stage leads to a sense of independence from the parent. Failure to complete this stage leads to obsessive-compulsive neuroses.

The phallic stage is from ages 3 to 5 years. In the phallic stage there is a focus on sexual interests and excitement in the genital area. The goal of this stage is to focus erotic interests in the genital area and lay the groundwork for gender identity. Poor resolution of this stage leads to the neuroses often associated with poor resolution of the oedipal complex. Successful resolution leads to a clear sense of sexual identity, curiosity without embarrassment, initiative without guilt, and mastery over things both internal and external.

The phallic stage is followed by latency, during which there is a decrease in sexual interest and energy. Latency lasts from age 5 years until puberty. It is a period of consolidating and integrating previous development in psychosexual functioning and developing adaptive patterns of functioning. At puberty there is an increase in sexual energy. This time is described as the genital stage. It lasts from about ages 11–13 years until adulthood. In this stage, libidinal drives are intensified. There is a regression in personality organization, allowing for resolution of prior conflicts and the solidification of the adult personality. The goal is the ultimate separation from the parents and the development of non-incestuous object relations. Failure to complete this stage can lead to multiple complex outcomes. Freud felt that one must pass successfully through all of these stages to develop normal functioning as an adult.

K&S Ch. 2

Question 2. A. Amaurosis fugax is a symptom of carotid artery territory ischemia. It presents as a sudden onset of transient loss of vision that manifests as a curtain or shade or veil usually over the central visual field. The duration of visual loss is generally brief, lasting about one to five minutes, and only infrequently exceeds thirty minutes in duration. When the episode

245

concludes, vision is generally returned to normal. The event is then truly termed a transient ischemic attack (TIA), because of a duration less than twenty-four hours. In some cases, there is permanent visual loss due to retinal infarction. Amaurosis fugax is the only feature that can distinguish a middle cerebral artery syndrome from a carotid artery syndrome. Vertebrobasilar territory ischemia would be expected to affect the cerebellum and/or brainstem. Classic posterior circulation ischemic symptoms include ataxia, nystagmus, vertigo, dysarthria, and dysphagia. An ipsilateral Horner's syndrome can occur if the descending oculosympathetic fibers are disrupted. Crossed weakness (ipsilateral facial paresis, contralateral limb paresis) is indicative of brainstem involvement above the level of the area of decussation of the pyramids in the medulla. Lenticulostriate territory ischemia affects the small penetrating branching arteries off of the middle cerebral artery that feed the striatum. Ischemia to this territory can produce lacunar infarcts of the internal capsule that result in a pure contralateral motor hemiparesis.

Anterior cerebral artery ischemia would be expected to produce a contralateral hemiparesis of the leg preferentially, because the cortical homuncular representation of the leg is situated parasagittally in the postcentral motor cortex.

Middle cerebral artery territory ischemia can take many different forms. If the lesion is in the dominant hemisphere, aphasia may result. Nondominant ischemia can result in hemineglect, anosognosia, visual and tactile extinction, aprosody of speech and contralateral limb apraxia.

B&D Ch. 57

Question 3. A. Norepinephrine (NE) is made in the locus caeruleus. Serotonin is made in the dorsal raphe nuclei. Dopamine is made in the substantia nigra. Acetylcholine is made in the nucleus basalis of Meynert.

K&S Ch. 3

Question 4. D. The onset of back pain, followed by leg weakness and urinary incontinence is a classic manifestation of bilateral spinal cord pathology. In this case, the correct syndrome is a transverse myelitis because the deficits are closely preceded by an influenza vaccination. Transverse myelitis is a segmental inflammatory syndrome of the bilateral spinal cord. It is believed to be immunologic in origin and often follows an infection or vaccination, or is the direct result of demyelination due to multiple sclerosis (MS). Up to 40% of cases have no identifiable origin. The classic presentation is the rapid onset of bilateral leg weakness that presents with a clear-cut sensory level below the level of the lesion. Pain and temperature sensation are usually affected, but often proprioception and vibration sensation are spared. Urinary and/or bowel incontinence are common findings. MRI of the spine is the imaging modality of choice. If both the spine and the brain show demyelination on MRI imaging the likelihood of the myelitis being the first manifestation of MS is greater than 50%. If the condition is proven to be a result of inflammation or demyelination, then high dose intravenous steroids are the initial acute treatment of choice.

Spinal cord metastases causing an acute cord compression would be expected to cause a similar presentation to myelitis as noted above, but one would expect the history to reveal some sort of primary cancer, such as that of the lung or prostate, that would precede the onset of spinal cord symptoms. Only about 15% of primary CNS tumors originate in the spinal cord. Emergent MRI must be performed to characterize the lesion. Treatment of acute cord compression due to metastatic lesions involves intravenous steroids, radiation therapy, and possible surgical decompression.

Vacuolar myelopathy is found almost uniquely in AIDS patients, and is similar to the condition noted in vitamin B12 deficiency. AIDS myelopathy is noted in about one-quarter of AIDS patients. The clinical picture is similar to that of myelitis or cord compression, but the timeline is usually much slower and more progressive, evolving over many months. The pathophysiology of AIDS-related vacuolar myelopathy may be due to viral release of cytokines that are neurotoxic in nature, or abnormalities in vitamin B12 utilization. Vitamin B12 levels are often normal in these cases. Antiretroviral therapy may not reverse the symptoms. Acute disseminated encephalomyelitis (ADEM) is a monophasic demyelinating syndrome that follows a systemic infection or vaccination. It differs from transverse myelitis, because ADEM involves the whole CNS and is not simply localized to a segment of the spinal cord. ADEM usually results in multifocal signs and symptoms that include an encephalopathy. Brainstem and cerebral involvement are noted, as well as symptoms localizing to the spinal cord.

B&D Ch. 59&60

Question 5. B. If different doctors can look at the same case and make the same diagnosis, the diagnosis is said to be reliable. In other words, it is consistent. Accuracy of the diagnosis is called validity. Descriptive validity means that the disorder has features that are characteristic enough to separate it from other disorders. Predictive validity means that the diagnosis allows the doctor to predict clinical course and treatment response. Construct validity means the diagnosis is based on underlying pathophysiology and the use of biologic markers to confirm the disease.

K&S Ch. 4

Question 6. C. Horner's syndrome results from an interruption to the sympathetic fibers supplying the pupil, upper eyelid, facial sweat glands and facial blood vessels. The classic symptom triad is that of ptosis, miosis, and anhydrosis. Horner's syndrome can be seen as part of the lateral medullary stroke syndrome (Wallenberg's syndrome), carotid occlusion or dissection, high spinal cord lesions, neoplasms like Pancoast's tumor that affect the cervical ganglia, or intracranial hemorrhage. If the condition affects only the eye and not the sweat glands, the lesion usually localizes to the territory of the internal carotid artery. The other answers to this question need no explanation as they are simply nonsense distracters.

B&D Ch. 83

Question 7. A. This question lists side effects that may be found with amphetamines. All of the answer choices except choice A, are central nervous system depressants and would be predicted to have effects opposite to many of those listed in the question, although there may be some similarities with certain symptoms. Amphetamine is a sympathomimetic.

K&S Ch. 12

Question 8. D. Prosopagnosia is the inability to recognize familiar faces. It is associated classically with bilateral occipital-temporal lesions. It is often associated with agraphia and achromatopsia (inability to recognize colors and hues). It is almost always associated with visual field deficits. Anosognosia, the denial of disease or hemiparesis, is seen with lesions of the non-dominant hemisphere. Simultanagnosia is the inability to perceive a scene with multiple parts to it. The patient is only able to see and recognize individual elements of a multi-part scene, and cannot interpret the overall picture. Astereognosis refers to the inability to recognize and identify items by weight, texture and form alone, when the items are held in the hand. It is a form of tactile agnosia. Aprosodia is a deficit in the emotional aspect of expressive or receptive speech.

B&D Chs. 11,12&57

Question 9. E. With PCP use hypertension is often seen, not hypotension. Other symptoms include paranoia, nystagmus, catatonia, convulsions, hallucinations, mood lability, loosening of associations, violence, mydriasis,

ataxia, and tachycardia. Treatment consists of haloperidol every 2–4 hours until the patient is calm. PCP can be detected in the urine up to eight days after ingestion.
K&S Ch. 12

Question 10. B. Bell's palsy (VII nerve palsy) is a severe, acute, unilateral, complete facial paresis that evolves over 24–48 hours. The condition is often accompanied by pain behind the ear. Taste impairment and hyperacusis are frequent associated symptoms. The incidence is about 20 in 100 000. The syndrome is believed to be of viral etiology, and herpes simplex virus is thought to be the most frequent viral pathogen responsible for the condition. About 80–85% of patients improve completely within three months. Incomplete paralysis at onset is a better prognostic sign than complete paralysis. Treatment with acyclovir and prednisone is often administered, but remains controversial due to the etiological uncertainty of the disorder. The paralysis of Bell's palsy involves the entire face, whereas the facial paresis of a hemispheric stroke spares the upper third of the face (the brow and upper eyelid).
B&D Ch. 76

Question 11. A. This question focuses on Piaget's stages of cognitive development. Object permanence develops during the sensorimotor stage. There are several other questions on Piaget in this book. If you did not get this question correct, go back and review those questions and answer explanations. Know Piaget well!
K&S Ch. 2

Question 12. A. Syringomyelia refers to the constellation of signs and symptoms produced by a syrinx, a cavitation of the central spinal cord. The cavitation may be contiguous with a dilated central spinal canal, or it may be separate from a central canal. Most syringes occur in the cervical spinal cord. Most of those that develop from a central spinal canal are associated with an Arnold-Chiari type I or type II malformation. The classic presentation is that of a dissociated suspended sensory deficit usually in a cape or shawl pattern over the arms and upper trunk. There is impairment of pain and temperature sensation and preserved light touch, vibration and proprioception. These sensory deficits are combined with lower motor neuron signs (flaccidity, muscular atrophy, fasciculations) at or about the level of the lesion, as well as spinal long tract signs below the level of the lesion. Pain often accompanies a syrinx and can manifest as headache, neck pain, radicular pain, and segmental dysesthesia. MRI of the spine is the imaging modality of choice to best evaluate a syrinx.
B&D Ch. 79

Question 13. E. Urinary retention is a side effect of the belladonna alkaloids, but not of glue and benzene products. All of the other answer choices are possibilities for a patient sniffing glue daily for over six months. In addition to those contained in the question, side effects include slurred speech, ataxia, hallucinations, and tachycardia with ventricular fibrillation. This grouping of substances includes glue, benzene, gasoline, paint thinner, lighter fluid, and aerosols.
K&S Ch. 12

Question 14. D. Opsoclonus-myoclonus is a paraneoplastic movement disorder that is also called "dancing eyes-dancing feet" syndrome. It is seen most often in infants ages 6 to 18 months and in 50% or more of cases is associated with an infantile neuroblastoma. In adults, lung cancer is a common cause of this disorder. It can also be noted as a result of postviral encephalitis, multiple sclerosis, thalamic hemorrhage, and hyperosmolar coma. The condition presents as multifocal myoclonus and rapid

dancing movements of the eyes. It is caused by lesions to the pause cells in the pons. Steroids or adrenocorticotropic hormone are effective treatment for this particular type of myoclonus. The other conditions noted in this question are distracters that are not related to opsoclonus-myoclonus.
B&D Ch. 16

Question 15. D. Social phobia is characterized by a fear of one or more social or performance situations in which the person is exposed to unfamiliar people or possible scrutiny by others. The individual is afraid of acting in a way that would be embarrassing. Exposure to the situation almost always causes anxiety, and the person is aware that the fear is excessive. In this question, fear of scrutiny is the most definitive symptom of social phobia. The other choices could provoke anxiety in someone with some type of anxiety disorder but are neither necessarily limited to nor considered major diagnostic criteria for social phobia.
K&S Ch. 16

Question 16. E. The Ramsay-Hunt syndrome is a herpetic cranial neuritis that affects the facial (VII) and acoustic (VIII) nerves. The pathogen is of course the varicella-zoster virus (herpes zoster; chicken pox virus). The clinical presentation is that of a painful facial palsy, vertigo, ipsilateral hearing loss and vesicles in the external auditory canal and sometimes on the pinna. The infection is presumed to localize to the geniculate ganglion. Treatment is symptomatic. Recovery is often worse than in idiopathic Bell's palsy. The other answer choices are distracters.
B&D Chs. 59&75

Question 17. D. All of the answer choices given are true except for D. In cases of body dysmorphic disorder, medical, dental, or surgical treatment fails to solve the patient's preoccupation. The disorder consists of a preoccupation with an imagined defect in appearance. If a slight physical anomaly is present the concern is markedly excessive. The cause of this disorder is unknown, onset is usually slow, and marked impairment in functioning occurs. There is an association with mood disorders and in some studies as many as 50% of patients benefited from treatment with a serotonin-selective reuptake inhibitor. The body part of concern may change over the course of the disorder. Differential diagnosis should include anorexia, gender identity disorder, and conditions that can result in brain damage such as neglect syndromes.
K&S Ch. 17

Question 18. B. Glioblastoma multiforme is the most common primary brain tumor in about 50% or more of patients over 60 years of age. Average survival is about one year after diagnosis with radiation therapy. Anaplastic astrocytoma has a bimodal peak in incidence in the first and third decades. Ependymomas make up about 5% of all brain tumors. They are the third most common CNS tumors in children. Meningiomas make up about 20–25% of all brain tumors. They are more likely to occur after 50 years of age, and occur about twice as frequently in females as in males. About 80% of meningiomas turn out to be benign. Acoustic neuromas are considered to be schwannomas (nerve sheath tumors). The peak incidence of acoustic neuromas is in the fourth and fifth decades.
B&D Ch. 58

Question 19. D. Neuroimaging studies in obsessive-compulsive disorder (OCD) patients have demonstrated abnormalities in the caudate, thalamus, and orbitofrontal cortex. Functional neuroimaging by positron emission tomography (PET) scanning has demonstrated increased metabolism in the basal ganglia (predominantly in the caudate), the frontal lobes and the cingulate gyrus. CT and MRI of the brains of patients with OCD have demonstrated bilaterally smaller caudate nuclei than those seen in normal controls.

K&S Ch. 16

Question 20. D. Anton's syndrome is considered to be an agnosia characterized by cortical blindness. The lesion localizes to the bilateral occipital lobes, usually due to strokes, particularly in the calcarine cortex (Brodmann's area 17) and visual association cortex. The hallmark of the syndrome is that patients deny that they are blind and they confabulate. Patients may also suffer from visual hallucinations.

B&D Ch. 14

Question 21. D. Signs of impending violence, or predictive factors for violence include alcohol and drug intoxication, recent acts of violence, command auditory hallucinations, paranoia, menacing behavior, psychomotor agitation, carrying weapons, frontal lobe disease, catatonic excitement, certain manic or agitated depressive episodes, violent ideation, male gender, ages 15–24 years, low socioeconomic status, and few social supports.

K&S Ch. 34

Question 22. A. Riluzole (Rilutek) is a glutamate antagonist and is FDA-approved in the treatment of amyotrophic lateral sclerosis (ALS). It has demonstrated mild to moderate improvement in the survival rate of ALS. It may also help patients remain in a milder disease state for a longer period of time. The medication comes in 50 mg tablets which are started at one per day at night and increased to twice daily after one to two weeks, if tolerated. Side effects include gastrointestinal upset, dizziness, fatigue, and liver enzyme elevation. The other answer choices are distracters.

B&D Ch. 80

Question 23. B. Conversion disorder consists of one or more neurological symptoms that can not be explained by a medical condition. The symptoms are thought to be unconsciously produced in response to psychological conflict. Pseudoseizures can be common symptoms of conversion disorder. Conversion disorder can be associated with passive-aggressive, antisocial, histrionic, and dependent personality disorders. In obsessive-compulsive disorder a patient has intrusive unwanted thoughts that cause them to repeat a ritual or action to remove the anxiety associated with that thought. Nothing like that is described in this question. Somatization disorder presents as a patient who has a number of medical complaints involving several organ systems that can not be otherwise explained by a known medical condition. That is not the case in this question. Social phobia presents as a patient who has a fear of being in social situations or meeting new people. That has nothing to do with this question. Panic disorder presents as a patient who has recurrent and unexpected panic attacks. This patient is having pseudoseizures, not panic attacks.

K&S Chs. 16&17

Question 24. B. Primary central nervous system lymphoma occurs in AIDS patients in about 5% of cases. These lymphomas are most often of B-cell origin. Patients can present with a gradual onset of any of the following symptoms: headache, aphasia, hemiparesis, altered mental status, behavioral changes, and ataxia. Constitutional symptoms like fever and weight loss are generally absent. Diagnosis is established by MRI brain imaging. PCR testing on CSF revealing Epstein-Barr virus DNA helps to corroborate the diagnosis. Treatment with antiretroviral polypharmacy can help slow progression. None of the other tumor types mentioned in the answer choices are particularly associated with AIDS.

B&D Ch. 59

Question 25. E. The development of the central nervous system is a very important area of study, as abnormal development is implicated in several clinical conditions, including schizophrenia. The central and peripheral nervous systems arise from the neural tube. The neural tube gives rise to the ectoderm, which becomes the peripheral nervous system, whereas the neural tube itself becomes the central nervous system. The second trimester of gestation is the peak of neuronal proliferation, with 250 000 neurons born each minute. Migration of neurons, guided by glial cells, peaks during the first 6 months of gestation. Synapse formation occurs at a high rate from the second trimester through age 10, but peaks around 2 years (toddler period) with as many as 30 million synapses forming per second. The nervous system is also actively myelinating its axons starting prenatally, and continuing through childhood, finishing in the third decade of life.
K&S Ch. 3

Question 26. E. AIDS dementia complex is a late complication of AIDS, particularly when the HIV infection is untreated and CD4 cell counts are low. Symptoms include poor attention and concentration, bradyphrenia, forgetfulness, poor balance, uncoordination, personality changes, apathy, and depression. Focal neurologic deficits are usually absent, such as hemiparesis or aphasia. Treatment involves administration of antiretroviral therapy.
B&D Ch. 59

Question 27. E. All of the answer choices given are correct, with the exception of increased bone density. Anorexic patients tend to suffer from osteoporosis. They also have cachexia, loss of muscle mass, reduced thyroid metabolism, loss of cardiac muscle, arrhythmias, delayed gastric emptying, bloating, abdominal pain, amenorrhea, lanugo (fine baby-like hair), and abnormal taste sensation.
K&S Ch. 23

Question 28. A. Central nervous system toxoplasmosis is the most frequent CNS opportunistic infection in the AIDS patient. It is noted in 10% or more of AIDS patients. The infection is caused by the parasite *Toxoplasma gondii*. Cerebral toxoplasmosis in the AIDS patient results most often from a resurgence of a previously acquired infection. The infection usually occurs in late-stage AIDS, when CD4 cell counts are less than 200/μL. CNS toxoplasmosis presents clinically with headache and focal neurological deficits with or without fever. Other possible manifestations include aphasia, seizures, and hemiparesis. In cases with significant progression, patients can develop confusion and lethargy that lead to coma. The diagnosis is made on the basis of CT or MRI brain imaging revealing a single lesion or multiple ring-enhancing lesions. Therapy is undertaken with pyrimethamine and sulfadiazine, or with clindamycin in sulfa-allergic patients. The other answer choices occur less frequently in AIDS patients. Cryptococcal meningitis, another important opportunistic infection in AIDS, as well as the other three answer choices, are explained elsewhere in this volume.
B&D Ch. 59

Question 29. D. All choices given are correct, except for hyperkalemia. In purging, it is common to see a hypokalemic, hyperchloremic alkalosis. In addition, one may also see hypomagnesemia, pancreatic inflammation, increased serum amylase, esophageal erosion, and bowel dysfunction.
K&S Ch. 23

Question 30. C. HIV-associated vacuolar myelopathy is the most common cause of spinal cord pathology in AIDS patients, and is seen in one-quarter to one-half of patients on autopsy. The disorder usually occurs in late-stage AIDS. The clinical picture is that of spasticity, gait instability, lower extremity

251

weakness, loss of proprioception and vibration sensation, and sphincter dysfunction. Neurologic examination reveals a spastic paraparesis, hyper-reflexia and Babinski's signs. It is unusual to note a clear-cut sensory level on the trunk. Vitamin B12 levels are usually normal. Viral neurotoxic cytokines may contribute to the pathophysiology of the disease.
Distal sensory polyneuropathy is the most common peripheral nerve syndrome that complicates AIDS. It is seen in about one-third of AIDS patients. The clinical presentation is that of diminished ankle jerk reflexes, decreased pain, temperature, and vibration sensation, and possible paresthesia or numbness of the feet. The disorder is usually symmetrical. The condition frequently presents with lower extremity neuropathic pain. Treatment involves antiretroviral therapy and manage-ment of the pain with tricyclic antidepressants, anticonvulsants, or even narcotic analgesics if needed.
Neurosyphilis, progressive multifocal leukoencephalopathy, and HTLV-1 myelopathy are all explained elsewhere in this volume.
B&D Ch. 59

Question 31. E. Central serous chorioretinopathy is a disease leading to detachment of the retina and has nothing to do with anxiety. Carcinoid syndrome can mimic anxiety disorders and is accompanied by hypertension, and elevat-ed urinary 5-HIAA. Hyperthyroidism presents with anxiety in the con-text of elevated T3, T4 and exophthalmos. Hypoglycemia presents with anxiety and fasting blood sugar under 50 mg/dL. Signs and symptoms of diabetes may also be present with hypoglycemia (polyuria, polydypsia, and polyphagia). Hyperventilation syndrome presents with a history of rapid deep respirations, circumoral pallor, and anxiety. It responds well to breathing into a paper bag.
K&S Ch. 16

Question 32. E. Progressive multifocal leukoencephalopathy (PML) is a demyelinating disorder affecting AIDS patients with low CD4 counts. It results from an opportunistic infection by the JC virus, a form of human papilloma virus. It occurs in about 5% of patients with AIDS. Demyelination occurs pref-erentially in the subcortical white matter of the parietal and/or occipital lobes. Clinical presentation can involve hemiparesis, aphasia, sensory deficits, ataxia, and visual field deficits. Mental status may deteriorate progressively over time. MRI often reveals multiple or coalesced non enhancing white matter lesions in the parietal or occipital lobes. CSF assay for the JC virus DNA by PCR can help confirm the diagnosis. There is no specific treatment for PML and mean survival is about two to four months after diagnosis. Antiretroviral therapy can reconstitute immune function, but often proves to be too little too late. The other answer choices in this question are distracters and are explained elsewhere in this volume.
B&D Ch. 59

Question 33. D. The distinction between social phobia and avoidant personality disorder can sometimes be confused. In a situation where the patient is afraid of almost all social situations, then avoidant personality disorder should be considered. Social phobia presents with a fear of one or more social situ-ations. Avoidant personality disorder is defined by a pervasive pattern of social inhibition, feelings of inadequacy, and hypersensitivity to negative evaluation. This can be shown by avoiding activities involving interper-sonal contact, unwillingness to get involved with people unless certain of being liked, showing fear in intimate relationships for fear of ridicule, preoccupation with criticism or rejection in social situations, viewing self as socially inept and being inhibited in new social situations or afraid to take risks for fear of embarrassment.
K&S Ch. 27

252

Question 34. D. Prion diseases are also known as transmissible spongiform encephalopathies. Prions are proteinaceous and infectious particles that are unlike bacteria or viruses. Prions are unique in that they can be passed on through heredity (chromosome 20), acquired by infection, or acquired spontaneously. Kuru is the prion disease endemic to the cannibalistic Fore people. The clinical presentation is that of progressive cerebellar ataxia. The progressive disease course generally leads to death in about twelve months from initial onset.

Gerstmann-Sträussler-Scheinker syndrome is an inherited form of prion disease. Symptoms begin to manifest in about the third or fourth decade. The disease is the slowest of the spongiform encephalopathies and can progress over several years. The clinical presentation depends on which mutation in the PRNP gene is acquired by the patient. The syndrome varies in nature and presents with any combination of ataxia, Parkinson's plus-like symptoms, or a progressive dementia.

Fatal familial insomnia occurs between ages 35 and 60 years. It presents with progressive insomnia and sympathetic autonomic hyperactivity, such as hyperhidrosis, tachycardia, hyperthermia, or hypertension. Mild cognitive impairment is usually noted. Other symptoms can include ataxia, tremor, myoclonus, confusion, or hallucinations.

Creutzfeldt-Jakob disease can be sporadic, iatrogenic or familial. CSF evaluation of 14-3-3 and Tau proteins is the diagnostic test of choice to confirm the disease. The classic sporadic disease usually affects those between ages 50 and 75 years. The downward clinical course is rapid and progresses towards death over 6 months to 2 years. The disease has three stages. Stage one presents with neuropsychiatric symptoms that can include fatigue, sleep disturbance, memory and concentration deficits, and personality changes. Stage two presents with generalized cognitive deficits, as well as significant psychiatric symptoms such as psychosis and hallucinosis. The third and final stage that precedes death is characterized by profound and severe dementia, with myoclonus and choreoathetosis. Treatment of the spongiform encephalopathies is palliative and symptomatic. There is no known cure for these diseases.

Devic's disease, also known as neuromyelitis optica, is believed to be a variant of multiple sclerosis (MS). The presentation is that of cervical myelopathy and bilateral optic neuropathy. In certain patients, the two conditions occur simultaneously, but in others, they occur at separate intervals, pointing more directly to a diagnosis of MS. Devic's disease is a disease of demyelination and has nothing to do with prions.
B&D Chs. 59&60

Question 35. E. Bipolar II disorder is characterized by at least one major depressive episode and at least one hypomanic episode during the patient's lifetime. There are no full manic episodes in bipolar II disorder. If criteria for a manic episode are met then the correct diagnosis is bipolar I disorder. Psychotic features can be found in bipolar I disorder but not in bipolar II disorder.
K&S Ch. 15

Question 36. A. Carotid artery occlusion presents with the triad of headache, ipsilateral Horner's syndrome, and contralateral hemiparesis. A resultant cerebral infarct can increase intracranial pressure and thereby cause headache. The Horner's syndrome itself can result in headache because of interruption of ascending sympathetic tracts from the superior cervical ganglion to the intracranial vessels and dura which are pain-sensitive structures. Pontine hemorrhage is a neurologic emergency as it can lead to rapid death if the bleed is large. This hemorrhage type accounts for about 5% of all intracranial hemorrhages. Large bleeds in the basal tegmentum of the pons result in a clinical presentation characterized by quadriplegia, coma, decerebrate posturing, respiratory rhythm anomalies (apneustic breathing), pinpoint reactive pupils, hyperthermia, horizontal ophthalmoplegia, and ocular bobbing. The likely etiology of these bleeds is the rupture of small tegmental pontine penetrating arteries that originate from the trunk of the basilar artery.

Cerebral aneurysmal rupture results in a sudden explosive headache ("the worst headache of my life"), obtundation, nausea, vomiting, meningeal signs, neck pain, and photophobia. Aneurysms are discussed in further detail elsewhere in this volume, as are giant cell arteritis and the Wallenberg's syndrome.

B&D Chs. 57 & 75

Question 37. C. Analysis of variance is a set of statistical procedures which compares two groups and determines if the differences are due to experimental influence or chance. Other answer choices were covered in Test Three.

K&S Ch. 4

Question 38. B. The condition described in this question is of course that of a Bell's palsy (VII nerve palsy). Bell's palsy is characterized by a sudden, severe, unilateral infranuclear (i.e., involving both the upper and lower parts of the face) facial paresis. In serious cases, the brow droops, with widening of the palpebral fissure, and the eyelid cannot close completely. When the patient tries to close the affected eye with effort, the lid remains partially opened and the globe turns up and out. This sign is known as Bell's phenomenon. The incidence is about 20 per 100 000, with a peak in the third decade. The disorder is believed to be viral in origin and is thought to be most often due to occult herpes simplex infection. The facial paresis is often preceded by pain behind the ipsilateral ear, which may resolve. The facial paresis results soon thereafter and may evolve over one to two days, with maximal deficit within the first 72 hours. Eighty to eighty-five per cent of patients recover fully within three months.

A 7 to 10-day course of oral acyclovir with an oral prednisone taper may shorten the course of the disorder, but studies have not demonstrated a clear-cut benefit to this approach.

Borrelia burgdorferi, the spirochete responsible for Lyme disease can result in a unilateral, or even bilateral Bell's palsy. This is often accompanied by an aseptic meningitis, which when combined with facial diplegia is termed Bannwarth's syndrome. Facial diplegia from Lyme disease is much less common than idiopathic Bell's palsy and the history should point to deer tick exposure in the outdoor setting at some time directly preceding the onset of symptoms.

Epstein-Barr virus, West Nile virus, and varicella zoster virus infections do not usually result in a Bell's palsy. Other conditions that can cause a VII nerve palsy include Guillain-Barré syndrome, sarcoidosis, and facial nerve tumors or metastases.

B&D Ch. 76

Question 39. E. This question gives a clear description of autism. In autism the child displays a lack of ability to use and read nonverbal gestures, failure to develop appropriate peer relationships, lack of sharing enjoyment with other people, and lack of emotional reciprocity. They also show communication deficits such as delays in language development (not seen in Asperger's), inability to sustain conversation, repetitive or idiosyncratic use of language, and lack of make-believe play. They exhibit repetitive or stereotyped patterns of behavior such as preoccupation with areas of interest that are abnormal either in intensity or focus, adherence to inflexible ineffective routines, repetitive motor mannerisms, or persistent preoccupation with parts of objects. Some of the above mentioned symptoms appear before three years of age.

K&S Ch. 41

Question 40. D. This question points to a diagnosis of rabies virus infection. Rabies virus is transmitted to humans most often by wild animals such as bats, foxes, and raccoons, or by nonimmunized dogs. The incubation period is about one to two months. There is a prodromal period characterized by paresthesias, headache, and fever, which can then progress to generalized neurologic compromise, coma, and death. During the progressive phase of the illness, 80% or more of patients exhibit hydrophobia, which manifests as pharyngeal and nuchal spasms that are triggered by swallowing, smells, tastes, or sounds. These spasms can last up to several minutes in duration. The condition usually progresses to an encephalitis that is often accompanied by high fever that can rise up to 107°F, as well as autonomic hyperactivity, seizures, agitation and psychosis. Treatment begins with postexposure prophylaxis with rabies vaccine and antirabies immunoglobulin in patients who have never received immunization. West Nile virus infection is an arbovirus infection that is endemic to many parts of the world. Mosquito bites from the genus *Culex* are frequent vectors of transmission of the virus to humans. Most infections in humans are asymptomatic. In about 20% of affected patients, the infection presents as a febrile condition after an incubation period of a few days to up to two weeks. Only 1 in 150 patients goes on to develop a meningitis or encephalitis picture. The infection may progress to the development of a demyelinating or axonal neuropathy. Diagnosis is made by detection of IgM antibodies in cerebrospinal fluid, or IgM and IgG antibodies in serum. Treatment is generally supportive. Patients with serious symptoms may respond to intravenous administration of anti-West Nile virus immunoglobulin.

Acute tetanus results from infection with the bacterium *Clostridium tetani*. This bacterium releases tetanospasmin, also known as tetanus toxin, which blocks GABA and glycine in the inhibitory interneurons in the spinal cord, and causes the characteristic muscle contractions that are seen in tetanus. The bacterial spores can live for years in dust and soil and when an open wound is inoculated with dirt that contains the spores, they can release the toxin that causes the disease. The toxin is taken up into the anterior horn cells by retrograde axonal transport. Trismus, or lockjaw, is a primary symptom of the disorder in over 75% of cases. Risus sardonicus, a sustained involuntary grimace resulting from uncontrollable facial muscle spasm, is another characteristic of tetanus. Laryngospasm can lead to respiratory compromise and death if the disorder is untreated. Cardiac arrest can also result from dysautonomia. Treatment begins with airway protection and intubation if there is respiratory compromise. Tetanus immune globulin given in a single intramuscular dose of 500 units neutralizes blood-borne toxin. Prevention of the disease by vaccination with anti-tetanus antibody vaccine following a dirty open wound is the cornerstone of disease management.

Clostridium botulinum is a bacteria that secretes a potent neurotoxin that blocks acetylcholine release at the neuromuscular junction and thus prevents neuromuscular transmission. The bacteria infects humans by its presence in tainted food or by wound contamination from dirt or soil containing the organism. Classic symptoms of botulism include dysphagia, dysarthria, ptosis, and diplopia. These symptoms rapidly progress to limb paralysis and eventually to paralysis of respiratory muscles that can lead to death if the condition is untreated. Gastrointestinal symptoms of nausea, vomiting, and diarrhea, often present with neurologic compromise after a 12 to 36-hour incubation period following ingestion of the toxin. Infants who consume unpasteurized honey may ingest spores and can present with weak cry, lethargy, floppiness, poor suck, and constipation. Diagnosis can be established by wound or stool culture. Electromyography and nerve conduction studies can reveal characteristic anomalies compatible with presynaptic neuromuscular blockade. Treatment is supportive, particularly with respect to airway protection, and trivalent equine antitoxin administration can reverse the effects of circulating toxin.

Epstein-Barr virus (EBV) infection can be asymptomatic, or it can present as infectious mononucleosis, with splenomegaly, pharyngitis, and cervical lymphadenopathy. Less than 1% of EBV infections present with neurologic manifestations, which can include meningitis, transverse myelitis, sensory polyneuropathy, or Guillain-Barré syndrome. EBV can be detected in the CSF of patients with AIDS-related primary CNS lymphoma.

B&D Ch. 59

Question 41. D. The three receptor types associated with glutamate are AMPA, kainate, and N-methyl-D-aspartate (NMDA). Acetylcholine is associated with the nicotinic and muscarinic receptors. Norepinephrine is associated with the alpha 1, alpha 2, and beta receptors. Serotonin is associated with the various 5-HT receptors. GABA is associated with the GABA receptor. Opioids are associated with the mu and delta receptors. Dopamine is associated with the D1, D2, D3, D4 receptors.

K&S Ch. 3

Question 42. B. This vignette depicts a patient with classic manifestations of Pick's disease. Pick's disease is one of the so-called frontotemporal dementias (FTDs). The frontal and temporal lobes are preferentially affected and pathological studies reveal localized "knife-edge" atrophy of these lobes, together with ballooned cells and intraneuronal inclusions, termed "Pick's inclusion bodies". These inclusions plus the finding of swollen neurons and gliosis have come to be termed Pick-type histology.

The clinical presentation can manifest either with predominant behavioral disturbance or with progressive language disturbance. In the first type, behavioral changes occur with poor judgment, inability to reason or plan, and impulsivity. Patients can display hyperorality and hypersexuality (similar to that in Klüver-Bucy syndrome) with both behavioral disinhibition and a lack of motivation.

Treatment is aimed at management of depression and behavioral problems. Antidepressant therapy with SSRI medication can be useful. Atypical antipsychotic agents may help with impulsivity and behavioral anomalies. The condition is invariably irreversible.

Hirano bodies are eosinophilic neuronal inclusions that can be seen in certain neurodegenerative diseases such as Creutzfeldt-Jakob disease and Alzheimer's dementia. Lewy bodies are cytoplasmic inclusions found in the substantia nigra and cortex of many patients with idiopathic Parkinson's disease and in the cerebral cortex of patient's with Alzheimer's dementia and diffuse Lewy body disease. Neurofibrillary plaques and tangles are the neuropathologic hallmark of Alzheimer's dementia. Severe white-matter demyelination can occur in several distinct diseases, particularly in multiple sclerosis, Binswanger's disease, acute disseminated encephalomyelitis, and progressive multifocal leukoencephalopathy.

B&D Ch. 72

Question 43. A It is thought that a child's temperament at an age as young as 8 months is a function of his genes. At such a young age environmental factors play a small role in the child's temperament. As the child gets older, environmental factors will play a larger and larger role. Temperament has been examined by researchers and divided into several components. These include activity level, rythmicity (of hunger, feeding, elimination etc.), approach or withdrawal, adaptability, intensity of reaction, responsiveness, mood, distractibility, and attention span. There is a genetic component to why these vary among individuals, as well as the influence of parents, consequences of the child's behavior, and other environmental influences.

K&S Ch. 2

Question 44. A. The neuropathological hallmark of idiopathic Parkinson's disease is the finding of characteristic Lewy bodies in surviving neurons in the pars reticulata of the substantia nigra in the midbrain. The substantia nigra itself is depigmented, pale and demonstrates gliosis and neuronal loss. Lewy bodies have a pale halo and an eosinophilic center.
Hirano bodies are eosinophilic neuronal inclusions that can be seen in certain neurodegenerative diseases such as Creutzfeldt-Jakob disease and Alzheimer's dementia.
Amyloid and neuritic plaques are noted in Alzheimer's dementia. Amyloid may also be found in the cerebrovascular wall. Mesial temporal sclerosis is the pathological hallmark of brain tissue in those with temporal lobe epilepsy. The entorhinal cortex and hippocampi are characterized by neuronal loss and gliosis. Atrophy of the head of the caudate nucleus is found in Huntington's disease, but it does not correlate with the severity of the disease.
B&D Chs. 72,73&77

Question 45. C. This question gives a description of someone who has schizotypal personality disorder. Schizotypal personality disorder is composed of a pervasive pattern of personal and social deficits characterized by ideas of reference, odd beliefs or magical thinking, unusual perceptual experiences, paranoid ideation, inappropriate affect, eccentric appearance, lack of close friends, and excessive social anxiety that has a paranoid flair.
K&S Ch. 27

Question 46. B. Fibromyalgia does not present with psychosis. Fibromyalgia is a controversial syndrome characterized by diffuse muscular and soft-tissue pain with multiple tender "trigger" points. The patient must have tenderness to palpation at eleven or more of eighteen specific tender points. Other clinical manifestations can include weakness, paresthesias, sleep disturbance, mood disturbance, headache, fatigue, muscle or joint stiffness, and dizziness. Neurological examination and all laboratory and clinical investigations are usually within normal limits. The cause of the disorder is not known. Treatment involves a good physician-patient relationship, exercise, avoiding a sedentary lifestyle and possibly the use of tricyclic antidepressants.
B&D Ch. 79

257

Question 47. C. Pancreatic cancer has been associated with a high rate of depression. Patients present with apathy, decreased energy, and anhedonia. It should be a consideration in the clinician's mind whenever seeing middle-aged depressed patients. Cancer in general brings about many psychological reactions in patients. Fear of death, fear of abandonment and disfigurement, loss of independence, denial, anxiety, guilt, financial worries, and disruption in relationships all play a role. Of patients with cancer, 50% often have comorbid psychiatric diagnoses with adjustment disorder, major depressive disorder, and delirium being the most common.
K&S Ch. 28

Question 48. C. This vignette depicts a classic neurologic emergency: acute epidural spinal cord compression (ESCC). In this case, the causative agent is likely to be a spinal metastasis from the patient's prostate cancer. Metastases from primary carcinoma of the breast, lung and prostate each make up 20% of the cause of ESCC. Back pain is the most frequent presenting feature in over 80% of cases. The back pain is usually progressive and increases with tumor growth over a period of up to two months before the onset of neurological deficits. Motor weakness is noted in about 80% of cases, and it predicts the post-treatment outcome much of the time. Sensory deficits are noted in about 75% of cases. Metastatic ESCC causes a spastic paraparesis or paraplegia with a sensory level that is usually several levels below the actual lesion. Bowel and bladder incontinence, urinary retention, or constipation, are observed in a majority of patients. Sagittal screening MRI imaging of the entire spine is the initial test of choice, if available, because only MRI and myelography can immediately identify and characterize the nature of the lesion and guide treatment. Treatment is undertaken acutely with parenteral corticosteroids and subacutely with radiation therapy. Decompressive laminectomy can be performed, but radiotherapy has of late produced results as good as a surgical approach. Chemotherapy is generally ineffective, because metastases causative of ESCC are usually not chemosensitive.

B&D Ch. 58

Question 49. D. It is important to be able to distinguish conduct disorder from other childhood psychiatric diagnoses. In conduct disorder the patient shows a pattern whereby the rights of others and societal rules are violated. This presents as bullying other children, using weapons, physical fighting, cruelty to animals, stealing, fire setting, destroying property, truancy, or running away from home. Patients with ADHD can have many behavioral problems, but those problems are a result of inattention, hyperactivity, and impulsivity. ADHD does not show a pattern where the child is intentionally or malevolently being violent or destructive. Any such acts happen as a result of hyperactivity and poor impulse control. In depression children can become very irritable, withdrawn, and not wish to socialize. They may even act out as a result of how badly they are feeling. However this is different than a long-standing pattern of actively trying to carry out violence or do property damage regardless of mood state. In bipolar disorder children may break rules and have behavioral difficulties during manic and depressive episodes. However there will be a clear cycling pattern to their moods (and other symptoms), which corresponds to the times when their behaviors become problematic. One of the other important distinctions to make is between conduct disorder and oppositional defiant disorder (ODD). In ODD there is a pattern of negativistic, hostile, or defiant behavior directed at adults or authority figures. In conduct disorder the negative behavior is directed at all others regardless of whether they are authority figures or not. ODD behaviors are therefore more targeted and have less of a wide-ranging destructive nature than those of conduct disorder.

K&S Ch. 44

Question 50. A. Subacute combined degeneration is the result of a deficiency in vitamin B12 (cobalamin). Cobalamin deficiency manifests as macrocytic anemia, atrophic glossitis, and neurologic deficits. Neurologic symptoms include lesions to the lateral and posterior columns of the spinal cord (subacute combined degeneration), peripheral neuropathy, optic atrophy, and brain lesions. Spinal cord symptoms present as posterior column deficits, which can manifest as upper motor neuron limb weakness, spasticity, and Babinski's signs. Peripheral neuropathy can present as paresthesias and large fiber sensory impairment (loss of proprioception and vibration sensation). Cerebral symptoms present as behavioral changes, forgetfulness, and in severe cases, dementia and stupor. Sensory ataxia is demonstrated by a positive Romberg sign. There can also be a diffuse hyper-reflexia with absent ankle jerk reflexes. Deficiencies of vitamins B6, niacin, and folic acid are explained elsewhere in this volume.

B&D Chs. 63&82

Question 51. D. Victims of childhood incest often develop depressive feelings mixed with guilt, shame, and a feeling of permanent damage. Teens that undergo sexual abuse often show poor impulse control, self-destructive behavior, and suicidal behavior. Adults abused as children often have posttraumatic

stress disorder and dissociative disorders. Incest is most often perpetrated by fathers, stepfathers or older siblings. It is defined as sexual relations between two people who are related or who society has deemed inappropriate to be sexually involved. Most reported cases involve father-daughter incest. In addition to depression, children involved in incest may present to the doctor with complaints of abdominal pain, genital irritation, separation anxiety disorder, phobias, or school problems.
K&S Ch. 32

Question 52. B. This question presents the classic lacunar stroke syndrome called pure motor hemiparesis. This lacunar syndrome classically localizes to the contralateral internal capsule. Two other possible locations of such a lacunar stroke are the contralateral basis pontis or corona radiata. The pure motor stroke presents without cortical deficits. There are no sensory or visual deficits. Aphasia, agnosia and apraxia, are all absent in a pure motor stroke. If both the thalamus and internal capsule are involved, one would expect to see a combined sensory-motor stroke, which manifests not only as a contralateral motor hemiparesis, but also as a contralateral hemisensory loss. The lesion localizes to ischemia in the territory of the small penetrating lenticulostriate arteries that originate off the proximal middle cerebral artery.
B&D Ch. 57

Question 53. D. The amino acid neurotransmitters include GABA, glutamate, and aspartate. GABA is the main inhibitory neurotransmitter of the brain. Glutamate is the main excitatory neurotransmitter of the brain. The benzodiazepines, barbiturates and several anticonvulsants work through the action of GABA-A and not GABA-B. Lioresal, a muscle relaxant, works through GABA-B. The street drug PCP works primarily through the glutamate receptor. Cocaine works by blocking reuptake of serotonin, norepinephrine, and dopamine. It is also believed to increase glutamate in the nucleus accumbens, accounting for its habit-forming effects. Histamine is a biogenic amine neurotransmitter.
K&S Ch. 3

Question 54. D. Choreoathetosis is not a feature of Parkinson's disease (PD). The classic cardinal clinical features of idiopathic Parkinson's disease are akinesia (or bradykinesia), rigidity, resting tremor, and loss of postural reflexes. Tremor is an oscillating 3 to 5 Hz, seen more in the hands where it resembles pill-rolling, but also in the face, chin and the lower extremities. Bradykinesia refers to slowness of voluntary movements that make it difficult for the patient to dress, eat and maintain personal hygiene. Bradykinesia becomes most evident when a patient attempts to perform rapid alternating movements. Rigidity is often manifested as a cogwheeling when the extremities are passively mobilized. Loss of postural reflexes is also a hallmark of idiopathic PD, and is responsible for the many falls sustained by patients with the disease. Other associated clinical features include masked facies, decreased blink, micrographia, seborrhea, weight loss, constipation, and dysphagia. Gait is classically altered and patients walk with "petits pas" (small steps) and a shuffling gait. When they turn around, they turn "en bloc" (without swinging the hips and shoulders, much like a robot). Other autonomic features include orthostatic hypotension, sweating disorder, and urinary frequency. Other symptoms include sleep disturbance, restless legs, fatigue, anxiety, depression, cognitive and behavioral disturbances. These associated features are not present in every case, and are seen less frequently than the cardinal symptoms.
B&D Ch. 77

Question 55. E. Reading disorder is characterized by reading achievement being substantially below what is expected for the child's age, intelligence, and

259

education. It interferes with academic achievement and activities of daily living that require reading skills. In the question given, the child's difficulties are all in situations where she may be asked to read. When children refuse to go to school, separation anxiety disorder should also be considered. In this case however, the child likes to stay with friends and grandparents, so separation from her parents is not the issue. Children with reading disorder become depressed and demoralized. The diagnosis must be made with a standardized reading test, and pervasive developmental disorders, attention-deficit/hyperactivity disorder, and mental retardation must be ruled out. Treatment consists of understanding the child's deficits and developing an educational program to remedy them. The child must be given coping strategies such that they are not overwhelmed and discouraged. Coexisting emotional and behavioral problems should also receive treatment.

K&S Ch. 39

Question 56. A. Myoclonus is not typically a symptom of botulism toxin poisoning. Botulism results from the ingestion of *Clostridium botulinum*, a bacteria that extrudes an exotoxin into the circulation and that blocks acetylcholine release at the neuromuscular junction. The bacteria infects humans by its presence in tainted food or by wound contamination from dirt or soil containing the organism. Classic symptoms of botulism include dysphagia, dysarthria, ptosis, diplopia, and urinary retention. Other systemic symptoms include dry mouth and lethargy. Pupillary reflexes are usually impaired. These symptoms rapidly progress to limb paralysis and eventually to paralysis of respiratory muscles that can lead to death if the condition is untreated. Gastrointestinal symptoms of nausea, vomiting, and diarrhea, often present with neurologic compromise after a 12 to 36-hour incubation period following ingestion of the toxin. Infants who consume unpasteurized honey may ingest spores and can present with weak cry, lethargy, floppiness, poor suck, and constipation. Diagnosis can be established by wound or stool culture. Electromyography and nerve conduction studies can reveal characteristic anomalies compatible with presynaptic neuromuscular blockade. Treatment is supportive, particularly with respect to airway protection, and trivalent equine antitoxin administration can help reverse the effects of circulating toxin.

B&D Ch. 84

Question 57. D. This question gives a clear case of oppositional defiant disorder (ODD). In ODD a child shows a pattern of negativistic, hostile, and defiant behavior directed at adults or authority figures. This behavior may include temper tantrums, arguing with adults, actively defying adults' requests or rules, deliberately annoying people, blaming others for their mistakes or misbehavior, being easily annoyed by others, being angry and resentful, or being spiteful or vindictive. The child in question should not meet criteria for conduct disorder to be diagnosed with ODD. The primary treatment for ODD is therapy for the child, and parental training to give parents management skills. Often behavioral therapy will be used to reinforce good behavior while ignoring or not reinforcing bad behavior.

K&S Ch. 44

Question 58. E. Balint's syndrome is a rare stroke syndrome resulting from ischemic lesions to the bilateral parietal-occipital lobes, or the occipital lobes alone. The condition is often a complication of vascular dementia and can occur after a series of strokes to the area involved. It can sometimes be the result of a "top of the basilar syndrome". The "top of the basilar syndrome" results from rostral basilary artery occlusion that is often embolic in origin. This results in infarction to the midbrain, thalamus and parts of the temporal and occipital lobes. "Top of the basilar syndrome" presents with delirium, peduncular hallucinosis (brainstem-induced visual

260

hallucinations), obtundation, and memory deficits. There may be a gaze palsy, skew deviation of the eyes, ocular bobbing, impaired convergence, or convergence-retraction nystagmus.
Balint's syndrome presents with ocular apraxia (the inability to scan extrapersonal space appropriately with the eyes), optic ataxia (dysmetric or saccadic jerks that can impede vision and ocular focus), and deficits in visual attention. Simultanagnosia may also be noted, which is an inability to perceive a scene with multiple parts to it. The patient is only able to see and recognize individual elements of a multi-part scene, and cannot interpret the overall picture. The optic tracts and radiations are usually spared so visual fields are generally normal. Balint's syndrome can be accompanied by a complete or partial Gerstmann's syndrome if the dominant parietal lobe is affected in the area of the angular gyrus (Gerstmann's syndrome is explained elsewhere in this volume). Balint's syndrome may also result in visuoconstructional apraxia (the inability to put things in their proper place or order). The other answer choices are explained in other questions in this volume, and examination candidates are strongly recommended to review these lobar syndromes as they appear frequently on standardized tests.
B&D Chs. 57&72

Question 59. D. Although there are no specific behaviors that prove that sexual abuse has taken place, children that have been abused often behave in certain patterns. If very young children have detailed knowledge of sexual acts, they have usually witnessed or participated in sexual behavior. They express their sexual knowledge through play and may initiate sexual behavior with other children. Abused children can also be very aggressive. Other signs of sexual abuse include bruising, pain or itching of the genitals, genital or rectal bleeding, recurrent urinary tract infections, or the presence of sexually transmitted disease.
K&S Ch. 32

Question 60. D. Anton's syndrome is considered to be an agnosia characterized by cortical blindness. The lesion localizes to the bilateral occipital lobes, usually due to strokes, particularly in the calcarine cortex (Brodmann's area 17) and visual association cortex. The arterial territory involved is that of the bilateral posterior cerebral arteries (PCAs). The hallmark of the syndrome is that patients are unaware or deny that they are blind and they confabulate. Patients may also suffer from visual hallucinations. Prosopagnosia is the inability to recognize familiar faces. It is associated classically with bilateral occipital-temporal lesions. It is often associated with agraphia and achromatopsia (inability to recognize colors and hues). It is almost always associated with visual field deficits. Aphasia is a disorder of speech and language that can be expressive, receptive, or both. Aphasia occurs following lesions to the dominant hemisphere. Prosopagnosia often occurs following lesions of the occipitotemporal region. The lesion is usually either bilateral or on the right side. Apraxia is the inability to perform simple motor tasks that have been previously learned. Motor apraxia can result from lacunar infarcts to the internal capsule or pons, or from non-dominant hemispheric strokes. Hiccups are often the result of phrenic nerve irritation. This is frequently caused by medication side effects such as dopa repletion therapy in Parkinson's disease.
B&D Chs 14&72

Question 61. D. Dependent personality disorder (DPD) is the least likely of the answer choices given to present with violence. Patients with dependent personality disorder subordinate their needs to those of others, get others to assume responsibility for major areas of their life, lack self-confidence, and are uncomfortable when alone. They have an intense need to be taken care of that leads them to be clingy, submissive, and fear separation. They can not make decisions without an excessive amount of advice from others. Because of their submissiveness patients with DPD are less likely to become violent than patients with other disorders. People with the other personality disorders listed can be aggressive, outrageous, and at odds with others. Some patients with these disorders may have a clear history of violence. Treatment of dependent personality disorder consists of therapy to modify the patient's interpersonal interactions, and medication to deal with comorbid anxiety and depression.

K&S Ch. 27

Question 62. B. Chronic abuse of *n*-hexane or other hydrocarbon inhalants (glue, paint thinner) can lead to distal sensorimotor polyneuropathy. The first manifestation is usually numbness and distal paresthesia, which is subsequently followed by distal motor weakness. If inhalants continue to be abused, the motor weakness can worsen and can spread to involve the proximal muscles of both the arms and the legs. At low to moderate doses, the inhalants cause dysarthria, uncoordination, euphoria, and relaxation. Higher doses and more chronic exposure can lead to hallucinosis, psychosis, and seizures, as well as more systemic end-organ damage such as renal failure, bone marrow suppression, and hepatic failure.

B&D Ch. 64

Question 63. D. Delusional disorder is characterized by a fixed false belief that is non-bizarre (i.e., may be possible...such as being poisoned, infected, followed, or having a disease). It is differentiated from schizophrenia by the lack of positive symptoms (no auditory or visual hallucinations, no thought disorganization). Tactile or olfactory hallucinations may be present. Apart from the direct impact of the delusion, the patient does not have a marked impairment in functioning. In the case of somatic delusions, the person believes he has some physical defect or medical condition. Treatment consists of antipsychotics in addition to psychotherapy.
The other answer choices do not fit the question stem. The patient does not have a neurological deficit, so conversion disorder is incorrect. He does not have auditory or visual hallucinations, and does not have significant negative symptoms and functional impairment, so schizophrenia is unlikely. There is no mention of depressive symptoms. This would not be considered hypochondriasis because hypochondriasis presents with an unreasonable obsession with a perceived medical problem that could be real. This cases clearly presents a delusion that has no possible basis in reality, which would push it out of the realm of hypochondriasis.

K&S Ch. 14

Question 64. C. Stimulants such as cocaine typically lower the seizure threshold when abused to intoxication. In moderate doses, cocaine and the stimulants can produce wakefulness, alertness, mood elevation, diminished appetite, and increased performance in certain tasks. The stimulants can also result in psychosis and paranoia. There is also an increased risk of myocardial infarction with cocaine use. Systemic problems such as dehydration, rhabdomyolysis, and hyperthermia can also be noted. The most common neurologic adverse effect of cocaine and the stimulants is headache. In certain cases, the stimulants can produce myoclonus, encephalopathy, and seizures. Cocaine is the stimulant that is most likely to induce seizures. Smoking and intravenous administration of cocaine are more likely to induce seizures than intranasal use. Ischemic and hemorrhagic strokes can also result from cocaine use. Cocaine is the most significant cause of drug-induced stroke and accounts for about 50% of all cases. The mechanism of cocaine-induced stroke is believed to involve vasoconstriction, acute hypertension, and vasospasm.

Opioid ingestion and intoxication can produce a state of euphoria or dysphoria. Other possible adverse effects include hallucinations, dry mouth, nausea, vomiting, constipation, and urinary retention. Examination usually reveals pupillary constriction during acute intoxication. Autonomic disturbance such as hypotension and hypothermia can also be noted. Seizures are rare with opioid intoxication. Overdose can result in coma and respiratory compromise. Opioids do not usually cause seizures or lower the seizure threshold.

Phencyclidine (PCP) intoxication produces hallucinosis, dysphoria, and paranoia. Agitation, catatonia, and bizarre behavior are also common. At higher doses, PCP use can lead to stupor and coma. In overdose, rhabdomyolysis may result from agitation and dysautonomia such as fever, hypertension, and sweating. PCP can lower the seizure threshold, but less frequently than cocaine.

Tetrahydrocannabinol (THC), the primary active ingredient in marijuana, causes euphoria, depersonalization, and relaxation. Other effects of the drug include sleepiness, paranoia, and anxiety. High doses of THC can result in hallucinosis, panic, and even paranoia. Seizures are not generally noted with THC intoxication.

Alcohol has intoxicating effects that can cause sedation, memory impairment, uncoordination, dysarthria, euphoria, dysphoria, sleepiness, and acute confusion. Alcohol intoxication does not lower the seizure threshold, it in fact is protective against seizures, because of its agonistic effects at the GABA-A receptor. Alcohol withdrawal can lower the seizure threshold because of rapid desaturation of the GABA-A receptor, in much the same way as the benzodiazepines.

B&D Ch. 64

Question 65. E. Mark, who has major depressive disorder, has the highest likelihood of completing suicide. About 95% of those who attempt or commit suicide have some form of psychiatric disorder. Major depressive disorder accounts for 80% of suicides, schizophrenia accounts for 10%, and dementia or delirium for 5%. Of those who have problems with alcohol, 15% attempt suicide, but the numbers are less than for those with depression. Personality disorders may contribute to suicide attempts, but numbers do not surpass those for depression, and often the two overlap. Mental retardation is not a significant risk factor for suicide. Always keep in mind that the best predictor of future suicidal behavior is past suicidal behavior.

K&S Ch. 34

Question 66. D. Meige's syndrome denotes the combination of blepharospasm (involuntary eyelid blinking) and oromandibular dystonia. Patients have involuntary contraction of the eyelids as well as the lower facial muscles in the area of the jaw, tongue, or neck. The treatment of choice is chemodenervation of the hyperactive muscles by Botulinum toxin type A injection. The tongue requires careful injection in these cases as it can fall back and occlude the airway if it is weakened too severely. The other answers are simply distracters.

B&D Ch. 17

Question 67. D. The Tarasoff rule came as a result of the Tarasoff court case. In this case it was decided that a physician or therapist who has reason to believe that a patient might injure or kill someone must notify the potential victim, their family or friends, and the authorities.

The Durham rule is no longer used, but said that an accused is not responsible if his or her unlawful actions were the result of mental disease or defect.

The M'Naughten rule comes from British law, stating that a patient is guilty by reason of insanity if they have a mental disease such that they were unaware of the nature, quality, and consequences of their actions, and were incapable of realizing that their actions were wrong.

Ford vs Wainwright was a case that sustained the need for a patient to be competent in order to be executed. Also worthy of note is that psychiatrists are ethically bound not to participate in state mandated executions in any way.

Respondeat superior is a legal concept stating that a person at the top of a hierarchy is responsible for the actions of those at the bottom of the hierarchy.

K&S Ch. 57

Question 68. A. Scanning speech is essentially a form of dysphasia that causes a cerebellar "dysmetria" of the speech pattern. It is also known as ataxic dysarthria. Lesions of the cerebellum such as strokes, degeneration, or tumor can cause this condition. Speech rhythm is usually irregular and choppy. This can also be accompanied by slow, labored speech pattern.

B&D Ch. 12

Question 69. B. As many as 40% of mothers may experience mood or cognitive symptoms during the postpartum period. Postpartum blues (or maternity blues) is a normal state of sadness, dysphoria, tearfulness, and dependence which may last for several days and is the result of hormonal changes and the stress of being a new mother.

Postpartum depression is more severe and involves neurovegetative signs and symptoms of depression and potential suicidality.

Postpartum psychosis can involve hallucinations and delusions, as well as thoughts of infanticide.

There is no DSM-recognized specific phobia regarding being a parent. The fear of the responsibility associated with parenthood may play a part in postpartum blues or postpartum depression, but is not a distinct entity.

K&S Ch. 30

Question 70. D. Aphemia is a motor speech disorder characterized by near muteness with normal reading, writing, and comprehension. Some experts consider aphemia to be the equivalent of pure speech apraxia; however, this remains a controversy. Aphemia is likely to result from lesions to the primary motor cortex or Broca's area. Patients are first mute, then they become able to speak with hesitancy and phonemic substitutions.

Aphasia is simply any acquired disorder of language. Aphasias can take multiple forms, including expressive, receptive, conduction, global, or transcortical varieties.

Agnosia is the inability to recognize and identify objects. Agnosias imply that the patient is able to see, hear, or touch the object to be identified and that the patient does not have a sensory or perceptual deficit that could impair perception of the object.

Apraxia is the inability to perform a skilled, learned, purposeful motor behavior, in the absence of other deficits that may impair motor functioning. Abulia resembles akinetic mutism. Patients display severe apathy, with affective blunting, amotivation, and immobility. There is an absence of spontaneous speech and movement. Patients retain awareness of their environment.

B&D Chs. 5&12

Question 71. B. The N-methyl-D-aspartate (NMDA) receptor is one of the best known glutamate receptors. It has been found to play a role in learning and memory, as well as in psychopathology. The other glutamate receptors are known as the non-NMDA glutamate receptors. The NMDA receptor allows sodium, potassium, and calcium to pass through. It opens when bound by two glutamate molecules and one glycine molecule at the same

time. The receptor can be blocked by physiological concentrations of magnesium, and bound by PCP and PCP-like substances.
K&S Ch. 3

Question 72. C. Stupor refers to a state of unresponsiveness from which arousal only occurs with vigorous and repeated stimulation. It is on the continuum between alertness and coma. Alert patients are awake and in a normal state of arousal. Lethargic patients are sleepy but awake and arousable to alertness with stimulation. Coma implies a state of unarousable unresponsiveness. The persistent vegetative state follows coma. Patients lose cognitive functioning, but retain vegetative, or autonomic functioning (such as cardiac function, respiration, and blood pressure maintenance).
B&D Ch. 5

Question 73. E. Of the various somatoform disorders, the one with the best prognosis is conversion disorder. The somatoform disorders are characterized by physical symptoms suggestive of a medical condition but are not fully explained by a medical condition or substance abuse. The symptoms are not intentionally produced as in factitious disorders or malingering. Somatization disorder consists of complaints from various organ systems and has a poor prognosis. In hypochondriasis the patient is falsely convinced that he has a serious disease, often based on the misinterpretation of bodily symptoms or functions. Hypochondriasis has a fair to good prognosis. Conversion disorder is the development of one or more neurological deficits that can not be explained by a known medical disorder. Psychological factors are often associated with the onset of the deficit. The prognosis is excellent. Somewhere from 90–100% of patients with conversion disorder are in remission within less than a month. Body dysmorphic disorder is characterized by the false belief or exaggerated perception that a body part is defective. The prognosis is usually poor and the disease is chronic. Pain disorder is marked by pain in one or more sites that is not fully accounted for by a medical condition. The prognosis is guarded and variable.
K&S Ch. 17

Question 74. B. All of these answer choices are at least partly untrue, except for answer choice B. Comatose patients require a head CT scan prior to lumbar puncture (LP), in order to assess if there is a presence of a mass lesion or acute hemorrhage that could result in transtentorial or cerebellar herniation if a LP were to be performed.
Not every patient with Guillain-Barré syndrome (GBS) should be hospitalized in an intensive care unit. Mild forms of the disease can be monitored in a regular inpatient setting and bedside respiratory peak-flow monitoring can be assessed frequently to screen for acute respiratory compromise that could lead to death. Patients with GBS who deteriorate rapidly, or show signs of poor oxygenation, can be transferred to an intensive care or pulmonary unit for close monitoring, and intubation can be undertaken if deemed clinically necessary. The rule of "20-30-40" is a guide for determining if intensive care unit admission is needed. A vital capacity of less than 20 mL/kg, or a decline by 30% from baseline, or a maximal inspiratory pressure less than 30 cmH$_2$O, or expiratory pressure less than 40 cmH$_2$O, all indicate the need for ICU admission and close monitoring of respiratory status.
A positive grasp reflex is usually a pathological sign in an adult. It is a normal infantile reflex that is present at birth and usually disappears by six months of age. Persistence or redevelopment of the reflex in adulthood would be indicative of frontal lobe pathology and the grasp reflex is considered one of the frontal-release signs.
Cerebellar hemispheric lesions produce movement deficits that affect the ipsilateral side of the body to the lesion. This is due to the double-crossing

of pathways. Ascending cerebello-cortical tracts decussate in the midbrain and proceed to the contralateral cortex. Descending corticospinal tracts (the pyramidal tracts) decussate in the medulla to project to the contra-lateral body.

Bell's palsy is believed to be the result of a herpes simplex infection that affects the Gasserian ganglion. *Borellia burgdorferi*, the spirochete responsible for Lyme infection, can indeed cause facial diplegia, but is a much rarer infection than that caused by the herpes simplex virus.

B&D Ch. 82

Question 75. D. The American Psychiatric Association considers it unethical for a psychiatrist to accept a patient's estate after death. It is considered an exploitation of the therapeutic relationship. It is acceptable to accept a token bequest that you were unaware was in the will when the patient was alive. All of the other acts listed are ethical. Psychiatrists can not participate in executions (often asked on exams). Abandoning patients without arranging for follow up care is unethical. It is unethical to release information about a patient to another party without the patient's permission. It is unethical to pay another doctor for sending you referrals. You can rent other doctors space in your office. And it is ethical to charge a fee for supervision.

K&S Ch. 58

Question 76. A. The amygdala is necessary for the recall of emotional contexts of specific events and the experience of fear, pleasure, or other emotions associated with these events. Declarative or episodic memory (also known as short-term memory) requires the intact functioning of the hippocampus and parahippocampal areas (nucleus basalis of Meynert) of the medial temporal lobe for storage and retrieval of information. The other answers are distracters.

B&D Ch. 6

Question 77. C. Desipramine is the least anticholinergic of the tricyclic antidepressants (TCAs). Anticholinergic side effects are common with patients on TCAs, but tolerance develops over time. Amitriptyline, imipramine, trimipramine, and doxepin are the most anticholinergic. Amoxapine, nortriptyline and maprotiline are less so. Anticholinergic side effects include dry mouth, blurred vision, constipation, and urinary retention. Because of this last side effect desipramine would be the best choice for someone with prostatic hypertrophy. One should always keep in mind the potential for severe anticholinergic effects to lead to a delirium.

K&S Ch. 36

Question 78. D. Children are expected to reach developmental milestones at the appropriate age. Standardized examination candidates should memorize these milestones, as questions concerning this material come up on many different examinations. Here are the milestones that need to be remembered:

- 2 months of age: cooing, smiling with social contact, holding head up 45°
- 4 months of age: laughing/squealing, sustaining social contact, grasping objects, weight bearing on legs
- 6 months of age: imitating speech sounds, single syllables, prefers mother, enjoys mirror, transferring objects hand to hand, raking grasp, sitting up with support
- 8 months of age: jabbering, playing peek-a-boo, patty-cake, waving bye-bye, sitting without support, creeping or crawling
- 12 months of age: speech specific to "dada/mama," playing simple ball games, able to adjust body to dressing, standing alone, able to use thumb-finger pincer grasp

- 14 months of age: one to two-word vocabulary, indicating desires by pointing, hugging parents, walking alone, stooping and recovering
- 18 months of age: six-word vocabulary, able to feed self, walking up stairs while hand is held, imitating scribbling
- 24 months of age: combining words, 250-word vocabulary, helping to undress, listening to picture stories, running well, making circular scribbles, copying a horizontal line
- 30 months of age: knows full name, refers to self as "I", pretending in play, helping put things away, climbing stairs alternating feet, copying a vertical line
- 36 months of age: counting three objects correctly, knowing age and sex, helping in dressing, riding a tricycle, standing briefly on one foot, copying a circle
- 48 months of age: telling a story, counting four objects, playing with other children, using toilet alone, hopping on one foot, using scissors to cut out pictures, copying a square and a cross
- 60 months of age: naming four colors, counting ten objects, asking about word meanings, domestic role playing, skipping, copying a triangle

B&D Ch. 7

Question 79. A. This question is a case of exhibitionism. Exhibitionism is a paraphilia in which the patient has a recurrent urge to expose their genitals to strangers. Sexual arousal is brought about by the event. Cases are almost always men exposing themselves to women. Medroxyprogesterone acetate has been shown to be helpful in some cases, and is useful in any sexual disorder in which the patients are extremely hypersexual to the point of being out of control or dangerous. Other drugs such as antipsychotics and antidepressants have not been shown to be particularly useful in such cases. Some patients may improve with the sexual side effects of a serotonin-selective reuptake inhibitor, but it would not be the first choice for treatment.

K&S Ch. 21

Question 80. B. The clinical vignette described in this question involves a classic presentation of Hoover's sign. Hoover's sign is positive when a patient suspected of a hysterical or psychogenic hemiparesis does not give effort in the contralateral (unaffected) lower extremity when asked to push down on the bed with the paretic (affected) lower extremity. The examiner places a hand under the patient's heel on the unaffected side to feel if the patient is pushing down towards the bed in an attempt to give a full effort at raising the affected leg. In a real hemiparesis, the patient would be expected to make every effort to brace himself with the unaffected leg while trying to raise the paretic leg.

Hoffman's sign is the equivalent to a Babinski's sign, but it is noted in the upper extremity. The sign is positive when a flick of the distal phalange of the index or middle finger results in an adduction of the ipsilateral thumb. The sign, when present, indicates contralateral cortico-spinal tract damage that affects the upper extremity.

Lasegue's sign is present when straight-leg raising in a recumbent position results in reproduction of pain or paresthesia in the sciatic distribution. The sign can either be ipsilateral or crossed. The positive sign points to sciatic nerve compression due to mechanical interruption of the nerve trajectory, most often due to an intervertebral disc bulge or herniation at the lumbar or sacral level.

Romberg's sign is positive when a patient is asked to stand up straight with eyes closed and subsequently loses his balance. The presence of Romberg's sign usually signals a deficit localizing either to the posterior columns of the spinal cord (i.e., loss of proprioception and/or vibration sensation in the legs), or to cerebellar pathology, or both.

Gegenhalten refers to "clasp-knife" type rigidity that can be observed in the extremities in several types of disorders that can include stroke, multiple sclerosis, and catatonia.

B&D Ch. 25

Question 81. E. Clomipramine is one of the tricyclic antidepressants. It has been useful in the treatment of patients with premature ejaculation, depression, panic, obsessive-compulsive disorder, phobias, and pain disorder. It has no use in treating psychosis. It carries with it the cardiac, autonomic, neurologic, sedative, and anticholinergic effects found with many of the tricyclic antidepressants. All tricyclic antidepressants should be avoided during pregnancy.

K&S Ch. 35

Question 82. C. The only true emergency in neurology that requires immediate MRI imaging is acute epidural spinal cord compression (ESCC). If MRI is unavailable, the alternate imaging modality of choice is a spinal myelogram. The cause of spinal cord compression can be an intervertebral disk, metastatic carcinoma, or epidural hematoma. Metastases from primary carcinoma of the breast, lung and prostate each make up 20% of the cause of ESCC. Back pain is the most frequent presenting feature in over 80% of cases. The back pain is usually progressive and increases with tumor growth over a period of up to two months before the onset of neurological deficits. Motor weakness is noted in about 80% of cases, and it predicts the post-treatment outcome much of the time. Sensory deficits are noted in about 75% of cases. Metastatic ESCC causes a spastic paraparesis or paraplegia with a sensory level that is usually several levels below the actual lesion. Bowel and bladder incontinence, urinary retention, or constipation, are observed in a majority of patients. Sagittal screening MRI imaging of the entire spine is the initial test of choice, if available, because only MRI and myelography can immediately identify and characterize the nature of the lesion and guide treatment. Treatment is undertaken acutely with parenteral corticosteroids and subacutely with radiation therapy. Decompressive laminectomy can be performed, but radiotherapy has of late produced results as good as a surgical approach. Chemotherapy is generally ineffective, because metastases causative of ESCC are usually not chemosensitive. The other answers are clearly distracters and are discussed individually elsewhere in this volume.

B&D Ch. 58

Question 83. C. The legal concept of parens patriae allows the state to intervene and act as a surrogate parent for those who are unable to care for themselves or who may harm themselves.
Actus reus means voluntary conduct. Mens rea means evil intent. Durable power refers to durable power of attorney, where a patient selects who they want to make decisions for them should they become incompetent to make those decisions for themselves. Respondeat superior is the concept that a person at the top of a hierarchy is responsible for the actions of those at the bottom of the hierarchy.

K&S Ch. 57

Question 84. B. Tiagabine (Gabitril) is the only agent that is a selective GABA reuptake inhibitor. It is FDA-approved as adjunctive treatment of partial complex seizures. Recent warnings have suggested that it can actually worsen or cause seizures. Gabapentin (Neurontin) is a GABA modulating agent that does not directly affect GABA receptors. It is FDA-approved for adjunctive therapy of partial complex seizures and postherpetic neuralgia. Pregabalin (Lyrica) is FDA-approved for adjunctive therapy in partial complex seizures and in neuropathic pain. Its mechanism of action is similar to that of gabapentin: it binds to the alpha-2-delta subunit of the voltage-gated calcium channel. Vigabatrin is not available on the US market. It is an irreversible inhibitor of GABA transaminase (the enzyme that metabolizes GABA) that is approved abroad in the adjunctive therapy of partial complex seizures. Lioresal (Baclofen) is a GABA-B agonist that is approved for spasticity in disorders such as stroke and multiple sclerosis.

B&D Ch. 73

Question 85. E. The trail-making test is a measure of executive function. The second part of the test consists of drawing lines between a series of letters and numbers in the correct order. For example, the patient would connect A-1-B-2-C-3 etc. The trail-making test is given as part of the Halstead-Reitan Test Battery.

K&S Ch. 5

Question 86. C. Memantine (Namenda) is an NMDA antagonist that is FDA-approved for the treatment of moderate to severe Alzheimer's dementia. It has a completely different mechanism of action to donepizil (Aricept), rivastigmine (Exelon), and galantamine (Reminyl), which are inhibitors of acetylcholinesterase that are FDA-approved for treatment of mild to moderate Alzheimer's dementia. There is now evidence to suggest that concomitant therapy with memantine and one of the cholinesterase inhibitors has measurable clinical advantages over therapy with either class of agent on its own. Neither of these two classes of agent attacks the true pathophysiology of Alzheimer's dementia, which is the formation of neurofibrillary plaques and tangles in the brain that lead to neuronal cell death. Memantine may reverse the process of apoptosis (preprogrammed cell death) that is believed to be intrinsic to the pathological basis of cell death in Alzheimer's dementia. Glutamate and NMDA hyperstimulation may lead to premature cell death by promoting calcium influx into neurons and this in turn leads to progression of Alzheimer's dementia. Memantine may slow disease progress by modulating and lessening the adverse effects of glutamate on the brain. The other answer choices are distracters and need no particular explanation.

B&D Ch. 72; also see www.namenda.com

Question 87. A. It is the GABA-A receptor that has binding sites for the benzodiazepines. There are three types of GABA receptors, GABA-A, B, and C. There are no GABA-D or GABA-E receptors. The benzodiazepines increase affinity of the GABA-A receptor for GABA. The GABA-A receptor is a chloride ion channel.

K&S Ch. 3

Question 88. A. Vagal nerve stimulation has been FDA-approved since 1997 for adjunctive treatment of refractory partial complex epilepsy in patients over 12 years of age. It recently obtained FDA-approval in intractable major depressive disorder. The modality involves the invasive implantation of an electric stimulating device inside the chest cavity. The stimulator is connected to a wire that wraps around the left vagal nerve (the right vagal nerve is not clinically important in the management of epilepsy). The stimulator is programmed to cycle on for 30 seconds and off for 5 minutes throughout the day. Seizure frequency is typically reduced by about 50%. Side effects can include hoarseness from irritation of the adjacent recurrent laryngeal nerve, and throat tingling and/or coughing during actual stimulation. Vagal nerve stimulation is not as of yet approved for use in any other psychiatric disorder apart from depression.

B&D Ch. 73

Question 89. D. It is true that some studies have shown the efficacy of using carbamazepine in the treatment of alcohol withdrawal to be equal to that of the benzodiazepines. Carbamazepine is approved in the US for temporal lobe and generalized epilepsy as well as trigeminal neuralgia. It is metabolized by the liver and excreted by the kidneys. It causes its own autoinduction by hepatic enzymes that makes it necessary over time to give more medication to achieve the same blood levels. It also affects the metabolism of several other drugs. Carbamazepine has been associated with a transient decrease in white blood cell count and has been associated with an inhibition of colony stimulating factor in the bone marrow. It has also been associated with severe blood dyscrasias such as aplastic anemia and agranulocytosis. A benign rash has been found in 10–15% of patients on carbamazepine, and a small percentage of these patients go on to develop serious rashes such as Stevens-Johnson syndrome, exfoliative dermatitis, erythema multiforme, or toxic epidermal necrolysis.

K&S Ch. 35

Question 90. E. Auscultation of the head that reveals a bruit is a classic hallmark of an arteriovenous malformation (AVM). Seizures are the presenting symptom of AVMs in about one-quarter to two-thirds of cases. Headaches occur in anywhere from 5 to 35% of cases. Hemorrhage from ruptured AVM tends to be intracerebral in location, rather than subarachnoid as in the case of a ruptured aneurysm. The other distracters are discussed elsewhere in this volume.

B&D Ch. 57

Question 91. D. The "Draw-A-Person" test is a projective test. It is administered by telling the patient to draw a person. Then the patient is asked to draw a person of the sex opposite that of the first drawing. The assumption is that the drawing of the patient's gender is representative of the self in the environment. The level of detail is also correlated with intelligence in children. The Halstead-Reitan battery is used to find the location and effects of certain brain lesions. It is not projective. The Stanford-Binet test is an intelligence test. The Wechsler-Bellvue test is a memory test. The Minnesota Multiphasic Personality Inventory (MMPI) is a self report inventory used to assess personality traits.

K&S Ch. 5

Question 92. B. The image depicts a classic colloid cyst of the third ventricle. This is a rare condition that presents in middle-aged adults. The cyst is a round, well-circumscribed lesion that is situated in the anterior aspect of the third ventricle. It appears as a "button nose" right in the middle of the ventricular system and this MRI image is a typical example of its appearance. Clinical presentation is that of intermittent headaches that result from increased intracranial pressure because of the ball-valve blockage of the passage of cerebrospinal fluid in the ventricular system. The blockage can even lead to brief intermittent drop attacks in certain patients. These cysts are composed of high concentrations of cholesterol and protein that give them their characteristic hyperintense appearance particularly on T2-weighted MRI brain imaging.

B&D Ch. 58

Question 93. C. Buprenorphine is a mixed opioid agonist/antagonist. It is used for the treatment of heroin addiction as an alternative to methadone. Aripiprazole is a mixed dopamine agonist/antagonist. Naltrexone is an opioid antagonist. Methadone is an opioid agonist. Gabapentin is an anticonvulsant, and is thus unrelated to the opioid receptors.

K&S Ch. 12

Question 94. D. Hallevorden-Spatz syndrome is a rare autosomal recessive disease of childhood onset that presents with the combination of dementia and parkinsonism. The classic neuropathologic hallmark of the disorder is a rusty-brown discoloration of the medial globus pallidus and pars reticulata of the substantia nigra on autopsy. The discoloration is due to the accumulation of iron in the basal ganglia. The disorder is caused by an enzymatic deficiency in cysteine dioxygenase. This leads to increased levels of cysteine in the brain, which chelates iron. Free iron deposits in the basal ganglia and leads to free radical formation, neuronal demise, and ultimately death. Other features of the syndrome include optic atrophy, pigmentary retinopathy, psychomotor retardation and clinical signs of corticospinal tract damage.

B&D Ch. 72

Question 95. C. Anterograde amnesia is most often associated with alcohol abuse. Keep the Wernicke-Korsakoff syndrome in mind. Wernicke's encephalopathy is an acute disorder characterized by ataxia, vestibular dysfunction, confusion, and eye movement abnormalities. Korsakoff's syndrome is a chronic amnestic syndrome that can follow Wernicke's. It presents with impaired recent memory and anterograde amnesia. The patient may or may not confabulate as well. Long term memory is usually not affected. Treatment for both of these conditions is thiamine administration. If not treated early, permanent damage can take place and Korsakoff's syndrome can become permanent.

K&S Ch. 12

Question 96. A. Subacute combined degeneration is the result of a deficiency in vitamin B12 (cobalamin). Cobalamin deficiency manifests as macrocytic anemia, atrophic glossitis, and neurologic deficits. Neurologic symptoms include lesions to the lateral and posterior columns of the spinal cord (subacute combined degeneration), peripheral neuropathy, optic atrophy, and brain lesions. Spinal cord symptoms present as posterior column deficits, which can manifest as upper motor neuron limb weakness, spasticity, and Babinski's signs. Peripheral neuropathy can present as paresthesias and large fiber sensory impairment (loss of proprioception and vibration sensation). Cerebral symptoms present as behavioral changes, forgetfulness, and in severe cases, dementia and stupor. Sensory ataxia is demonstrated by a positive Romberg sign. There can also be a diffuse hyper-reflexia with absent ankle jerk reflexes. Treatment is undertaken with parenteral B12 injections intramuscularly.

B&D Ch. 82

Question 97. C. The appropriate action to take in the case presented is to increase the carbamazepine dose and take follow up levels. This is because carbamazepine has an auto-induction phenomenon whereby it causes the induction of the hepatic enzymes which break it down. Thus, after starting at one dose, the enzymes are induced and break down more carbamazepine, thereby decreasing the serum level. The answer? Give more carbamazepine to bring serum levels back up. The informed clinician knows that this phenomenon will happen, and as such knows the patient is being honest. There is no need to switch to another medication if the carbamazepine was keeping the patient stable. Adding a serotonin-selective reuptake inhibitor would be a good way to flip the patient into overt mania, but not a good way to solve this problem. The patient in question has yet to meet criteria for hospitalization, so that would just be overly aggressive and unwarranted.

K&S Ch. 36

Question 98. A. Isoniazid (INH) exposure can cause a vitamin B6 (pyridoxine) deficiency. Most normal adults consume adequate amounts of vitamin B6 in their diets (1.5–2 mg daily). Hydralazine and penicillamine can also cause drug-induced vitamin B6 deficiency. These drugs interfere with vitamin B6 coenzyme activity. Vitamin B6 deficiency results in a distal sensorimotor peripheral neuropathy. Patients can develop distal

271

paresthesias, sensory loss and motor weakness after six months of INH therapy if not on vitamin B6 supplementation. Pyridoxine supplementation of 100 mg daily needs to accompany INH therapy to avoid this untimely deficiency.

Vitamin A deficiency is rare and can occur with malabsorption syndromes like sprue and biliary atresia. The earliest manifestation is night blindness. Hypervitaminosis A is associated with pseudotumor cerebri which manifests as headache and papilledema. The other answer choices are distracters that are explained elsewhere in this volume.

B&D Chs. 63&82

Question 99. A. The answer to this question is undoubtedly choice A. Although border-line patients make frequent suicidal gestures, they are extremely impulsive. As such it is the psychiatrist's job to assume that any gesture could be potentially life threatening and to take the threat seriously. Steps must be taken to protect these patients. Choices B and C are ridiculous and dangerous. Talking about suicide does not increase the risk that patients will try to harm themselves. Isolating them will offer them less support and increase their chances of harming themselves. Choice D is inappropriate because these patients can not be relied on to keep promises when they are in an impulsive, emotionally labile state. Giving these patients a benzodiazepine could potentially disinhibit them further and make it more likely that they would try to harm themselves.

K&S Ch. 33

Question 100. B. West Nile virus infection is an arbovirus (a form of flavivirus) infection that is endemic to many parts of the world. Mosquito bites from the genus *Culex* are frequent vectors of transmission of the virus to humans. Most infections in humans are asymptomatic. In about 20% of affected patients, the infection presents as a febrile condition after an incubation period of a few days to up to two weeks. Only one in 150 patients goes on to develop a meningitis or encephalitis picture. The infection may progress to the development of a demyelinating or axonal neuropathy. Diagnosis is made by detection of IgM antibodies in cerebrospinal fluid, or IgM and IgG antibodies in serum. Treatment is generally supportive. Patients with serious symptoms may respond to intravenous administration of anti-West Nile virus immunoglobulin.

Arenaviruses are rodent-borne and infect humans when a person comes into contact with infected rodent fecal matter. Lymphocytic choriomeningitis virus and Lassa fever virus are two examples of arenaviruses. Filoviruses are represented by the Ebola and Marburg viruses. The reservoir of these viruses is not known. Infection can cause a severe hemorrhagic encephalitis with myositis and muscle pain. Treatment is supportive. Body fluids of these patients are highly contagious. Retroviruses are represented by the well-known HIV, HTLV-1 and HTLV-2. The JC virus is a papovavirus and is the causative pathogen of progressive multifocal leukoencephalopathy that can develop in patients with advanced AIDS with low CD4 cell counts. JC virus can be detected in CSF by PCR amplification of its DNA.

B&D Ch. 59

Question 101. B. You, being the skillful physician that you are, would order a lithium level on this patient! Why? Because the side effects of lithium intoxication include gastrointestinal upset such as nausea, vomiting, and diarrhea. Lithium can cause tremor, nephrogenic diabetes insipidus, acne, muscular weakness, hypothyroidism, weight gain, edema, leukocytosis, psoriasis, hair loss and cardiac dysrythmias. When toxic it can also cause ataxia, slowed thinking, impaired memory, impaired consciousness, seizures, and death.

K&S Ch. 36

Question 102. E. This question asks the exam taker to correlate the neuroanatomical location of a certain type of neurons with the function of the neurotransmitter particular to those neurons. The best answer to this question is choice E, acetylcholine. The basal forebrain is the location of the nucleus basalis of Meynert, which is the structure containing a high density of cholinergic neurons. These neurons project to the limbic system and the cerebral cortex. Alzheimer's disease is a result of cholinergic neuronal demise predominantly in the nucleus basalis of Meynert.

Acetylcholine is synthesized from acetylcoenzyme A and choline by the enzyme choline acetyltransferase in the synaptic nerve terminal. Acetylcholine is then stored in vesicles in the synaptic bouton. Once released into the synapse, it is inactivated and metabolized by acetylcholinesterase and the resultant choline is taken back up into the presynaptic terminal for reutilization.

Acetylcholine is responsible for maintaining short-term memory, attention, executive functioning, and novelty-seeking, which are mediated through the nucleus basalis of Meynert. In Alzheimer's dementia, acetylcholine is depleted and memory and executive functioning are compromised as a result. The Alzheimer's agents donepizil, rivastigmine, and galantamine are all acetylcholinesterase inhibitors and can increase levels of circulating acetylcholine in the nucleus basalis and throughout the brain, thereby improving symptoms of dementia to a limited extent. The other neurotransmitters offered in this question are distracters. Each one is explained in other questions in this volume.
K&S Ch. 3

Question 103. E. The tricyclic antidepressants, venlafaxine, bupropion, and nefazodone block the reuptake of norepinephrine (and serotonin in some cases) into the presynaptic neuron. This leads to more norepinephrine in the synaptic cleft. Mirtazapine works by blocking presynaptic alpha-2 receptors, which stops feedback inhibition on the release of norepinephrine into the synaptic cleft. This results in more norepinephrine released into the synapse.
K&S Ch. 3

Question 104. D. PCP exerts its hallucinogenic effects by antagonism of N-methyl-D-aspartate (NMDA) receptors which in turn prevents the influx of calcium ions into neurons. PCP also activates ventral tegmental dopamine which results in the reinforcing qualities of the drug. Tolerance to the physiologic effects of PCP can occur in humans, but dependence and physiologic withdrawal do not usually occur. PCP intoxication produces hallucinosis, dysphoria, and paranoia. Agitation, catatonia, and bizarre behavior are also common. At higher doses, PCP use can lead to stupor and coma. In overdose, rhabdomyolysis may result from agitation and dysautonomia such as fever, hypertension, and sweating. The other answer choices are simply distracters that need no explanation.
K&S Ch. 12

Question 105. B. The three best benzodiazepines for patients with liver dysfunction are temazepam, oxazepam, and lorazepam. This is an important little fact for the well-prepared test taker to know. They have short half lives, and do not have active metabolites. Other benzodiazepines are less desirable in patients with hepatic dysfunction.
K&S Ch. 36

Question 106. C. *Aspergillus* is a fungus that colonizes in the paranasal sinuses and can cause a hypersensitivity pneumonitis. Infection can originate from the lungs in immunocompromised patients. The fungus has a predilection for invading the posterior circulation and can cause vertebrobasilar strokes. The fungus causes a cerebral vasculitis by invasion of vessel walls. Sinus infection can extend to the brain by contiguous infiltration. Spinal cord compression can result from pulmonary Aspergillosis that extends to the thoracic vertebrae through the epidural space.

Histoplasma is a fungus that can cause an influenza-like infection with erythematous skin lesions and liver function abnormalities. In fewer than 20% of cases, there is a development of neurologic manifestations in the form of cerebritis, basilar meningitis, or CNS granuloma. Cerebral abscess is also a possible neurologic complication of histoplasmosis infection in about 40% of cases. Meningeal symptoms and signs of headache, fever and neck stiffness can also be noted in the neurologic form of the infection.

Candida albicans is one of the most common fungal organisms found in the human body. Neurologic infection is rare in immunocompetent hosts. In patients with immune compromise, candidal infection can manifest in the form of intracranial abscesses, vasculitis, and small vessel thrombosis. Candida can form mycotic intracerebral aneurysms that can rupture and cause parenchymal hemorrhage.

Pseudallecheria boydii is an uncommon fungal pathogen that can infect immunosuppressed patients. Clinical presentation is typically that of a meningitis or multiple brain abscesses.

Cryptococcus neoformans infection is discussed in detail elsewhere in this volume.

B&D Ch. 59

Question 107. C.   Adverse effects of fluoxetine that set it apart from other serotonin-specific reuptake inhibitors include headache, anxiety, and respiratory complaints. Other side effects include nausea, diarrhea, and insomnia. High blood pressure is found with patients on venlafaxine. Blurred vision can occur from anticholergic medications. Shuffling gait can occur as a result of parkinsonian side effects of antipsychotics. Loss of consciousness occurs with sedatives.

K&S Ch. 36

Question 108. B.   The GABA-A receptor (the most predominant GABA receptor) is a chloride channel. Such a useful little fact for the prudent student to know!

K&S Ch. 3

Question 109. D.   After making an error in psychodynamic psychotherapy, the best way to proceed is to briefly acknowledge that a mistake was made, and move on, focusing on the patient and their problems. Interpreting the patient's reaction can be seen as dismissive. It does not address the fact that the therapist made a mistake, not the patient. Ignoring the mistake will contaminate the patient's transference toward the therapist, potentially making him angry. Giving a long but clear explanation puts too much emphasis on the mistake. The emphasis should be on the patient and his behavior, not the therapist and hers. To profusely apologize is the wrong approach, as it is an over reaction to a minor mistake. The goal is to acknowledge the mistake and move on, spending as little time focusing on the therapist and her actions and more time on the patient and his actions. Mistakes are a normal part of therapy, as the therapist is human. Dealing with them in a way that maintains boundaries and therapeutic neutrality will be in the best interest of the patient and the therapy.

K&S Ch. 35

Question 110. C.   Identity diffusion is the failure to develop a cohesive self or self-awareness. Do not bother looking the other answer choices up. They are unrelated distracters, some of which are ludicrously unrelated to the question.

K&S Ch. 2

Question 111. C. Treatment of children with separation anxiety disorder should be multi-modal. It should involve individual therapy for the child, medication to reduce anxiety, family therapy and education, and return to school which is graded if necessary (i.e., start with one hour per day, then increase to two hours, then three hours etc.). The parental education should focus on giving the child consistent support but maintaining clear boundaries about the child's avoidant behaviors towards anxiety provoking situations.
K&S Ch. 48

Question 112. D. Naltrexone is an opioid antagonist that is often used as an adjunctive agent for alcohol abuse because it decreases craving and alcohol consumption. It is nowhere near 100% effective and its success is very much dependent on the patient's desire to stop drinking and the success of concurrent behavioral modification. It is not better than behavioral modification. Naltrexone has nothing to do with dopamine or the GABA receptor.
K&S Ch. 36

Question 113. D. The anticholinergic activity of many psychiatric drugs (including tricyclic antidepressants like imipramine) can cause urinary hesitancy, dribbling, and urinary retention. These side effects occur especially with older men who have enlarged prostates. Treatment usually consists of bethanechol 10–30 mg three to four times daily.
K&S Ch. 36

Question 114. B. The most important take home point from this question is that bipolar I disorder has equal prevalence for men and women. Major depression is more common in women than in men. There is no correlation between socioeconomic status and frequency of depression. There is a correlation between hypersecretion (not hyposecretion) of cortisol and increased depression. Only about 50% of those with major depressive disorder receive specific treatment.
K&S Ch. 15

Question 115. B. A child who is not speaking should first have her hearing checked. Phonological disorders are characterized by a child's inability to make age appropriate speech sounds. The child can not be diagnosed if the deficits are being caused by a structural or neurological problem, therefore these things must first be ruled out. Phonological disorder may present as substitutions of one sound for another, or omissions such as leaving the final consonant off of words. The treatment of choice is speech therapy, and recovery can be spontaneous in some children. Speech therapy is indicated if the child can not be understood, is over 8 years old, when self-image and peer relationships are being affected, when many consonants are misarticulated, and when the child is frequently omitting parts of words.
K&S Ch. 41

Question 116. E. State-dependent learning is the facilitated recall of information in the same internal state or environment in which the information was originally obtained. An example of this is when someone learns a behavior when intoxicated with a drug. Without the drug they can not recall the behavior. When the drug is given to them again they remember the behavior. The other answer choices relate to learning and conditioning. The most important of them have been covered in their own separate questions. Others are just distracters.
K&S Ch. 4

Question 117. C. This is a case of Wernicke's encephalopathy. Wernicke's, and its partner, Korsakoff's amnesia, are the result of thiamine deficiency often found in alcoholics. Wernicke's is an acute neurological disorder characterized by ataxia, confusion, vestibular dysfunction, and eye movement impairment. Wernicke's encephalopathy is reversible with treatment, but if it progresses into Korsakoff's amnesia, damage may be irreversible. Korsakoff's presents as impaired recent memory and anterograde amnesia. The treatment for these syndromes is thiamine, first intravenously in the case of an acute Wernicke's, then orally for as long as 3 to 12 months in the case of Korsakoff's amnesia. While other answer choices are good ideas, the primary goal is to prevent further brain damage by getting thiamine into the patient immediately.

K&S Ch. 12

Question 118. B   Niacin is an essential nutrient also called nicotinic acid. Niacin deficiency, termed pellagra, occurs in individuals who consume corn as their main carbohydrate staple. Corn lacks niacin and tryptophan (which can be converted in the body to niacin). Bread is now niacin fortified, which has diminished the widespread problem of pellagra in most countries. Pellagra causes the classic triad of the three Ds: dementia, dermatitis and diarrhea. Gastrointestinal problems present as diarrhea, anorexia, and abdominal discomfort. Skin manifestations present as a hyperkeratotic corporal rash over much of the body. The neurological manifestations can include depression, memory impairment, apathy, and irritability. A confusional state may result and may lead to stupor or coma. Oral doses of 50 mg three times daily of nicotinic acid can reverse the symptoms of pellagra.

The triad of neuropathy, retinopathy, and areflexia can result from a deficiency in vitamin E (α-tocopherol). Other manifestations can include ataxia, loss of proprioception and vibration sensation, nystagmus and external ophthalmoplegia.

The triad of neuropathy, ataxia, and dementia can result from vitamin B12 (cobalamin) deficiency. Symptoms present as paresthesias of the hands and feet, weakness, gait disturbance, depression, confusion, psychosis, peripheral neuropathy, and loss of position and vibration sensation. Myelopathic symptoms such as spastic paraparesis can occur, as well as visual disturbances as manifested by optic atrophy and visual loss. Treatment is undertaken with parenteral administration of vitamin B12 100 µg daily or 1000 µg twice weekly for two weeks.

Folate deficiency can result in a clinical picture that is similar in presentation to that of B12 deficiency. Elevated serum homocysteine is a surrogate marker for low folate levels. The deficiency can lead to neuropathy and/or spasticity due to spinal cord involvement. Treatment is initially undertaken with 1 mg of folate orally three times daily, followed by a maintenance dose of 1 mg daily. Answer choice A is a nonsense distracter and needs no explanation.

B&D Ch. 63

Question 119. C.   The best way to address a missed therapy session is to use neutral questioning to help explore why it happened. Ignoring the missed appointment is a mistake that can be misunderstood by the patient as the therapist not caring if she shows or not. Getting angry at the patient or punishing the patient is the wrong approach. It will only make the patient angry and less likely to reveal the emotional reasons for why the session was missed, and what meaning that has for the therapeutic relationship. In therapy, the patient's treatment of the therapist is a reflection of how he or she treats others in life as well. As such, aspects of the patient's behavior such as missed appointments should be noted and explored.

K&S Ch. 1

Question 120. D.   Tachycardia, not bradycardia, is a symptom of cannabis intoxication. All other answer choices are also symptoms. Orthostatic hypotension is usually only seen with high doses of cannabis.

K&S Ch. 12

Question 121. E. Akathisia is a subjective feeling of muscular tension caused by antipsychotic medication, which can cause restlessness, pacing, or an inability to stand still. Treatment consists of a beta adrenergic receptor antagonist such as propranolol. Other choices include anticholinergic medications such as benztropine. Benzodiazepines can be useful in some cases.
K&S Ch. 36

Question 122. C. Clonidine works by agonist activity at presynaptic alpha-2 receptors. This leads to a decrease in the amount of neurotransmitter released into the synaptic cleft leading to decreased sympathetic tone and decreased arousal. In the case of opioid withdrawal the action of clonidine on the locus ceruleus is thought to be particularly important to the decrease in autonomic symptoms associated with withdrawal. Other answer choices are unrelated distracters.
K&S Ch. 36

Question 123. B. Blockade of muscarinic cholinergic receptors is a common side effect of many drugs. Blockade leads to blurred vision, dry mouth, constipation, and difficulty urinating. When there is excessive blockade of this receptor, a patient can develop confusion and delirium. Alzheimer's disease has been postulated to be in part, the result of too little cholinergic activity. As such, drugs like donepezil block the enzyme acetylcholinesterase (which breaks down acetylcholine) and thereby increase cholinergic activity. This has been shown to be useful in the treatment of dementia. This is the opposite of blockade of muscarinic cholinergic receptors which one would postulate, would worsen the symptoms of Alzheimer's.
K&S Ch. 3

Question 124. A. While all of the lab tests involved in this question can be elevated in alcohol abuse, the most likely test to pick up alcohol abuse is the gamma-glutamyl transferase (GGT). It is elevated in 80% of those with alcohol-related disorders. The other tests are elevated at lower rates than 80% and as such will not pick up as many alcohol disorders as the GGT.
K&S Ch. 12

Question 125. B. Pimozide (Orap) is a dopamine receptor antagonist which has been approved in the US for the treatment of Tourette's disorder. Haloperidol is also widely used for this indication. In Europe, pimozide is used as an antipsychotic medication for treatment of schizophrenia.
K&S Ch. 36

Question 126. C. The gene for amyloid precursor protein is found on chromosome 21. Amyloid precursor protein is broken down to form beta amyloid protein, which is a major component of senile plaques in Alzheimer's disease.
K&S Ch. 10

Question 127. D. Heinz Kohut developed the school of self-psychology. Central to his theories of personality development is the idea that when parents mirror a child's behavior this functions as a form of empathy, which is necessary for personality development and the formation of healthy self-esteem. When this parental empathy is lacking, the sense of self does not develop properly and personality disorders develop. Patients then need others to fulfill functions that the self would normally handle. Oedipal conflict is a classic part of Freud's theories in which, greatly simplified, a child competes with the parent of the same sex for the attention of the parent of the opposite sex. The concept of the good enough mother came from Winnicott. He describes a holding environment that develops, where the good enough mother allows the child's true self to develop. He also gave us the concept of the transitional object. The paranoid-schizoid position and the depressive position are found in the work of Melanie Klein. The

277

paranoid-schizoid position is a view of the world from the perspective of the infant, in which the whole world is split into good and bad elements. The depressive position occurs when the infant is able to view the mother ambivalently as having both positive and negative aspects.

K&S Ch. 6

Question 128. D. When erythromycin and carbamazepine are given together the carbamazepine levels are increased.

K&S Ch. 36

Question 129. D. Valproic acid should be avoided during pregnancy because of its propensity to cause neural tube defects in the developing fetus. It should not be used by nursing mothers, as it is excreted in breast milk. Should the continuation of valproic acid in pregnancy be an absolute necessity, risk of neural tube defects can be reduced by giving the patient 1–4 mg of folic acid per day. However switching to another medication is the best choice.

K&S Ch. 36

Question 130. D. Increased appetite, weight gain, and increased sleep make this question a case of atypical depression. The treatment of choice for atypical depression is the monoamine oxidase inhibitors (MAOIs). As such phenelzine is the answer, as it is the only MAOI listed.

K&S Ch. 15

Question 131. C. Venlafaxine carries the potential side effect of increasing blood pressure. For this reason a baseline blood pressure should be taken for anyone starting venlafaxine, and regular monitoring of blood pressure is a good idea. Increased blood pressure has been found particularly with doses over 300 mg per day, and lower doses have shown less hypertension. As such, caution must be used when giving this drug to anyone with preexisting hypertension.

K&S Ch. 36

Question 132. D. Interpersonal therapy (IPT) was developed to treat depression. It focuses on interpersonal behavior and social interaction. Patients are taught to rate their interactions with others and become aware of their own behavior. The therapist may give direct advice, help make decisions, and clarify conflicts.

K&S Ch. 35

Question 133. E. Imprinting is the work of Konrad Lorenz. Imprinting implies that an animal has a critical period when it is sensitive to certain stimuli that elicit a specific behavioral response. For example, the baby goose has a period where it "imprints" on its mother and learns to follow her wherever she goes. If a person was the first moving object the goose saw it would imprint on that person and follow that person as if she were the mother. Nikollas Tinbergen conducted experiments both on animal behavior and on humans. He worked on measuring the power of certain stimuli to elicit specific behaviors from animals. He studied displacement activities, where in times when the urge to fight or flee would be equal, the animal would do some other activity to diffuse the tension. Humans also do this in times of stress. He described innate release mechanisms whereby animals have a specific response that is triggered by a releaser. A releaser is an environmental stimulus that prompts the specific response. Tinbergen also worked with human autistic children. He observed both the behavior of autistic children and normal children and postulated that in autistic children certain stimuli that are comforting to a normal child arouse fear in the autistic child. He postulates that this is part of what leads to the behavioral pattern found in autistic children.

K&S Ch. 4

Question 134. E. The hippocampus is one of the most important structures in the formation of memory. Other areas important to memory include some of the diencephalic nuclei and the basal forebrain. The amygdala also plays a role by rating the emotional content of memories thereby leading to stronger recall of more emotionally charged memories.
K&S Ch. 3

Question 135. E. This is a difficult question unless you know all of the involved scales. It is easier if you know that the brief psychiatric rating scale (BPRS) is a scale used for schizophrenia and psychosis. This is the take-home point. The other scales listed all are mood disorder scales. Will the Montgomery-Asberg scale end up on a standardized test near you? Probably not. But the BPRS probably will, so remember it. It is a good idea to be familiar with the most common psychiatric rating scales such as the BPRS, Hamilton, and GAF (global assessment of functioning – axis V). We will not print the full scales in this text, but it is worth your time to be familiar with them.
K&S Ch. 9

Question 136. C. Sleep terror disorder is characterized by recurrent episodes of awakening and screaming during the first third of the night. The patient has intense fear, autonomic arousal, sweating, tachycardia, and rapid breathing. The patient is unresponsive to efforts of others to comfort him. There are no dreams recalled and there is amnesia for the event. Small doses of diazepam are often useful to stop the episodes.
K&S Ch. 24

Question 137. C. Thioridazine (Mellaril) is one of the older typical antipsychotics that is not used as frequently since the advent of the atypicals. It is very sedating, causes orthostatic hypotension, has anticholinergic side effects, and has low rates of extrapyramidal symptoms. One of its more notable side effects is retrograde ejaculation, in addition to impotence. Patients on thioridazine can be told that retrograde ejaculation is not dangerous, but they will produce milky-white urine following orgasm.
K&S Ch. 36

Question 138. C. Donepezil is an acetylcholinesterase inhibitor. All other answer choices are distracters. Donepezil is used to treat mild to moderate Alzheimer's disease. By blocking acetylcholinesterase, the drug leads to increased acetylcholine in the synaptic cleft which has been proven to slow decline in Alzheimer's disease.
K&S Ch. 36

Question 139. B. Different cultures may present with culture-bound psychiatric syndromes, or different aspects of a certain disorder may be more prevalent in one culture than in another. With regard to depression, Chinese culture often presents with more somatic complaints and less focus on mood symptoms. Very often Chinese patients will come to the primary care physician or emergency room with somatic symptoms that are somewhat non-specific and are found to be driven by an underlying depressive disorder. Cultures have differences in how they view many things, including definitions of what constitutes health and sickness.
K&S Ch. 4

Question 140. A. The amphetamines in general exert their effects through the dopaminergic system. However, ecstasy is a "designer amphetamine" which acts through both the dopaminergic and serotonergic systems. Had dopamine been given as an answer choice it would also have been acceptable. The other neurotransmitters listed are unrelated to ecstasy.
K&S Ch. 12

Question 141. C. The field of child psychiatry developed out of the growth of child guidance centers in the early 1900s. Other answer choices are just distracters. Choice A happened after the early 1900s. Choice B happened before the early 1900s. Choice E took place in 1996 and is a bill relating to HIV testing. Choice D is unrelated to the US, as Freud lived in Vienna.
K&S Ch. 36

Question 142. A. Sarcoidosis is a granulomatous disease that affects multiple organ systems. Neurological manifestations occur in about 5% of sarcoidosis patients. Up to 20% of neurologic manifestations present as a peripheral neuropathy. Cranial neuropathies, and in particular facial nerve palsy, are the most common manifestation of neurosarcoidosis, occurring in up to 75% of cases. The treatment of choice is systemic corticosteroid or immunosuppressive therapy. The diagnosis is established clinically, but can often be confirmed by muscle biopsy or an elevated level of angiotensin converting enzyme (ACE) in the CSF. Other possible neurologic manifestations include cauda equina syndrome, mononeuropathy multiplex, peripheral sensorimotor polyneuropathy, diffuse meningoencephalitis, uveitis, and polyradiculoneuropathy resembling Guillain-Barré syndrome.
B&D Chs 55&82

Question 143. D. Trazodone is an antidepressant which is frequently used for insomnia. It is associated with priapism, which is a prolonged erection in the absence of sexual stimulation. Priapism is a potential medical emergency which can be treated by intracavernosal injection of epinephrine. Untreated priapism can also lead to impotence. Patients who start to develop priapism on trazodone should be switched to another medication.
K&S Ch. 36

Question 144. C. Low levels of cerebrospinal fluid serotonin are associated with increased aggression. Increased levels of dopamine are associated with increased aggression.
K&S Ch. 4

Question 145. C. Mirtazapine is an antidepressant medication which works by antagonism of presynaptic alpha-2 adrenergic receptors leading to potentiation of serotonergic and noradrenergic neurotransmission. Mirtazapine is sedating, particularly at low doses, which is good for depressed patients with insomnia. It lacks the anticholinergic side effects of the tricyclics, and lacks the anxiogenic side effects of the serotonin-selective reuptake inhibitors. Mirtazapine is also notable for its lack of sexual side effects.
K&S Ch. 36

Question 146. D. Sleep changes characteristic of the elderly include both decrease in REM sleep and decrease in slow wave sleep. This is a useful little fact for the test-taker to remember.
K&S Ch. 24

Question 147. D. A score of 70 on the global assessment of functioning (GAF) corresponds with "some difficulty in social, occupational, or school functioning, but generally functioning well, has some meaningful interpersonal relationships". A persistent failure to maintain personal hygiene is a GAF of 10. Major impairment in several areas is a GAF of 40. Superior functioning in all areas is a 100. No friends, unable to keep a job is a GAF of 30. It is a good idea to be familiar with the most common psychiatric rating scales such as the BPRS, Hamilton, and GAF (global assessment of functioning-axis V). We will not print the full scales in this text, but it is worth your time to be familiar with them.
K&S Ch. 9

Question 148. C. Kleine-Levin syndrome is a rare condition. (But not so rare on standardized tests!) It is marked by periods of hypersomnia with periods of normal sleep in between. During the periods of excessive sleep the patients wake up and experience apathy, irritability, confusion, voracious eating, loss of sexual inhibitions, disorientation, delusions, hallucinations, memory impairment, incoherent speech, excitation, and depression. The onset of the illness usually hits between 10 and 20 years of age, and it goes away by the time the patient is in his forties.
K&S Ch. 24

Question 149. C. David has obsessive-compulsive personality disorder. Obsessive-compulsive personality disorder (OCPD) presents as a pervasive pattern of preoccupation with orderliness, perfectionism, and control. This preoccupation comes at the expense of openness, efficiency, and flexibility. The OCPD patient's perfectionism interferes with task completion. These patients are inflexible regarding moral and ethical issues. They devote time to work at the expense of leisure activities. They are reluctant to delegate tasks to others. They are characteristically rigid and stubborn. OCPD patients often can not discard old or worn-out objects even when they have no value. They will not give tasks to others without reassurance that the tasks will be done their way. They are miserly in spending and view money as something to be hoarded for catastrophes. David is not presenting with prominent anxiety symptoms, so generalized anxiety disorder is incorrect. He does not have obsessive thoughts, and compulsions to stop those thoughts, so obsessive-compulsive disorder is incorrect. If David had schizoid personality disorder we would see that he had no friends or close contacts and that this does not bother him. In this question David has few friends because he spends all of his time working. If David had avoidant personality disorder he would have a pattern of social inhibition, feelings of inadequacy, and hypersensitivity to negative evaluation. That pattern is not described in this question.
K&S Ch. 27

Question 150. E. Cognitive behavioral therapy is founded on the principle that people make assumptions that affect their thoughts. Their thoughts then affect their mood. The goal of the therapy is therefore to uncover assumptions and thoughts that may be both faulty and automatic and determine how they contribute to changes in mood. Then the therapy aims to correct these faulty thoughts and stop them from being automatic.
The other answer choices are all appropriate pieces of psychodynamic therapy and psychoanalysis. They are not however part of cognitive behavioral therapy.
K&S Ch. 35